Veterinary Science: Theory and Case Studies

Veterinary Science: Theory and Case Studies

Edited by Peter Jones

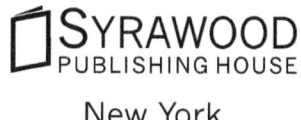

SYRAWOOD
PUBLISHING HOUSE

New York

Published by Syrawood Publishing House,
750 Third Avenue, 9th Floor,
New York, NY 10017, USA
www.syrawoodpublishinghouse.com

Veterinary Science: Theory and Case Studies
Edited by Peter Jones

International Standard Book Number: 978-1-68286-727-3 (Hardback)

Cataloging-in-Publication Data

Veterinary science : theory and case studies / edited by Peter Jones.
     p. cm.
Includes bibliographical references and index.
ISBN 978-1-68286-727-3
1. Veterinary medicine. 2. Veterinary medicine--Case studies.
3. Animals--Diseases. 4. Animal health. I. Jones, Peter.
SF745 .V48 2019
636.089--dc23

TABLE OF CONTENTS

PREFACE

Veterinary science is a branch of medicine that is concerned with the prevention, diagnosis and treatment of diseases and disorders in animals. It also deals with treating injuries in both domesticated or wild animals. Zoonotic disease control, food safety assurance and livestock health monitoring are significant areas of emphasis. Some of the commonly performed veterinary surgeries are in the areas of joint replacement, wound management, neurosurgery, oncological surgery, etc. Animal behavior and welfare are also closely studied and monitored under this field. This book consists of contributions made by international experts working in diverse areas of veterinary science. It traces the progress of this field and highlights some of its key concepts and applications. It is a vital tool for all researching and studying this discipline.

This book is the end result of constructive efforts and intensive research done by experts in this field. The aim of this book is to enlighten the readers with recent information in this area of research. The information provided in this profound book would serve as a valuable reference to students and researchers in this field.

At the end, I would like to thank all the authors for devoting their precious time and providing their valuable contribution to this book. I would also like to express my gratitude to my fellow colleagues who encouraged me throughout the process.

Editor

Understanding the Osteosarcoma Pathobiology: A Comparative Oncology Approach

Jyotika Varshney [1,2], Milcah C. Scott [1,3,4], David A. Largaespada [1,5] and Subbaya Subramanian [1,2,*]

Academic Editors: Duncan C. Ferguson and Margarethe Hoenig

[1] Masonic Cancer Center, University of Minnesota, Minneapolis, MN 55455, USA; varsh005@umn.edu (J.V.); scot0340@umn.edu (M.C.S.); larga002@umn.edu (D.A.L.)
[2] Department of Surgery, University of Minnesota Medical School, Moos Tower, 11-212420 Delaware Street, S.E.; MMC 195, Minneapolis, MN 55455, USA
[3] Animal Cancer Care and Research Program, University of Minnesota, St. Paul, MN 55455, USA
[4] Department of Veterinary Clinical Sciences, College of Veterinary Medicine, University of Minnesota, St. Paul, MN 55108, USA
[5] Department of Pediatrics, University of Minnesota, Minneapolis, MN 55455, USA
* Correspondence: subree@umn.edu

Abstract: Osteosarcoma is an aggressive primary bone tumor in humans and is among the most common cancer afflicting dogs. Despite surgical advancements and intensification of chemo- and targeted therapies, the survival outcome for osteosarcoma patients is, as of yet, suboptimal. The presence of metastatic disease at diagnosis or its recurrence after initial therapy is a major factor for the poor outcomes. It is thought that most human and canine patients have at least microscopic metastatic lesions at diagnosis. Osteosarcoma in dogs occurs naturally with greater frequency and shares many biological and clinical similarities with osteosarcoma in humans. From a genetic perspective, osteosarcoma in both humans and dogs is characterized by complex karyotypes with highly variable structural and numerical chromosomal aberrations. Similar molecular abnormalities have been observed in human and canine osteosarcoma. For instance, loss of *TP53* and *RB* regulated pathways are common. While there are several oncogenes that are commonly amplified in both humans and dogs, such as *MYC* and *RAS*, no commonly activated proto-oncogene has been identified that could form the basis for targeted therapies. It remains possible that recurrent aberrant gene expression changes due to gene amplification or epigenetic alterations could be uncovered and these could be used for developing new, targeted therapies. However, the remarkably high genomic complexity of osteosarcoma has precluded their definitive identification. Several advantageous murine models of osteosarcoma have been generated. These include spontaneous and genetically engineered mouse models, including a model based on forward genetics and transposon mutagenesis allowing new genes and genetic pathways to be implicated in osteosarcoma development. The proposition of this review is that careful comparative genomic studies between human, canine and mouse models of osteosarcoma may help identify commonly affected and targetable pathways for alternative therapies for osteosarcoma patients. Translational research may be found through a path that begins in mouse models, and then moves through canine patients, and then human patients.

Keywords: osteosarcoma; comparative oncology; microRNAs; prognosis; canine osteosarcoma

1. Introduction

Osteosarcoma is an aggressive primary bone tumor most prevalent in human patients. It mostly occurs during adolescence, with a second peak at middle age (older than 40) [1,2]. The tumor is characterized by increased production of osteoid (abnormal bone matrix) and by exceptionally complex karyotypes [3,4]. While the target cell for malignant transformation in the formation of osteosarcoma is not known with certainty, it is thought to be a mesenchymal stem cell (MSC) or a cell committed to the osteoblast lineage [5]. Evidence from mouse models indicates that any of several cell stages could serve as target cells for osteosarcoma development [6]. There are three common histologic types of osteosarcoma: osteoblastic, where tumor cells produce large amounts of tumor osteoid; chondroblastic, where tumor cells produce chondroid (cartilage) in addition to some amount of tumor osteoid; and fibroblastic, where tumor cells are predominantly fibroblasts and can produce both collagen and tumor osteoid [7]. The disease is highly metastatic, with distant spread mostly to lungs and other sites in bone, but osteosarcoma can also metastasize to lymph nodes and intra-abdominal organs [8,9]. The metastatic pattern (lungs, bones, lymph nodes) is similar for dogs and humans [10]. Osteosarcoma may present with macroscopic metastatic disease or metastatic disease can occur after therapy. In either case, prognosis is significantly worse once metastasis has been detected [11,12].

In canine patients, osteosarcoma is a disease primarily of adult dogs; the median age at diagnosis is approximately eight years, with a small peak of incidence in young animals (younger than 3 years) [10,13]. This differs from the situation in human patients where the peak age of incidence is in adolescence. Nevertheless, the natural history of the disease is similar in canine and human osteosarcoma patients [14]. Moreover, we have observed that genome wide expression profiles of canine osteosarcoma are indistinguishable from human pediatric osteosarcoma and more like human osteosarcoma than any other human cancer [14,15]. In dogs, there is generally a strong breed preference in the risk for cancer, such as osteosarcoma [16,17]. Many large breed dogs have an increased risk for osteosarcoma compared to other breeds [4,18,19]. The genetic determinants of osteosarcoma susceptibility in dogs are not fully elucidated, and it is possible that these factors will also be important in human osteosarcoma susceptibility. The development of treatment strategies in dogs and people has proven mutually beneficial for both species [20]. In fact, current treatment options are similar in both species.

Osteosarcoma is treated using surgery, radiation and chemotherapy. Surgical techniques have greatly improved with time, and in many cases limb salvage is feasible with low rates of local recurrence in humans [21]. Combination chemotherapies are vital for effective treatment of osteosarcoma [22]. However, despite decades of effort, nothing better than the most often used combination of three chemotherapeutic agents (*i.e.*, methotrexate, doxorubicin and cisplatin) has been found [22]. The adjuvant chemotherapy is generally administered prior to surgery and, according to many studies, the extent of necrosis observed in the primary tumor after surgical removal is correlated with the outcome. [21]. The goal of the adjuvant chemotherapy is to eliminate the micrometastases that are thought to be present in >80% of all patients at the time of diagnosis, thus preventing relapse [1]. New research is underway to define specific molecular targets that could be utilized to treat this disease, but their elucidation has been proven difficult. It is possible that osteosarcoma may also be treated using recently developed immunotherapies, such as immune checkpoint blockade or chimeric antigen receptor-engineered T cells [21].

Osteosarcoma is characterized by aneuploidy and extensive genetic instability [23]. Due to this extreme genetic instability, common causes of osteosarcoma development have largely been limited to implicating loss of *RB* and *TP53* regulated cellular activities and upregulation of *MYC* transcriptional activity reviewed by Morrow *et al.* [24]. Beyond these, few alterations are common or well accepted as osteosarcoma drivers. Gene amplification and protein overexpression of the *RUNX2* transcription factor, which is a regulator of bone renewal, has been proposed to drive osteosarcoma [25]. Conflicting data on activation of beta-catenin dependent transcription in osteosarcoma has been reported [26]. In addition, TGF-β signaling has been proposed to promote the acquisition of metastatic disease [27]. Notable, expression of Ezrin at high levels has been found in metastatic human and canine osteosarcoma and functionally validated in model systems as a driver of osteosarcoma metastasis [28]. Recently, a large scale *Sleeping Beauty* (SB) transposon-based forward genetic screen was carried out for osteosarcoma in mice [29]. From this screen, a large number of new candidate osteosarcoma proto-oncogene and tumor suppressors were reported. These included the candidate oncogenes *SEMA4D* and *SEMA6D*, which were partially functionally validated as well as tumor suppressors like *NF1*, *NF2* and *PTEN* [29]. Beyond protein encoding genes, several micro RNAs (miRNAs) and miRNA clusters have been suggested as drivers or suppressors of osteosarcoma development and progression [30]. What remains unclear is which common oncogenic drivers for osteosarcoma should be targeted and how they would be targeted. Unlike the case for other malignancies, osteosarcoma is genetically heterogeneous and common molecular targets may not be present.

Osteosarcoma is much more common in dogs than in people (greater than 15 times) and can be experimentally induced in mice via transgenesis. Perceivably, the opportunity to study osteosarcoma in three different species may make it possible to identify core genes and pathways, whose alterations are central to the osteosarcoma phenotype and that would make good targets for therapy. In the past, the main challenges were the development of improved surgical techniques for limb salvage, prevention of local recurrence and the identification of effective combination chemotherapies. Currently, a major pressing need is the development of new therapies to prevent the outgrowth of metastatic disease and to treat it once it has occurred. It is possible that germline or somatic mutations or tumor gene expression signatures identified through multi-species approaches could help predict which patients will respond well to current treatment regimes and which need to be referred for more intensive therapy or follow-up screening. However, much remains to be learned about what allows microscopic osteosarcoma lesions to resist chemotherapy and to suddenly break tumor dormancy and form a macroscopic mass. Until these questions are answered, we are not fully capable to help many human and canine osteosarcoma patients.

This review is an attempt to address many of the unanswered questions pertaining to osteosarcoma by focusing on recently acquired knowledge from a multi-species approach.

2. Human Osteosarcoma

Osteosarcoma in human patients is a rare tumor with a peak incidence in the second decade of life. The incidence is roughly 25 cases per 10 million per year in the United States [31]. A second wave of osteosarcoma is diagnosed in individuals between 70 and 80 years of age, often in association with Paget's disease. Paget's disease is an abnormality of bone homeostasis in which excessive bone reabsorption and reformation occur. Genetic and viral origins of Paget's disease have been suggested. While osteosarcoma is a rare manifestation of the disease, risk for osteosarcoma is increased. Osteosarcoma can occur in nearly any part of the skeleton, but commonly affects one of the long bones. As it occurs during a period of intense bone growth, there may be an association between this growth and sensitivity to osteoblast transformation [31]. Indeed, children with osteosarcoma are on average tall for their age [32]. Genetic studies also have suggested an association between the inheritance of certain forms of growth control genes and risk for osteosarcoma [33]. Other risk factors for human osteosarcoma include prior radiation therapy, male gender, and possibly African ancestry [34,35]. A genome-wide association study (GWAS) revealed possible risk alleles in the glutamate receptor, metaotropic 4 (*GRM4*) gene and a gene desert at chromosome 2p25.2 [36]. A recent GWAS also identified a potential high-risk allele for osteosarcoma metastasis at presentation within the transcriptional activator *NFIB* [37], a gene that was also identified as a potential tumor/metastasis suppressor in a transposon-based genetic screen in mice [29].

Some rare inherited cancer predisposition syndromes increase the risk for osteosarcoma. These rare cancers include Li-Fraumeni syndrome, hereditary retinoblastoma and Rothman-Thompson syndrome caused by germline mutations in *TP53*, *RB1*, and *RECQL4*, respectively [38]. Certain other cancer predisposition syndromes also seem to increase the risk of osteosarcoma development including Neurofibromatosis Type 1 syndrome, Werner's syndrome and Diamond-Blackfan anemia [24]. Patients with hereditary multiple osteochondromas, due to inheritance of mutations in the *EXT1* or *EXT2* genes, are predisposed to development of osteosarcoma also [24].

Human osteosarcoma is typically diagnosed due to swelling and pain often in the limbs. This can cause a limp if the involved limb is a leg or immobility of a joint. Pain may be constant or associated with exertion. In rare cases osteosarcoma will trigger a bone fracture. Diagnosis is made following a complete medical exam and imaging studies. Often an X-ray is done, followed by positron emission tomography or a bone scan. As osteosarcoma can often metastasize to the lungs, lung X-rays are utilized. A definitive diagnosis requires a biopsy. Staging of osteosarcoma is controversial. Most believe that all osteosarcoma should be considered high grade and treated as such although low grade osteosarcoma seems to be a distinct entity [38]. The only commonly accepted staging is localized *versus* metastatic disease.

Human osteosarcoma is commonly treated using surgery and chemotherapy [38]. Chemotherapy for roughly ten weeks that precedes surgery and the extent of necrosis in the surgically removed primary tumor has been suggested to be associated with long term risk for disease recurrence [38]. Chemotherapy is also given after surgery for a period of up to a year. Usually two or three chemotherapeutic agents are given for osteosarcoma treatment. Common combinations include high-dose methotrexate, doxorubicin and cisplatin (sometimes with ifosfamide); doxorubicin and cisplatin; ifosfamide and etoposide; ifosfamide, cisplatin (or carboplatin) and epirubicin [38]. Radiation therapy is used in some cases for non-resectable tumors [38].

The prognosis of human osteosarcoma is affected largely by the presence or absence of metastases. The 5-year survival rate for localized osteosarcoma is estimated to be between 50% and 60%. For metastatic disease the 5-year survival rate is 15% to 30% [39]. There is a better prognosis if metastatic osteosarcoma is present only in the lungs and is all metastatic lesions can be removed surgically [39]. That said, there is a dire need to develop therapies that can be used to treat patients who present with extensive metastatic disease or who recur with metastatic disease. At present, palliative care is often used in such cases or referral for clinical trials [38].

3. Canine Osteosarcoma

Canine osteosarcoma accounts for 80%–90% of canine primary bone tumors [40]. Dogs often present with a history of lameness or in some cases with a pathologic fracture of the affected bone. Diagnosis is based on clinical signs, imaging and biopsy. The metaphyseal region of long bones is the most common primary site with front limbs affected twice as often as rear limbs and the distal radius and proximal humerus being the two most common locations [41,42].

It is believed that external factors such as chemical carcinogens, ionization radiation, metallic implants to fix fractures and precedent skeletal disorders such as osteomyelitis and microscopic fractures can lead to canine osteosarcoma [10]. There are implications of genetic factors such as *TP53* and RB1 aberrations, as well as certain viruses and growth factor alterations [43]. Osteosarcoma can affect any breed of dog, but it is more commonly found in the larger breeds. Some breeds, such as the Scottish Deerhound, Great Dane, St. Bernard and Greyhound, are at high risk for developing primary bone tumors suggesting a genetic predilection [40]. In fact, the CDKN2A locus has been recently linked to osteosarcoma risk in dogs, and the risk allele is fixed in certain breeds like Rottweilers and Irish Wolfhounds [4].

Without treatment, the estimated survival for a dog with osteosarcoma is less than 3 months. On the other hand, survival times of approximately 1 year (or about 10% of a dog's lifetime) are achievable for 20%–50% of dogs with osteosarcoma treated using the current standard of care, and a small percentage of dogs can survive up to 5–6 years after diagnosis [44]. Standard of care for dogs is surgery (amputation of limb sparing surgery) with adjuvant chemotherapy [45]. The choice of chemotherapy drugs does not seem to influence survival, thus, toxicity, quality of life and cost tend to be the factors that guide treatment decisions [44]. Chemotherapy is only recommended when the primary tumor is removed and as of current, the drug of choice is carboplatin.

Many well-controlled studies show that a clinical response for osteosarcoma is only achievable with accepted standard of care. In very rare cases, dogs with osteosarcoma that receive palliative care may have prolonged (>1 year) survival, even in face of metastatic disease. Anecdotal benefits reported from herbal or "alternative" treatments, have not been reproducible, and no alternative therapies have been shown to have efficacy or provide consistent clinical benefit in controlled trials.

Metastatic bone cancer is the common cause of death or euthanasia, in 90% of dogs by 1 year [46]. Reducing the primary tumor's ability to metastasize and enhancing the antitumor activity of chemotherapy drugs and yet having minimal negative side effects is still a challenge for veterinary practitioners [10]. Treatment options for canine patients with metastases include pulmonary metastasectomy, but treatment for metastatic disease is only recommended if the primary tumor remains in complete remission [47]. The median survival after pulmonary metastasectomy can be up to 6 months; but without standard surgical procedure, survival outcome is usually less than 2 months [46].

4. Mouse Models of Osteosarcoma

The number of genetically engineered or other mouse models of osteosarcoma are fairly restricted. However, these have been useful for studies on the cell of origin for osteosarcoma development and gaining insight into new genes and pathways that influence osteosarcoma initiation, progression and the process of metastasis. Most of the reported models utilize Cre/LoxP mediated deletion of *Trp53* and/or *Rb1* (reviewed in [48]). A few other models have been created by transgenic overexpression of various oncogenes including *Fos* and SV40 large T antigen [49], or co-deletion of one copy of *Twist* and mutation of *Apc* [50]. Osteosarcoma can be induced with high efficiency in mice by osteoblast lineage specific deletion of the *Trp53* gene, although the latency and penetrance is greatly enhanced by co-deletion of both copies of the *Rb1* gene [51].These data are consistent with the centrality of *TP53* and *RB1* loss of function alterations in human osteosarcoma [23]. Mouse osteosarcoma induced by deletion of *Trp53* is genomically unstable, as is seen in human osteosarcoma [52].

Others have created mouse cell lines from spontaneously occurring osteosarcoma. In cases in which these osteosarcoma were induced on a uniform strain background, the osteosarcoma cells can be grown in syngeneic hosts by intravenous, subcutaneous, or orthotopic injections into the tibia (reviewed in [53]). Examples include the K12 and K7M2 derivative that is highly metastatic, and the Dunn along with its metastatic derivative LM8. These cell lines have been useful for testing the role of various components of the immune system on primary osteosarcoma tumor growth and osteosarcoma metastasis [54]. Such cell lines have also been used to create matched pairs of poorly and highly metastatic cell lines for study [53]. These have been useful for developing candidate genes and pathways that may regulate the process of metastasis, such as high-level expression of ezrin [28].

Quist *et al.* reported that osteosarcoma could be induced in mice via homozygous Cre/LoxP-mediated deletion of *Trp53* and *Rb1* in undifferentiated mesenchyme, pre-osteoblasts or infrequently cycling mature osteoblasts [6]. These data suggest that a variety of cell types could be targets for osteosarcoma development. This plasticity may also be the basis for the ready acquisition of new osteosarcoma phenotypes in patients, including chemo/radiotherapy resistance and the ability to readily colonize the lung.

From osteosarcoma mouse models, we have learned that osteosarcoma cells have a predilection to metastatic colonization of the lung, but, interestedly, have observed a metastatic potential spectrum across various cell lines. Intriguingly, in mouse models of Li-Fraumeni, the rate of lung metastasis is influenced by the nature of the p53 mutant allele used and when in the lifetime of the mouse Cre is used to induce mutation of the p53 gene [51]. The rate of spontaneous development of osteosarcoma and the frequency of lung metastasis is higher in mice heterozygous for the $Trp53^{R272H}$ allele than in mice heterozygous for the carry $Trp53^{R270H}$ allele [55].

Recently, a new mouse model of osteosarcoma was developed which utilizes the *Sleeping Beauty* (SB) transposon mutagenesis system [29]. In this project, a SB transposon vector designed to activate proto-oncogenes or inactivate tumor suppressor genes by insertional mutagenesis, was mobilized specifically in *Osx1+* cells using a tissue-specific mutagenesis approach. Mutagenesis by SB was able to induce osteosarcoma in otherwise wild type mice or accelerate osteosarcoma in mice with tissue-specific induction of the $Trp53^{R270H}$ allele. Transposon insertion mutations in specific regions of the genome are found recurrently in SB induced tumors and these regions are called "common insertion sites" or CIS [29]. CIS result from selection for insertions that occur within or near a cancer gene in the right position and the right orientation so as to give the cell a selective advantage and drive the development of a tumor. Thus, the identification of genes at or near CIS defines new candidate drivers of cancer development.

5. Conserved Drivers of Osteosarcoma

5.1. Genomic Alterations

It has been reported that genomic alterations are necessary for development of osteosarcoma in mouse models (*TP53*) and are accepted as being commonly shared in humans and dogs [13,29,56].

Highly chaotic karyotypes encompass a key feature that characterizes some mouse models used for osteosarcoma studies, and naturally occurring osteosarcoma in dogs, as well as in human patients. The average human osteosarcoma harbors roughly 30 coding alterations [23,57] while in dog osteosarcoma and mouse models, this figure is not known with certainty. Many of the candidate genes implicated in the pathogenesis and progression of osteosarcoma in people have also been characterized in the canine disease. Notable examples of these genes are *PTEN* (phosphatase and tensin homolog), *RB1* (retinoblastoma), and *TP53* (tumor protein 53), and *MET* (mesenchymal-epithelial transition factor).

Genetic alterations of the retinoblastoma susceptibility (*RB1*) gene have been implicated in the development and progression of osteosarcoma. In people, almost 70% of osteosarcomas have at least one *RB1* gene alteration and the percentage is similar in dog osteosarcomas [13]. We recently reported that an aberrant RB-E2F1 regulatory pathway is predictive of biological behavior [58]. Since our work, another group has reported that RB1 alterations may serve as a prognostic marker for the management of osteosarcoma patients [59].

Approximately 50% of human osteosarcomas have been reported to have somatic *TP53* deletions or point mutations detected using exon sequencing strategies [23]. However, a recent study that used whole genome sequencing of human osteosarcomas suggests that nearly all osteosarcoma tumors have p53 pathways lesions, which in many cases are translocations that break in the first intron of *TP53* gene [57]. Thus, it would appear that p53 pathway loss might be a requirement for osteosarcoma development in people. Clearly, germline *TP53* mutations, which cause Li-Fraumeni syndrome, predispose to osteosarcoma. However, it is unclear whether *TP53* mutations act as initiating mutations or progression mutations in sporadic osteosarcoma. In any case, p53 pathway alterations are common in genetically engineered mouse models as well as spontaneous canine and human osteosarcoma. Therefore, mouse models could be used to develop therapies that exploit p53 pathway alterations in patient osteosarcoma.

In humans and dogs, several oncogenes have been identified as possibly playing a role in osteosarcoma including *MET*, *FOS*, *IGF1R* (Insulin-Like Growth Factor 1 Receptor), *PVT1/MYC*, *RUNX2*, and *HER2*. Some of these changes involve copy number alterations. Consistent genome and chromosome copy number changes have been reported in canine and human osteosarcoma [17]. For instance, a high copy number gain of the *RUNX2* locus has been reported in both human and dog osteosarcoma [56].

Some of these genes, or the pathways they regulate, including the *PVT1/MYC* locus, *MET* signaling, and *IGF1R* have been implicated in genetically engineered mouse models of osteosarcoma [29,52].

Recurrent point mutations have been observed in osteosarcoma, but there are few beyond *RB1* and *TP53* that reach statistical significance. This is in part because too few samples have been sequenced. However, point mutations or deletions of several tumor suppressor genes, likely to be drivers of osteosarcomagenesis, were observed in a recent report of human osteosarcoma including *NF1*, *NF2* and *PTEN*, all of which were also recovered in a transposon-based screen for osteosarcoma in mice [29].

Overlap exists between other reported candidate human osteosarcoma genes after genome-wide copy number and whole exome sequencing were done [23], and also after transposon based screening in a mouse model including activation of *PI3KCA*, and *AKT1*, and inactivation of *ARID1A* [29].

5.2. Deregulation of Micrornas in Canine and Human Osteosarcoma

microRNAs (miRNAs) are small non coding RNAs that regulate more than 60% of the genome post transcriptionally. Several studies have identified deregulated miRNAs in osteosarcoma [60–66]. One of the earliest studies reported four differentially expressed miRNAs in a handful of osteosarcoma samples compared to controls [67]. Since these initial studies, additional research has shown that miRNA deregulation is potentially central to osteosarcoma development and progression [68]. Indeed, our group generated a Sarcoma MicroRNA Expression Database (S-MED) that represents 22 different sarcoma types, including osteosarcoma [69]. Through S-MED we found that osteosarcoma clustered separately from all other sarcoma types indicating the presence of potentially biologically important miRNAs. One of the unique miRNA signatures we found revealed the significant downregulation of around 50 miRNAs in the human 14q32 locus compared to the controls [65]. Most importantly, we have also shown a comparable decrease in expression of orthologous 14q32 miRNAs in canine osteosarcoma samples [65]. Interestingly we did not observe any copy number changes at the 14q32 locus, suggesting epigenetic changes at the locus. We confirmed that subset of these 50 miRNAs (miR-382, miR-369-5p, miR-544 and miR-134) could target the 3′ UTR of cMYC transcript. Additionally, overexpression of these miRNAs in osteosarcoma cells decreased the cMYC levels and induced apoptosis [65,70]. Also cMYC has been shown to transactivate a commonly known miRNA cluster, miR-17-92 [71]. We showed that restoration of the 14q32 miRNAs not only did decrease the cMYC levels but also significantly reduced the levels of mir-17-92 [70].

It was observed in other studies that miR-135b, -150, -370, -542-5p, -652, and -654 were highly expressed compared to osteoblasts [72–74]. Many of them play crucial roles in bone differentiation and key signaling pathways (miR-206 and -286) [75]. Additionally, miRNAs target *TP53*, which is an important tumor suppressor gene, was mutated in more than 60% osteosarcoma tumors [76]. One of the key miRNAs in the *TP53* pathway is miR-34, which is significantly downregulated in many osteosarcoma tumors that affects the cell cycle and proliferation [77–79].

The role of miRNAs in canine osteosarcoma remains to be fully elucidated. Since the discovery of miRNAs, there have been few studies that show a correlation between deregulation of miRNAs and canine osteosarcoma. A recent study investigated the role of miR-196a and its target Annexin V in human (143B, MG63) and canine (DAN) osteosarcoma cell lines to identify potential targets for new therapeutic agents in both the species [80]. They observed that miR-196a is downregulated in many of the canine osteosarcoma tumors compared to the normal bone, which is in contradiction with some earlier studies [66,81]. Further studies need to be performed on a larger cohort to establish that miR-196a is a potential therapeutic target and can impact multiple downstream targets in canine osteosarcoma.

A study led by Fenger *et al.*, sought to characterize miRNA expression in canine primary tumors among the major large breeds (greyhounds, rottweilers, golden retrievers and some mixed breeds) [43,82]. Using Nanominer software, they determined 189 miRNAs that were differentially expressed. Of these, miR-494 was highly expressed in all the breeds compared to normal canine osteoblasts.

As mentioned earlier, our group was among the first groups to observe a significant downregulation of around 50 miRNAs in the human 14q32 chromosomal region, which was highly conserved in the dog genome. Out of the 50 miRNAs, 2 miRNAs, miR-134 and mir-544, shared 100% conservation with the canine genome and mapped to the predicted synteny in canine osteosarcoma [14]. We have comprised a table of key miRNAs that play an important role in survival outcome and chemoresponse that can potentially lead to osteosarcoma diagnosis, subtyping and therapeutics in human and canine osteosarcoma (Table 1).

Table 1. miRNAs as potential markers for survival outcome and/ or chemosensitivity.

miRNAs Deregulated in OS	Expression Levels Compared to the Controls	Overall Function	References
miR-382	Down-regulated	Poor survival outcome and metastasis marker	[70,83]
miR-154	Down-regulated	Poor survival outcome	[70]
miR-33a	Up-regulated	Chemoresistance	[84]
miR-34c	Down-regulated	Chemoresistance	[85]

5.3. Epigenetic Changes in Osteosarcoma

Most forms of human cancer have changes in the epigenome compared to the normal cellular counterparts from which they are derived. Indeed, changes to the epigenome seem to be a ubiquitous feature of cancer. Epigenetic changes are revealed in alterations to the pattern of DNA methylation, histone modifications and nucleosome remodeling (reviewed in [24]). Osteosarcoma, like other forms of human cancer, seems to have many such epigenome changes compared to normal osteoblasts, the presumptive target cell for transformation. Several studies have analyzed the epigenome in a genome-wide manner, albeit with low numbers of cases [86,87]. These studies confirm that specific methylation events are heterogeneous among different cases of human osteosarcoma and that these differences may help explain differences in the clinical behavior of different osteosarcomas. These genome wide studies in human osteosarcoma have been restricted to the study of DNA methylation. Work on other chromatin modification remains to be done. The study of genome wide epigenetic changes has not been undertaken on a large scale in genetically engineered mouse models or canine osteosarcoma samples.

Many studies in osteosarcoma have focused on methylation of specific genes or gene regions. These studies suggest that certain genes and genetic pathways are subject to control by DNA methylation and attendant modifications to the histone code. Among these are alterations to the RB and p53 pathways. While these specific genes are not frequent targets of methylation based gene silencing, genes in these pathways have been reported as targets for pathogenic methylation. Specifically the *CDKN2A* locus, encoding the cyclin dependent kinase inhibitor p16^{INK4a} and the Mdm2 inhibitor p14^{Arf}, has been reported [88,89]. Several genes that are targets of p53, or modulate p53 activity, have been shown to be methylated and silenced in osteosarcoma cell lines or xenograft tumors including *CDKN1A*, *HIC1* and *GADD45* [90–92]. Many other tumor suppressor genes are silenced by promoter hypermethylation in osteosarcoma cell lines including *RASSF1A*, *TIMP3*, DAPK1 and others (review in Morrow and Khanna, Critical Reviews in Oncogenesis, 2015). Methylation and silencing of tumor suppressive miRNA genes has also been observed as specific events in human osteosarcoma cell lines and primary tumors. Promoter hypomethyation, and probable overexpression, of oncogenes is less well studied in osteosarcoma, but several reports have been made suggesting such a mechanism, notably for the metastasis promoting gene *IRX1* and the growth factor gene *IGF2* [93,94]. Several candidate osteosarcoma oncogenes found in a transposon-based forward genetic screen in mice are also hypomethylated and overexpressed in human osteosarcoma compared to normal osteoblasts, including *SEMA4D*, *RAF1* and *PAK1* [29]. Some of these epigenetic changes, including aberrant repression and activation, are associated with loss of imprinting control at specific loci in osteosarcoma cells [95–97].

Genome wide studies of epigenetic alterations in human osteosarcoma need to incorporate many more samples before we learn to what extent they may explain molecular subtypes and clinical behavior of different cases. No such studies have been reported for canine osteosarcomas or mouse models either. When they are, they will allow cross-species comparisons that could help reveal the most meaningful alterations. Despite these limitations, it is apparent that osteosarcoma development is accompanied by changes to the epigenome that drive progression and confer specific cancer phenotypes. Published data does suggest that epigenome targeted therapies, including histone deacetylase inhibitors and

DNA demethylating agents, can alter gene expression and inhibit osteosarcoma growth and/or metastasis [93,98]. Indeed, one study suggests that osteosarcoma cell lines can be reprogrammed using induced pluripotency genes and that the accompanying epigenetic changes reduce tumorigenic potential [99]. Taken together, these data suggest that modification of osteosarcoma epigenomes will be a useful therapeutic approach.

6. Advantages of A Multi-Species, Comparative Osteosarcoma Study Approach

Using comparative genetic studies in multiple organisms, it is possible to understand more about the inherited and somatically acquired genetic alterations that are informative of osteosarcoma risk and clinical behavior, especially metastasis. It is reasonable that genetic alterations that are present in human, dog, and mouse osteosarcomas represent the most likely true drivers of osteosarcoma progression, based on the concept of convergent evolution. Singly, mouse models offer opportunities to discover new genes and pathways important in disease initiation and progression. Dogs bring many other advantages to the table. Notably, since they show remarkable intra-breed homogeneity, which, together with noticeable interbreed heterogeneity, the dog offers distinctive opportunities to understand the genetics underlying osteosarcoma. Taken all together, an interspecies approach offers a possibly broader view and understanding of osteosarcoma since, for example, what is found to be altered at the genetic level in one species may be epigenetically silenced altered in another, but would be hard to pick out based on changes to gene expression alone.

Findings from mouse models and naturally occurring osteosarcoma in dogs need to be translated into therapeutic approaches in a clinically relevant model. Advantages of clinical trials in dogs are numerous and include that there are many more cases of canine osteosarcoma than human osteosarcoma [100,101]. In addition, disease progression in dogs, even with standard of care, is rapid so that assessments of improvement can be made in comparatively short periods of time [102].

It has been shown that histological response is not a good predictor (St. Jude, CTOS 20th Annual Meeting) in human osteosarcoma patients, and so there is an urgent need for informative biomarkers. The 14q32 locus is a new and promising marker, which was discovered by our group through a comparative species approach [65].

7. Conclusions

In more than 70% of osteosarcoma patients, current standard-of-care therapies ultimately fail to prevent relapse and metastasis. This dismal outcome has not improved over the past three decades, indicating a desperate need for novel drugs and treatment strategies. As osteosarcoma is genetically heterogeneous, successful therapies will need to target conserved pathobiology. In this review, we discussed the presence of multiple conserved signaling mechanisms as well as some of the approaches for understanding osteosarcoma pathobiology. Recent studies highlight the role of microRNAs in regulation of these conserved signaling pathways. In addition, we have just begun to understand the roles of the regulatory small RNAs and long-noncoding RNAs (lncRNAs). Further, intricacy in gene regulations does not end with identification of regulatory RNAs and its interacting partners. Molecular intricacy is also heavily dependent on our understanding of the implications of other layers of gene regulation such as role for competing endogenous RNAs along with pseudogenes, circular RNAs and lncRNAs. Acquiring such breadth and depth of knowledge is critical for developing therapies that will prevent bypass mechanisms of resistance to therapies. Moreover, cell non-autonomous functions of secreted factors such as exosomes are currently being investigated. In addition, emerging concepts of immune regulation by cancer and recent advancements in immunotherapy hold promise for treating and better outcomes in osteosarcoma.

Acknowledgments: We thank Jaime Modiano and Aaron Sarver for helpful discussions and Anne Sarver for assisting in manuscript preparation. Due to the space restrictions we could not cite many other significant contributions made by numerous researchers and laboratories in this potentially important and rapidly progressing field. Subbaya Subramanian and David A. Largaespada are supported by research grants funded by American

Cancer Society Grant (RSG 13-381-01-RMC), the Sobiech osteosarcoma fund, Children's cancer research funds, the Wyckoff Rein in Sarcoma Foundation.

Author Contributions: Jyotika Varshney and Subbaya Subramanian developed the concept for the review. Milcah C. Scott and David A. Largaespada provided input in the canine osteosarcoma and epigenetics of osteosarcoma.

References

1. Moore, D.D.; Luu, H.H. Osteosarcoma. *Cancer Treat Res.* **2014**, *162*, 65–92. [PubMed]
2. Ottaviani, G.; Jaffe, N. The epidemiology of osteosarcoma. *Cancer Treat Res.* **2009**, *152*, 3–13. [PubMed]
3. Letson, G.D.; Muro-Cacho, C.A. Genetic and molecular abnormalities in tumors of the bone and soft tissues. *Cancer Control* **2001**, *8*, 239–251. [PubMed]
4. Karlsson, E.K.; Sigurdsson, S.; Ivansson, E.; Thomas, R.; Elvers, I.; Wright, J.; Howald, C.; Tonomura, N.; Perloski, M.; Swofford, R.; *et al.* Genome-wide analyses implicate 33 loci in heritable dog osteosarcoma, including regulatory variants near CDKN2A/B. *Genome Biol.* **2013**, *14*, R132. [CrossRef] [PubMed]
5. Mutsaers, A.J.; Walkley, C.R. Cells of origin in osteosarcoma: Mesenchymal stem cells or osteoblast committed cells? *Bone* **2014**, *62*, 56–63. [CrossRef] [PubMed]
6. Quist, T.; Jin, H.; Zhu, J.F.; Smith-Fry, K.; Capecchi, M.R.; Jones, K.B. The impact of osteoblastic differentiation on osteosarcomagenesis in the mouse. *Oncogene* **2015**, *34*, 4278–4284. [CrossRef] [PubMed]
7. Yoshida, H.; Adachi, H.; Hamada, Y.; Aki, T.; Yumoto, T.; Morimoto, K.; Orido, T. Osteosarcoma. Ultrastructural and immunohistochemical studies on alkaline phosphatase-positive tumor cells constituting a variety of histologic types. *Acta Pathol. Jpn.* **1988**, *38*, 325–338. [CrossRef] [PubMed]
8. Dirik, Y.; Cinar, A.; Yumrukcal, F.; Eralp, L. Popliteal lymph node metastasis of tibial osteoblastic osteosarcoma. *Int. J. Surg. Case Rep.* **2014**, *5*, 840–844. [CrossRef] [PubMed]
9. Jeffree, G.M.; Price, C.H.; Sissons, H.A. The metastatic patterns of osteosarcoma. *Br. J. Cancer* **1975**, *32*, 87–107. [CrossRef] [PubMed]
10. Morello, E.; Martano, M.; Buracco, P. Biology, diagnosis and treatment of canine appendicular osteosarcoma: Similarities and differences with human osteosarcoma. *Vet. J.* **2011**, *189*, 268–277. [CrossRef] [PubMed]
11. Gill, J.; Ahluwalia, M.K.; Geller, D.; Gorlick, R. New targets and approaches in osteosarcoma. *Pharmacol. Ther.* **2013**, *137*, 89–99. [CrossRef] [PubMed]
12. Jaffe, N. Osteosarcoma: Review of the past, impact on the future. The American experience. *Cancer Treat Res.* **2009**, *152*, 239–262. [PubMed]
13. Modiano, J.F.; Breen, M.; Lana, S.E.; Ehrhart, N.; Fosmire, S.P.; Thomas, R.; Jubala, C.M.; Lamerato-Kozicki, A.R.; Ehrhart, E.J.; Schaack, J.; *et al.* Naturally occurring translational models for development of cancer therapy. *Gene Ther. Mol. Biol.* **2006**, *10*, 31–40.
14. Scott, M.C.; Sarver, A.L.; Gavin, K.J.; Thayanithy, V.; Getzy, D.M.; Newman, R.A.; Cutter, G.R.; Lindblad-Toh, K.; Kisseberth, W.C.; Hunter, L.E.; *et al.* Molecular subtypes of osteosarcoma identified by reducing tumor heterogeneity through an interspecies comparative approach. *Bone* **2011**, *49*, 356–367. [CrossRef] [PubMed]
15. Paoloni, M.; Davis, S.; Lana, S.; Withrow, S.; Sangiorgi, L.; Picci, P.; Hewitt, S.; Triche, T.; Meltzer, P.; Khanna, C. Canine tumor cross-species genomics uncovers targets linked to osteosarcoma progression. *BMC Genom.* **2009**, *10*, 625. [CrossRef] [PubMed]
16. Schiffman, J.D.; Breen, M. Comparative oncology: What dogs and other species can teach us about humans with cancer. *Philos. Trans. R. Soc. Lond. B Biol. Sci.* **2015**, *370*. [CrossRef] [PubMed]
17. Thomas, R.; Wang, H.J.; Tsai, P.C.; Langford, C.F.; Fosmire, S.P.; Jubala, C.M.; Getzy, D.M.; Cutter, G.R.; Modiano, J.F.; Breen, M. Influence of genetic background on tumor karyotypes: Evidence for breed-associated cytogenetic aberrations in canine appendicular osteosarcoma. *Chromosome Res.* **2009**, *17*, 365–377. [CrossRef] [PubMed]

18. McNeill, C.J.; Overley, B.; Shofer, F.S.; Kent, M.S.; Clifford, C.A.; Samluk, M.; Haney, S.; van Winkle, T.J.; Sorenmo, K.U. Characterization of the biological behaviour of appendicular osteosarcoma in Rottweilers and a comparison with other breeds: A review of 258 dogs. *Vet. Comp. Oncol.* **2007**, *5*, 90–98. [CrossRef] [PubMed]

19. Dobson, J.M. Breed-predispositions to cancer in pedigree dogs. *ISRN Vet. Sci.* **2013**, *2013*, 941275. [CrossRef] [PubMed]

20. Paoloni, M.; Khanna, C. Translation of new cancer treatments from pet dogs to humans. *Nat. Rev. Cancer* **2008**, *8*, 147–156. [CrossRef] [PubMed]

21. Isakoff, M.S.; Bielack, S.S.; Meltzer, P.; Gorlick, R. Osteosarcoma: Current treatment and a collaborative pathway to success. *J. Clin. Oncol.* **2015**, *33*, 3029–3035. [CrossRef] [PubMed]

22. Ferrari, S.; Serra, M. An update on chemotherapy for osteosarcoma. *Expert Opin. Pharmacother.* **2015**, *16*, 2727–2736. [CrossRef] [PubMed]

23. Perry, J.A.; Kiezun, A.; Tonzi, P.; van Allen, E.M.; Carter, S.L.; Baca, S.C.; Cowley, G.S.; Bhatt, A.S.; Rheinbay, E.; Pedamallu, C.S.; *et al.* Complementary genomic approaches highlight the PI3K/mTOR pathway as a common vulnerability in osteosarcoma. *Proc. Natl. Acad. Sci. USA* **2014**, *111*, 5564–5573. [CrossRef] [PubMed]

24. Morrow, J.J.; Khanna, C. Osteosarcoma genetics and epigenetics: Emerging biology and candidate therapies. *Crit. Rev. Oncog.* **2015**, *20*, 173–197. [CrossRef] [PubMed]

25. Li, N.; Luo, D.; Hu, X.; Luo, W.; Lei, G.; Wang, Q.; Zhu, T.; Gu, J.; Lu, Y.; Zheng, Q. RUNX2 and osteosarcoma. *Anticancer Agents Med. Chem.* **2015**, *15*, 881–887. [CrossRef] [PubMed]

26. Tian, J.; He, H.; Lei, G. Wnt/beta-catenin pathway in bone cancers. *Tumour Biol.* **2014**, *35*, 9439–9445. [CrossRef] [PubMed]

27. Lamora, A.; Talbot, J.; Bougras, G.; Amiaud, J.; Leduc, M.; Chesneau, J.; Taurelle, J.; Stresing, V.; Le Deley, M.C.; Heymann, M.F.; *et al.* Overexpression of smad7 blocks primary tumor growth and lung metastasis development in osteosarcoma. *Clin. Cancer Res.* **2014**, *20*, 5097–5112. [CrossRef] [PubMed]

28. Khanna, C.; Wan, X.; Bose, S.; Cassaday, R.; Olomu, O.; Mendoza, A.; Yeung, C.; Gorlick, R.; Hewitt, S.M.; Helman, L.J. The membrane-cytoskeleton linker ezrin is necessary for osteosarcoma metastasis. *Nat. Med.* **2004**, *10*, 182–186. [CrossRef] [PubMed]

29. Moriarity, B.S.; Otto, G.M.; Rahrmann, E.P.; Rathe, S.K.; Wolf, N.K.; Weg, M.T.; Manlove, L.A.; LaRue, R.S.; Temiz, N.A. A Sleeping Beauty forward genetic screen identifies new genes and pathways driving osteosarcoma development and metastasis. **2015**, *47*, 615–624. [CrossRef] [PubMed]

30. Chang, L.; Shrestha, S.; LaChaud, G.; Scott, M.A.; James, A.W. Review of microRNA in osteosarcoma and chondrosarcoma. *Med. Oncol.* **2015**, *32*, 613. [CrossRef] [PubMed]

31. Geller, D.S.; Gorlick, R. Osteosarcoma: A review of diagnosis, management, and treatment strategies. *Clin. Adv. Hematol. Oncol.* **2010**, *8*, 705–718. [PubMed]

32. Mirabello, L.; Pfeiffer, R.; Murphy, G.; Daw, N.C.; Patino-Garcia, A.; Troisi, R.J.; Hoover, R.N.; Douglass, C.; Schuz, J.; Craft, A.W.; *et al.* Height at diagnosis and birth-weight as risk factors for osteosarcoma. *Cancer Causes Control* **2011**, *22*, 899–908. [CrossRef] [PubMed]

33. Savage, S.A.; Woodson, K.; Walk, E.; Modi, W.; Liao, J.; Douglass, C.; Hoover, R.N.; Chanock, S.J. Analysis of genes critical for growth regulation identifies Insulin-like Growth Factor 2 Receptor variations with possible functional significance as risk factors for osteosarcoma. *Cancer Epidemiol. Biomark. Prev.* **2007**, *16*, 1667–1674. [CrossRef] [PubMed]

34. Miller, R.W. Contrasting epidemiology of childhood osteosarcoma, Ewing's tumor, and rhabdomyosarcoma. *Natl. Cancer Inst. Monogr.* **1981**, *56*, 9–15. [PubMed]

35. Jawad, M.U.; Cheung, M.C.; Min, E.S.; Schneiderbauer, M.M.; Koniaris, L.G.; Scully, S.P. Ewing sarcoma demonstrates racial disparities in incidence-related and sex-related differences in outcome: An analysis of 1631 cases from the SEER database, 1973–2005. *Cancer* **2009**, *115*, 3526–3536. [CrossRef] [PubMed]

36. Savage, S.A.; Mirabello, L.; Wang, Z.; Gastier-Foster, J.M.; Gorlick, R.; Khanna, C.; Flanagan, A.M.; Tirabosco, R.; Andrulis, I.L.; Wunder, J.S.; *et al.* Genome-wide association study identifies two susceptibility loci for osteosarcoma. *Nat. Genet.* **2013**, *45*, 799–803. [CrossRef] [PubMed]

37. Mirabello, L.; Koster, R.; Moriarity, B.S.; Spector, L.G.; Meltzer, P.S.; Gary, J.; Machiela, M.J.; Pankratz, N.; Panagiotou, O.A.; Largaespada, D.; *et al.* A Genome-wide scan identifies variants in NFIB associated with metastasis in patients with osteosarcoma. *Cancer Discov.* **2015**, *5*, 920–931. [CrossRef] [PubMed]

38. Gorlick, R.; Khanna, C. Osteosarcoma. *J. Bone Miner. Res.* **2010**, *25*, 683–691. [CrossRef] [PubMed]

39. Hameed, M.; Dorfman, H. Primary malignant bone tumors—Recent developments. *Semin. Diagn. Pathol.* **2011**, *28*, 86–101. [CrossRef] [PubMed]

40. Anfinsen, K.P.; Grotmol, T.; Bruland, O.S.; Jonasdottir, T.J. Breed-specific incidence rates of canine primary bone tumors—A population based survey of dogs in Norway. *Can. J. Vet. Res.* **2011**, *75*, 209–215. [PubMed]

41. Liptak, J.M.; Dernell, W.S.; Straw, R.C.; Rizzo, S.A.; Lafferty, M.H.; Withrow, S.J. Proximal radial and distal humeral osteosarcoma in 12 dogs. *J. Am. Anim. Hosp. Assoc.* **2004**, *40*, 461–467. [CrossRef] [PubMed]

42. Boerman, I.; Selvarajah, G.T.; Nielen, M.; Kirpensteijn, J. Prognostic factors in canine appendicular osteosarcoma—A meta-analysis. *BMC Vet. Res.* **2012**, *8*, 56–56. [CrossRef] [PubMed]

43. Fenger, J.M.; London, C.A.; Kisseberth, W.C. Canine osteosarcoma: A naturally occurring disease to inform pediatric oncology. *ILAR J.* **2014**, *55*, 69–85. [CrossRef] [PubMed]

44. Szewczyk, M.; Lechowski, R.; Zabielska, K. What do we know about canine osteosarcoma treatment? Review. *Vet. Res. Commun.* **2015**, *39*, 61–67. [CrossRef] [PubMed]

45. Berg, J. Canine osteosarcoma: Amputation and chemotherapy. *Vet. Clin. N. Am. Small Anim. Pract.* **1996**, *26*, 111–121. [CrossRef]

46. Straw, R.C.; Withrow, S.J.; Powers, B.E. Management of canine appendicular osteosarcoma. *Vet. Clin. North Am. Small Anim. Pract.* **1990**, *20*, 1141–1161. [CrossRef]

47. Gilson, S.D. Principles of surgery for cancer palliation and treatment of metastases. *Clin. Tech. Small Anim. Pract.* **1998**, *13*, 65–69. [CrossRef]

48. Guijarro, M.V.; Ghivizzani, S.C.; Gibbs, C.P. Animal models in osteosarcoma. *Front. Oncol.* **2014**, *4*, 189. [PubMed]

49. Ruther, U.; Komitowski, D.; Schubert, F.R.; Wagner, E.F. c-fos expression induces bone tumors in transgenic mice. *Oncogene* **1989**, *4*, 861–865. [PubMed]

50. Entz-Werle, N.; Choquet, P.; Neuville, A.; Kuchler-Bopp, S.; Clauss, F.; Danse, J.M.; Simo-Noumbissie, P.; Guerin, E.; Gaub, M.P.; Freund, J.N.; *et al.* Targeted apc;twist double-mutant mice: A new model of spontaneous osteosarcoma that mimics the human disease. *Transl. Oncol.* **2010**, *3*, 344–353. [CrossRef] [PubMed]

51. Walkley, C.R.; Qudsi, R.; Sankaran, V.G.; Perry, J.A.; Gostissa, M.; Roth, S.I.; Rodda, S.J.; Snay, E.; Dunning, P.; Fahey, F.H.; *et al.* Conditional mouse osteosarcoma, dependent on p53 loss and potentiated by loss of Rb, mimics the human disease. *Genes Dev* **2008**, *22*, 1662–1676. [CrossRef] [PubMed]

52. Rao, P.H.; Zhao, S.; Zhao, Y.J.; Yu, A.; Rainusso, N.; Trucco, M.; Allen-Rhoades, W.; Satterfield, L.; Fuja, D.; Borra, V.J.; *et al.* Coamplification of Myc/Pvt1 and homozygous deletion of Nlrp1 locus are frequent genetics changes in mouse osteosarcoma. *Genes Chromosomes Cancer* **2015**, *54*, 796–808. [CrossRef] [PubMed]

53. Mohseny, A.B.; Hogendoorn, P.C.; Cleton-Jansen, A.M. Osteosarcoma models: From cell lines to zebrafish. *Sarcoma* **2012**, *2012*, 417271. [CrossRef] [PubMed]

54. Merchant, M.S.; Melchionda, F.; Sinha, M.; Khanna, C.; Helman, L.; Mackall, C.L. Immune reconstitution prevents metastatic recurrence of murine osteosarcoma. *Cancer Immunol. Immunother.* **2007**, *56*, 1037–1046. [CrossRef] [PubMed]

55. Olive, K.P.; Tuveson, D.A.; Ruhe, Z.C.; Yin, B.; Willis, N.A.; Bronson, R.T.; Crowley, D.; Jacks, T. Mutant p53 gain of function in two mouse models of Li-Fraumeni syndrome. *Cell* **2004**, *119*, 847–860. [CrossRef] [PubMed]

56. Angstadt, A.Y.; Thayanithy, V.; Subramanian, S.; Modiano, J.F.; Breen, M. A genome-wide approach to comparative oncology: High-resolution oligonucleotide aCGH of canine and human osteosarcoma pinpoints shared microaberrations. *Cancer Genet.* **2012**, *205*, 572–587. [CrossRef] [PubMed]

57. Chen, X.; Bahrami, A.; Pappo, A.; Easton, J.; Dalton, J.; Hedlund, E.; Ellison, D.; Shurtleff, S.; Wu, G.; Wei, L.; *et al.* Recurrent somatic structural variations contribute to tumorigenesis in pediatric osteosarcoma. *Cell Rep.* **2014**, *7*, 104–112. [CrossRef] [PubMed]

58. Scott, M.C.; Sarver, A.L.; Tomiyasu, H.; Cornax, I.; van Etten, J.; Varshney, J.; O'Sullivan, M.G.; Subramanian, S.; Modiano, J.F. Aberrant RB-E2F transcriptional regulation defines molecular phenotypes of osteosarcoma. *J. Biol. Chem.* **2015**. [CrossRef] [PubMed]

59. Ren, W.; Gu, G. Prognostic implications of RB1 tumour suppressor gene alterations in the clinical outcome of human osteosarcoma: A meta-analysis. *Eur. J. Cancer Care* **2015**. [CrossRef] [PubMed]

60. Sampson, V.B.; Yoo, S.; Kumar, A.; Vetter, N.S.; Kolb, E.A. MicroRNAs and potential targets in osteosarcoma: Review. *Front. Pediatr.* **2015**, *3*, 69. [PubMed]

61. Zhang, J.; Yan, Y.G.; Wang, C.; Zhang, S.J.; Yu, X.H.; Wang, W.J. MicroRNAs in osteosarcoma. *Clin. Chim. Acta* **2015**, *444*, 9–17. [CrossRef] [PubMed]

62. Miao, J.; Wu, S.; Peng, Z.; Tania, M.; and Zhang, C. MicroRNAs in osteosarcoma: Diagnostic and therapeutic aspects. *Tumour Biol.* **2013**, *34*, 2093–2098. [CrossRef] [PubMed]

63. Zhou, G.; Shi, X.; Zhang, J.; Wu, S.; Zhao, J. MicroRNAs in osteosarcoma: From biological players to clinical contributors, a review. *J. Int. Med. Res.* **2013**, *41*, 1–12. [CrossRef] [PubMed]

64. Li, Y.; Zhang, J.; Zhang, L.; Si, M.; Yin, H.; Li, J. Diallyl trisulfide inhibits proliferation, invasion and angiogenesis of osteosarcoma cells by switching on suppressor microRNAs and inactivating of Notch-1 signaling. *Carcinogenesis* **2013**, *34*, 1601–1610. [CrossRef] [PubMed]

65. Sarver, A.L.; Thayanithy, V.; Scott, M.C.; Cleton-Jansen, A.M.; Hogendoorn, P.C.; Modiano, J.F.; Subramanian, S. MicroRNAs at the human 14q32 locus have prognostic significance in osteosarcoma. *Orphanet J. Rare Dis.* **2013**, *8*, 7. [CrossRef] [PubMed]

66. Namlos, H.M.; Meza-Zepeda, L.A.; Baroy, T.; Ostensen, I.H.; Kresse, S.H.; Kuijjer, M.L.; Serra, M.; Burger, H.; Cleton-Jansen, A.M.; Myklebost, O. Modulation of the osteosarcoma expression phenotype by microRNAs. *PLoS ONE* **2012**, *7*, e48086. [CrossRef] [PubMed]

67. Lulla, R.R.; Costa, F.F.; Bischof, J.M.; Chou, P.M.; de, F.B.M.; Vanin, E.F.; Soares, M.B. Identification of differentially expressed MicroRNAs in osteosarcoma. *Sarcoma* **2011**, *2011*, 732690. [CrossRef] [PubMed]

68. Varshney, J.; Subramanian, S. MicroRNAs as potential target in human bone and soft tissue sarcoma therapeutics. *Front. Mol. Biosci.* **2015**, *2*, 31. [CrossRef] [PubMed]

69. Sarver, A.L.; Phalak, R.; Thayanithy, V.; Subramanian, S. S-MED: Sarcoma microRNA expression database. *Lab. Investig. J. Tech. Methods Pathol.* **2010**, *90*, 753–761. [CrossRef] [PubMed]

70. Thayanithy, V.; Sarver, A.L.; Kartha, R.V.; Li, L.; Angstadt, A.Y.; Breen, M.; Steer, C.J.; Modiano, J.F.; Subramanian, S. Perturbation of 14q32 miRNAs-cMYC gene network in osteosarcoma. *Bone* **2012**, *50*, 171–181. [CrossRef] [PubMed]

71. Li, Y.; Choi, P.S.; Casey, S.C.; Dill, D.L.; Felsher, D.W. MYC through miR-17–92 suppresses specific target genes to maintain survival, autonomous proliferation, and a neoplastic state. *Cancer Cell* **2014**, *26*, 262–272. [CrossRef] [PubMed]

72. Schaap-Oziemlak, A.M.; Raymakers, R.A.; Bergevoet, S.M.; Gilissen, C.; Jansen, B.J.; Adema, G.J.; Kogler, G.; le Sage, C.; Agami, R.; van der Reijden, B.A.; *et al.* MicroRNA hsa-miR-135b regulates mineralization in osteogenic differentiation of human unrestricted somatic stem cells. *Stem. Cells Dev.* **2010**, *19*, 877–885. [CrossRef] [PubMed]

73. Wei, J.Q.; Chen, H.; Zheng, X.F.; Zhang, B.X.; Wang, Y.; Tang, P.F.; She, F.; Song, Q.; Li, T.S. Hsa-miR-654–5p regulates osteogenic differentiation of human bone marrow mesenchymal stem cells by repressing bone morphogenetic protein 2. *J. Southern Med. Univ.* **2012**, *32*, 291–295.

74. Fang, S.; Deng, Y.; Gu, P.; Fan, X. MicroRNAs regulate bone development and regeneration. *Int. J. Mol. Sci.* **2015**, *16*, 8227–8253. [CrossRef] [PubMed]

75. Inose, H.; Ochi, H.; Kimura, A.; Fujita, K.; Xu, R.; Sato, S.; Iwasaki, M.; Sunamura, S.; Takeuchi, Y.; Fukumoto, S.; *et al.* A microRNA regulatory mechanism of osteoblast differentiation. *Proc. Natl. Acad. Sci. USA* **2009**, *106*, 20794–20799. [CrossRef] [PubMed]

76. Feng, Z.; Zhang, C.; Wu, R.; Hu, W. Tumor suppressor p53 meets microRNAs. *J. Mol. Cell Biol.* **2011**, *3*, 44–50. [CrossRef] [PubMed]

77. Wang, Y.; Jia, L.S.; Yuan, W.; Wu, Z.; Wang, H.B.; Xu, T.; Sun, J.C.; Cheng, K.F.; Shi, J.G. Low miR-34a and miR-192 are associated with unfavorable prognosis in patients suffering from osteosarcoma. *Am. J. Transl. Res.* **2015**, *7*, 111–119. [PubMed]

78. Zhao, H.; Ma, B.; Wang, Y.; Han, T.; Zheng, L.; Sun, C.; Liu, T.; Zhang, Y.; Qiu, X.; Fan, Q. miR-34a inhibits the metastasis of osteosarcoma cells by repressing the expression of CD44. *Oncol. Rep.* **2013**, *29*, 1027–1036. [PubMed]

79. He, C.; Xiong, J.; Xu, X.; Lu, W.; Liu, L.; Xiao, D.; Wang, D. Functional elucidation of MiR-34 in osteosarcoma cells and primary tumor samples. *Biochem. Biophys. Res. Commun.* **2009**, *388*, 35–40. [CrossRef] [PubMed]

80. Pazzaglia, L.; Leonardi, L.; Conti, A.; Novello, C.; Quattrini, I.; Montanini, L.; Roperto, F.; del Piero, F.; di Guardo, G.; Piro, F.; *et al.* miR-196a expression in human and canine osteosarcomas: A comparative study. *Res. Vet. Sci.* **2015**, *99*, 112–119. [CrossRef] [PubMed]

81. Zhang, W.; Zhang, C.; Chen, H.; Li, L.; Tu, Y.; Liu, C.; Shi, S.; Zen, K.; Liu, Z. Evaluation of microRNAs miR-196a, miR-30a-5P, and miR-490 as biomarkers of disease activity among patients with FSGS. *Clin. J. Am. Soc. Nephrol.* **2014**, *9*, 1545–1552. [CrossRef] [PubMed]

82. Gardner, H.L.; Fenger, J.M.; London, C.A. Dogs as a model for cancer. *Annu. Rev. Anim. Biosci.* **2015**, in print. [CrossRef] [PubMed]

83. Xu, M.; Jin, H.; Xu, C.X.; Sun, B.; Song, Z.G.; Bi, W.Z.; Wang, Y. miR-382 inhibits osteosarcoma metastasis and relapse by targeting Y box-binding protein 1. *Mol. Ther.* **2015**, *23*, 89–98. [CrossRef] [PubMed]

84. Zhou, Y.; Huang, Z.; Wu, S.; Zang, X.; Liu, M.; Shi, J. miR-33a is up-regulated in chemoresistant osteosarcoma and promotes osteosarcoma cell resistance to cisplatin by down-regulating TWIST. *J. Exp. Clin. Cancer Res.* **2014**, *33*, 12. [CrossRef] [PubMed]

85. Xu, M.; Jin, H.; Xu, C.X.; Bi, W.Z.; Wang, Y. MiR-34c inhibits osteosarcoma metastasis and chemoresistance. *Med. Oncol.* **2014**, *31*, 972. [CrossRef] [PubMed]

86. Rosenblum, J.M.; Wijetunga, N.A.; Fazzari, M.J.; Krailo, M.; Barkauskas, D.A.; Gorlick, R.; Greally, J.M. Predictive properties of DNA methylation patterns in primary tumor samples for osteosarcoma relapse status. *Epigenetics* **2015**, *10*, 31–39. [CrossRef] [PubMed]

87. Kresse, S.H.; Rydbeck, H.; Skarn, M.; Namlos, H.M.; Barragan-Polania, A.H.; Cleton-Jansen, A.M.; Serra, M.; Liestol, K.; Hogendoorn, P.C.; Hovig, E.; *et al.* Integrative analysis reveals relationships of genetic and epigenetic alterations in osteosarcoma. *PLoS ONE* **2012**, *7*, e48262. [CrossRef] [PubMed]

88. Oh, J.H.; Kim, H.S.; Kim, H.H.; Kim, W.H.; Lee, S.H. Aberrant methylation of p14ARF gene correlates with poor survival in osteosarcoma. *Clin. Orthop. Relat. Res.* **2006**, *442*, 216–222. [CrossRef] [PubMed]

89. Park, Y.B.; Park, M.J.; Kimura, K.; Shimizu, K.; Lee, S.H.; Yokota, J. Alterations in the INK4a/ARF locus and their effects on the growth of human osteosarcoma cell lines. *Cancer Genet. Cytogenet.* **2002**, *133*, 105–111. [CrossRef]

90. Al-Romaih, K.; Sadikovic, B.; Yoshimoto, M.; Wang, Y.; Zielenska, M.; Squire, J.A. Decitabine-induced demethylation of 5′ CpG island in GADD45A leads to apoptosis in osteosarcoma cells. *Neoplasia* **2008**, *10*, 471–480. [CrossRef] [PubMed]

91. Badal, V.; Menendez, S.; Coomber, D.; Lane, D.P. Regulation of the p14ARF promoter by DNA methylation. *Cell Cycle* **2008**, *7*, 112–119. [CrossRef] [PubMed]

92. Chen, W.; Cooper, T.K.; Zahnow, C.A.; Overholtzer, M.; Zhao, Z.; Ladanyi, M.; Karp, J.E.; Gokgoz, N.; Wunder, J.S.; Andrulis, I.L.; *et al.* Epigenetic and genetic loss of Hic1 function accentuates the role of p53 in tumorigenesis. *Cancer Cell* **2004**, *6*, 387–398. [CrossRef] [PubMed]

93. Lu, J.; Song, G.; Tang, Q.; Zou, C.; Han, F.; Zhao, Z.; Yong, B.; Yin, J.; Xu, H.; Xie, X.; *et al.* IRX1 hypomethylation promotes osteosarcoma metastasis via induction of CXCL14/NF-kappaB signaling. *J. Clin. Investig.* **2015**, *125*, 1839–1856. [CrossRef] [PubMed]

94. Li, Y.; Meng, G.; Huang, L.; Guo, Q.N. Hypomethylation of the P3 promoter is associated with up-regulation of IGF2 expression in human osteosarcoma. *Hum. Pathol.* **2009**, *40*, 1441–1447. [CrossRef] [PubMed]

95. Ulaner, G.A.; Vu, T.H.; Li, T.; Hu, J.F.; Yao, X.M.; Yang, Y.; Gorlick, R.; Meyers, P.; Healey, J.; Ladanyi, M.; *et al.* Loss of imprinting of IGF2 and H19 in osteosarcoma is accompanied by reciprocal methylation changes of a CTCF-binding site. *Hum. Mol. Genet.* **2003**, *12*, 535–549. [CrossRef] [PubMed]

96. Li, Y.; Meng, G.; Guo, Q.N. Changes in genomic imprinting and gene expression associated with transformation in a model of human osteosarcoma. *Exp. Mol. Pathol.* **2008**, *84*, 234–239. [CrossRef] [PubMed]

97. Lee, D.F.; Su, J.; Kim, H.S.; Chang, B.; Papatsenko, D.; Zhao, R.; Yuan, Y.; Gingold, J.; Xia, W.; Darr, H.; *et al.* Modeling familial cancer with induced pluripotent stem cells. *Cell* **2015**, *161*, 240–254. [CrossRef] [PubMed]

98. Thayanithy, V.; Park, C.; Sarver, A.L.; Kartha, R.V.; Korpela, D.M.; Graef, A.J.; Steer, C.J.; Modiano, J.F.; Subramanian, S. Combinatorial treatment of DNA and chromatin-modifying drugs cause cell death in human and canine osteosarcoma cell lines. *PLoS ONE* **2012**, *7*, e43720. [CrossRef] [PubMed]

99. Zhang, X.; Cruz, F.D.; Terry, M.; Remotti, F.; Matushansky, I. Terminal differentiation and loss of tumorigenicity of human cancers via pluripotency-based reprogramming. *Oncogene* **2013**, *32*, 2249–2260. [CrossRef] [PubMed]

100. Maniscalco, L. Canine osteosarcoma: Understanding its variability to improve treatment. *Vet. J.* **2015**, *203*, 135–136. [CrossRef] [PubMed]

101. Rodriguez, C.O., Jr. Using canine osteosarcoma as a model to assess efficacy of novel therapies: Can old dogs teach us new tricks? *Adv. Exp. Med. Biol.* **2014**, *804*, 237–256. [PubMed]
102. Modiano, J.F.; Bellgrau, D.; Cutter, G.R.; Lana, S.E.; Ehrhart, N.P.; Ehrhart, E.; Wilke, V.L.; Charles, J.B.; Munson, S.; Scott, M.C.; *et al.* Inflammation, apoptosis, and necrosis induced by neoadjuvant fas ligand gene therapy improves survival of dogs with spontaneous bone cancer. *Mol. Ther.* **2012**, *20*, 2234–2243. [CrossRef] [PubMed]

Shape Variation in the Craniomandibular System and Prevalence of Dental Problems in Domestic Rabbits: A Case Study in Evolutionary Veterinary Science

Christine Böhmer [1,*] and Estella Böhmer [2]

[1]   UMR 7179 CNRS, Muséum National d'Histoire Naturelle, CP 55, 57 rue Cuvier, 75231 Paris CEDEX 05, France

[2]   Chirurgische und Gynäkologische Kleintierklinik ,Tierärztliche Fakultät, Ludwig-Maximilians-Universität München, Veterinärstr 13, 80539 München, Germany; e.boehmer@lmu.de

*   Correspondence: boehmer@vertevo.de

Academic Editor: Patrick Butaye

Abstract: In contrast to wild lagomorphs, pet rabbits exhibit a noticeably high frequency of dental problems. Although dietary habits are considered as a major factor contributing to acquired malocclusions, the exact causes and interrelationships are still under debate. In this regard, an important aspect that has not been considered thoroughly to date is the effect of diet-induced phenotypic plasticity in skull morphology. Therefore, we conducted a geometric morphometric analysis on skull radiological images of wild and pet rabbits in order to quantify intraspecific variation in craniomandibular morphology. The statistical analyses reveal a significant morphological differentiation of the craniomandibular system between both groups. Furthermore, the analysis of covariance shows that the force-generating modules (cranium and mandible) vary independently from the force-receiving module (hypselodont teeth) in pet rabbits, which is in contrast to their wild relatives. Our findings suggest that the phenotypic changes in domestic rabbits impact mastication performance and, consequently, oral health. An adequate close-to-nature nutrition throughout the whole life and especially beginning early parallel to weaning (phase of increased phenotypic plasticity) is necessary to ensure a normal strain on the teeth by promoting physiological lateral gliding movements and avoiding direct axial loads.

Keywords: masticatory apparatus; axial load; malocclusion; reference lines; Lagomorpha; evolutionary morphology; phenotypic plasticity

1. Introduction

All breeds of domestic rabbits descend from the European rabbit *Oryctolagus cuniculus*, which is a member of the family Leporidae (rabbits and hares). A remarkable peculiarity in veterinary medicine is the prevalence of dental problems among small herbivorous pet animals in general and rabbits in particular [1–3]. In pet rabbits, almost 90% of reported patients suffer from malocclusion caused by pathological tooth changes [1,4,5], in contrast to previous surveys that under-reported the frequency of dental problems: 30% [6], 38% [2]. Since obvious clinical evidence typically appears fairly late in the course of the dental disease, dental radiology is crucial for proper diagnosis [1,7–9]. Species-specific reference lines superimposed on radiographs enable objective interpretation of malocclusion in small pet animals [1,4,10,11]. Despite its proven usefulness in most domestic rabbits with a malocclusion, the anatomical reference lines appear to be not suitable for use in wild rabbits. This indicates intraspecific variation in skull morphology of the European rabbit (*Oryctolagus cuniculus*) and requires exploration in order to quantify morphological trends among domestic and wild rabbits.

It is well known that the evolution of wild species into domestic forms by artificial selection has resulted in changes in behavior and morphology [12,13] and various fields of research have improved our understanding of animal domestication [14,15]. Recent molecular approaches offered insights into the genotypic variation underpinning morphological and behavioral traits e.g., [16–19]. However, as of yet, the genetic changes associated with animal domestication are still not fully understood because most domestic animals are genetically diverse and there are multiple genetic pathways producing domestic traits [20–22]. Comparative morphometric analyses revealed variation in the morphology of wild and domestic animals and related it to allometry and differences in the timing of developmental processes i.e., heterochrony) e.g., [13,23–26]. Most obvious morphological changes under domestication can be seen in the skull, but it appears that not all cranial areas vary equally (modularity) [27–29]. For instance, a modular separation of the nasomaxillary complex versus the neurocranium has been noted in the skull of canids [27,30]. A similar pattern of modularity has been reported for the skull of felids and the functional implications have been related to respiratory dysfunction [29]. In rabbits, domestication has resulted in changes in morphology as well, notably in skull shape. However, both domestic and wild rabbits have continuously growing, high-crowned teeth (hypselodont) and, thus, dentition is not basically affected by the domestication process (Figure 1A,B). This indicates at least two distinct modules in the cranium of *O. cuniculus*. Yet, the covariation among distinct modules in the skull of rabbits and the link between morphological variation and functional implications (in particular mastication) remains largely unknown.

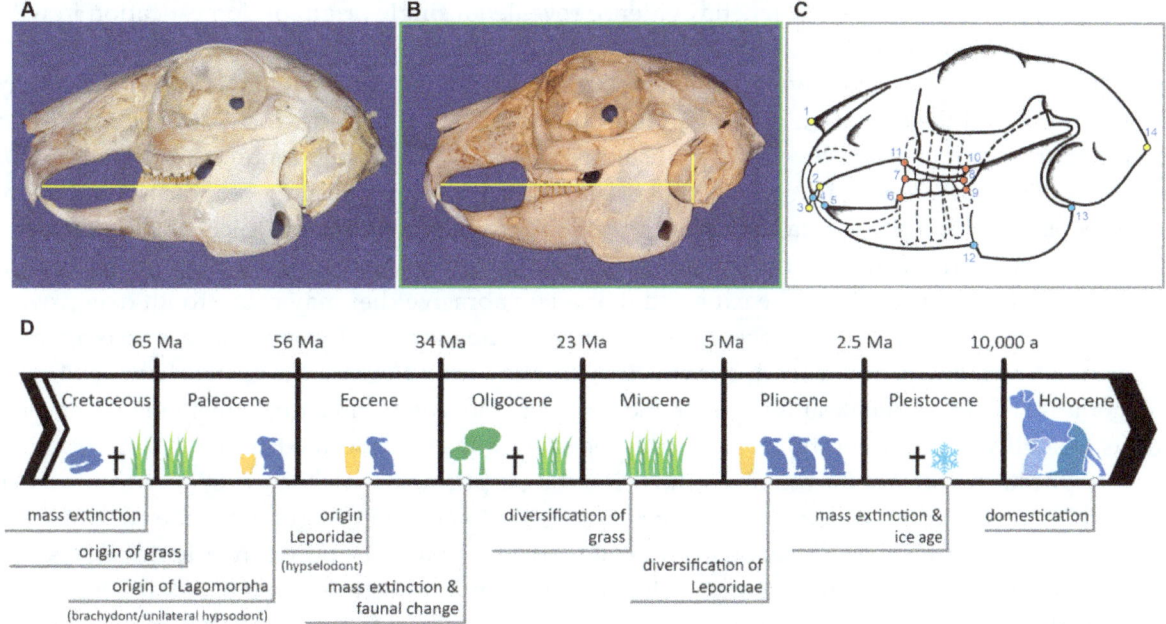

Figure 1. Morphology and evolution. (**A**) Craniomandibular morphology at occlusal resting pose in wild rabbit and (**B**) domestic rabbit in lateral view (scaled to same height). In pet rabbits without pathological changes of the skull or teeth, the species-specific reference line (yellow) begins at the rostral end of the hard palate immediately caudal to the second incisor and extends caudally to pass through the tympanic bulla at approximately one-third of its height (according to [4]); (**C**) Schematic representation of the 2D landmark set used in the present study (refer to Table 1 for description of landmarks). The color coding indicates the three landmark sub-sets representing the distinct modules: cranium (yellow), mandible (blue) and cheek teeth (red); (**D**) Simplified timeline of major evolutionary events concerning the origin of lagomorphs.

A major factor contributing to the alarming situation with regard to dental problems in pet rabbits is the feeding behavior [31,32], which strongly depends on the human pet owner and mostly differs from the natural diet of their wild relatives [31]. However, from an evolutionary perspective, teeth are an adaptation to feeding [33–36], and since a dynamic relation exists between diet, the masticatory apparatus and oral health, it is reasonable that differences in diet affect the dentition and may be causative for pathological tooth changes. The skeleton and teeth of domestic rabbits reflect their phylogenetic heritage and, thus, it is important to consider the evolutionary history of *O. cuniculus* in order to understand the significant role of the highly specialized masticatory apparatus in rabbits including their hypselodont teeth.

The evolutionary history of Leporidae dates back to the Eocene [37] and is linked to the global tectonic and environmental changes during the Cenozoic Era [38] (Figure 1D). Originating from Asia, the radiation of leporids across Europe and North America began in particular after the major turnover in terrestrial ecosystems at the Eocene-Oligocene boundary (about 34 Ma) [39]. During the Eocene-Oligocene transition (EOT), a change from warm-humid forests with large-sized perissodactyls as dominant mammals to dry-temperature forest-steppe with open grasslands and with small rodents and lagomorphs as the dominant group occurred [39]. Leporids reached the highest diversity during the Pliocene (5–2.5 Ma) expanding to Africa and South America [38,40] and by this time the oldest evidence of the European rabbit genus *Oryctolagus* is noted in the fossil record, associated with an arid, warm savannah-type fauna [40]. The global cooling during the Pleistocene (2–5 Ma-10,000 a) caused a severe decline in leporid diversity and many genera became extinct [40]. *Oryctolagus* persists until today, but with only one species (*O. cuniculus*) left, and the last glacial period confined it to the Iberian Peninsula and southern France [40]. About 1500 years ago, rabbit domestication was initiated [14,41] and historical records as well as genetic evidence revealed a single origin of domestication in wild populations from France [42].

Due to the interaction between climate and vegetation, the global climate change in the early Cenozoic affected the evolution of the herbivorous rabbits. In this context, a main factor limiting the life span of mammals in the wild is tooth abrasion e.g., [43]. Hypselodont teeth compensate for intensive abrasion (resulting in loss of dental tissue) during food intake and food processing and are regarded as an evolutionary adaptation to the high abrasiveness of plants which is a consequence of an increased silica content (intrinsic by phytoliths in grasses, extrinsic by dust ingested with grass) [33,34,44,45]. Thus, it can be expected that a less abrasive diet may cause tooth overgrowth terminating in malocclusion. However, there is evidence showing that hypselodonty is accompanied by a regulatory mechanism for tooth growth compensating for differences in dental abrasion [46–48]. This topic is still under debate and although the dentition and skull form a functional unit, the specific effects of skull shape in domestic rabbits in this regard have been neglected to date.

Despite its importance for veterinary medicine, it is surprising to note that we still lack knowledge about the patterns of morphological changes in the skull and dentition of a number of domestic animals including rabbits. Here, we quantify skull morphology in *O. cuniculus* in order to address the following questions: (1) how does the entire skull morphology vary between wild and domestic rabbits; (2) to what extent is morphological variation in the skull modular and (3) what are the implications for the masticatory apparatus of domestic rabbits. Ultimately, we seek to provide an explanation for the high abundance of dental problems in pet rabbits from an evolutionary perspective. This will not only improve our understanding of the relation between morphology and pathologies in domestic animals, but is also an important case study of Evolutionary Veterinary Science (EvoVetSci).

2. Materials and Methods

2.1. Data Set and Radiographic Screening

In this case study, we examine the skulls of 12 mature European wild rabbits and 12 mature domestic rabbits belonging to the species *O. cuniculus*. The wild rabbits originate from southern Germany and Austria (victims of traffic accidents). The sex is unknown. Due to the aforementioned prevalence of dental problems among domestic rabbits (almost 90%), the sample is somewhat limited, but sufficient to yield a reasonable signal. The pet rabbit sample represents no specific breed with erect ears in order to avoid extreme phenotypes characteristic of certain breeds. The specimens are radiographed for medical reasons and not for the purpose of this study. Only specimens with adult dentition and without pathologies are included. Skull radiographs (laterolateral view) of anesthetized specimens are obtained with the mouth closed or open about one millimeter [4].

2.2. Shape Analysis

Landmark-based geometric morphometrics was used to quantify skull morphology and to analyze phenotypic differences. A total of 14 landmarks (LMs) in two dimensions were taken on laterolateral radiological images of the skull (Table 1, Figure 1C). The homologous osteological points were chosen in order to describe the skull morphology considering the species-specific reference lines by Böhmer and Crossley [4] that enable objective interpretation of malocclusion in small pet animals. Sets of landmarks were subsequently separated into three distinct modules: cranium (LM 1, 2, 3 and 14), mandible (LM 4, 5, 12 and 13), and cheek teeth (LM 6, 7, 8, 9, 10 and 11) (Figure 1C). Using the software tpsDig2 [49], type I and type II landmarks (sensu [50]) were digitized onto the skulls in lateral view. The digitalization of the landmarks was performed by a single author (EB) in order to prevent inter-observer measurement errors. The placement of the landmarks were repeated three times for each individual. The assessment of intra-observer variance revealed that the error is low ensuring reproducibility of the measurements. In order to superimpose geometries and to isolate size and shape, a generalized Procrustes analysis (GPA) was conducted using the software Morphologika^2 [51]. Next, a relative warp (RW) analysis was performed in the same software. The RW analysis summarized the multi-dimensional information and constructed a morphospace in which shape variation can be quantified. With the applied settings, this method is equivalent to a principal components analysis. The shape differences were visualized with thin-plate splines.

Table 1. Definition of landmarks (LM) (type I and II (sensu [50])) applied to laterolateral radiological images of the skull in wild and domestic rabbits.

LM	Type	Definition
1	II	most anterior point of nasal bone
2	I	intersection between second maxillary incisor (I2) (peg tooth) and maxillary bone
3	II	most anterior tip of first maxillary incisor (I1)
4	II	most anterior tip of first mandibular incisor (i1)
5	I	intersection between first mandibular incisor (i1) and mandibular bone
6	I	anterior intersection between mandible and first mandibular cheek tooth (p2)
7	II	most anterior point of occlusal plane between maxillary and mandibular first cheek tooth (P2, p2)
8	II	most posterior point of occlusal plane between maxillary and mandibular last molar (M3, m3)
9	I	posterior intersection between mandible and last mandibular molar (m3)
10	I	posterior intersection between maxillary bone and last maxillary molar (M3)
11	I	anterior intersection between maxillary bone and first maxillary cheek tooth (P2)
12	II	antegonial notch of mandible
13	II	most posterior dorsal point of angular process
14	II	most posterior point of occipital protuberance

All subsequent analyses and statistical tests were performed using the software PAST [52]. In order to test if shape variation is a function of size, a multivariate regression analysis (log centroid size against RWs) was performed. Log transformed centroid size, the sum of squared distances of each landmark from the centroid of the skull, was used as a measure of size and RWs as a measure of shape [53]. A discriminant analysis was performed in order to test for significance of differences between the shapes of wild and domestic rabbits. Therefore, the RWs were subjected to a Hotelling's T^2 test. The Procrustes distances of both groups (wild vs. domestic rabbits) from group mean shape were calculated as a measure of disparity (i.e., morphological diversity) [54].

2.3. Integration and Modularity

Modular covariation of the shape between cranium, mandible and cheek teeth is investigated using two-block partial least squares (2-block PLS) analysis [55] in the software PAST [52]. The program analyzes two blocks of shape data as separate configurations. Therefore, the data from the single Procrustes fit for the entire structure (skull) is divided into three subsets with equal number of landmark coordinates in order to analyze the modules against each other: module 1 (cranium) against module 2 (mandible), module 1 against module 3 (cheek teeth), and module 2 against module 3.

3. Results

The collected 2D LM coordinates of the analyzed specimens are available in supplementary Table S1.

3.1. Patterns of Morphological Diversification

About 95% of the total variance in the sample is explained by the first nine RWs (Table 2). The first three RWs account for more than 75% of the total variance in the sample (RW 1: 56.60%, RW 2: 13.24%, RW 3: 9.91%) and the morphospace constructed from RW 1 and RW 2 provides a reasonable approximation of the shape variation (Figure 2A). Wild and domestic rabbits are clearly separated along RW 2 and to a lesser extent along RW 1. The scatter plot reveals that the majority of wild rabbits fall in quadrant four, whereas almost all domestic rabbits lie in quadrant one and two, respectively.

Table 2. Variance and cumulative variance percentages per relative warp (RW).

RW	Variance (%)	Cumulative Variance (%)
RW 1	54.60	54.60
RW 2	13.24	67.83
RW 3	9.91	77.74
RW 4	5.25	83.00
RW 5	3.72	86.72
RW 6	2.80	89.52
RW 7	2.67	92.19
RW 8	2.14	94.33
RW 9	1.40	95.73

The Hotelling's T^2 test on the first nine RWs reveals that the mean difference values are significantly high (p-value < 0.001), predicting major differences between both groups. Figure 3 shows the result of the discrimination analysis. There is no significant difference between the morphological disparity (MD) of both groups: MD (wild rabbits) = 0.46 and MD (domestic rabbits) = 0.40 (t-test: p-value > 0.05).

In total, the geometric morphometric analysis thus indicates a distinct morphological differentiation between wild and domestic rabbit skulls.

3.2. Allometry: Size and Shape

The variance of log centroid size in wild and domestic rabbits is significantly different ($p < 0.05$). Means of log centroid size do not differ significantly between both groups ($p > 0.05$). Thus, the skull of pet rabbits reveals a larger variation in size than their wild counterparts. However, the average size is similar in both groups.

Allometry of the skull accounts partly for a portion of shape variation among rabbits. The multivariate regression of the shape variables (RW 1–9) on log centroid size shows that shape variation associated with RW 1, 3 and 5 to 9 are not a function of size (Table 3). There is an allometric relationship with RW 2 and RW 4 ($p < 0.05$). The amount of shape variation accounted for by the regressions is about 16.88% and 51.10%, respectively (Table 3). The plot of RW 2 against log centroid size reveals a separation of wild rabbits associated with negative RW 2 values and smaller log centroid size and domestic rabbits related with positive RW 2 values and larger log centroid size (Figure 4). The latter vary slightly in size, whereas wild rabbits are all of same size (Figure 4).

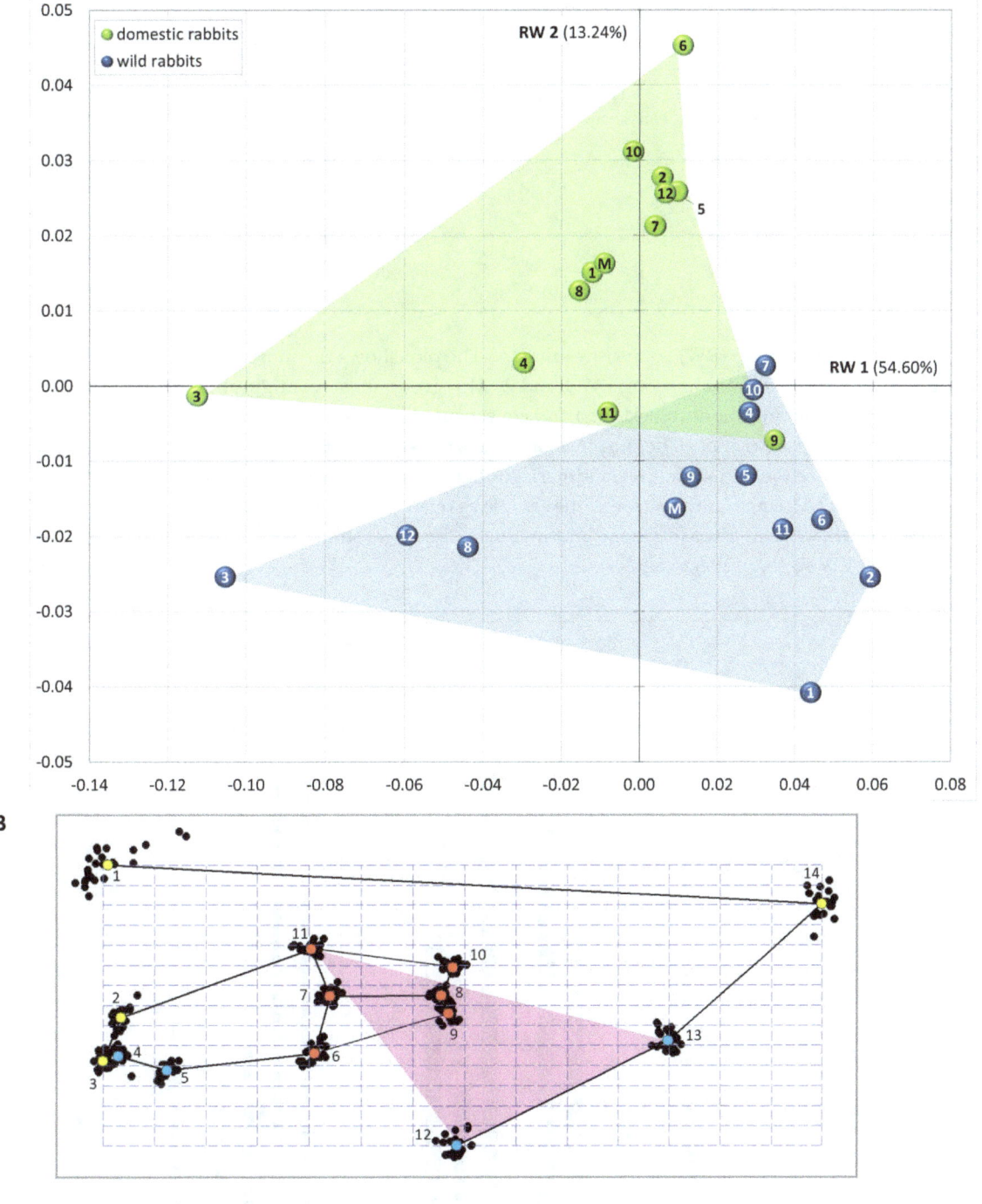

Figure 2. *Cont.*

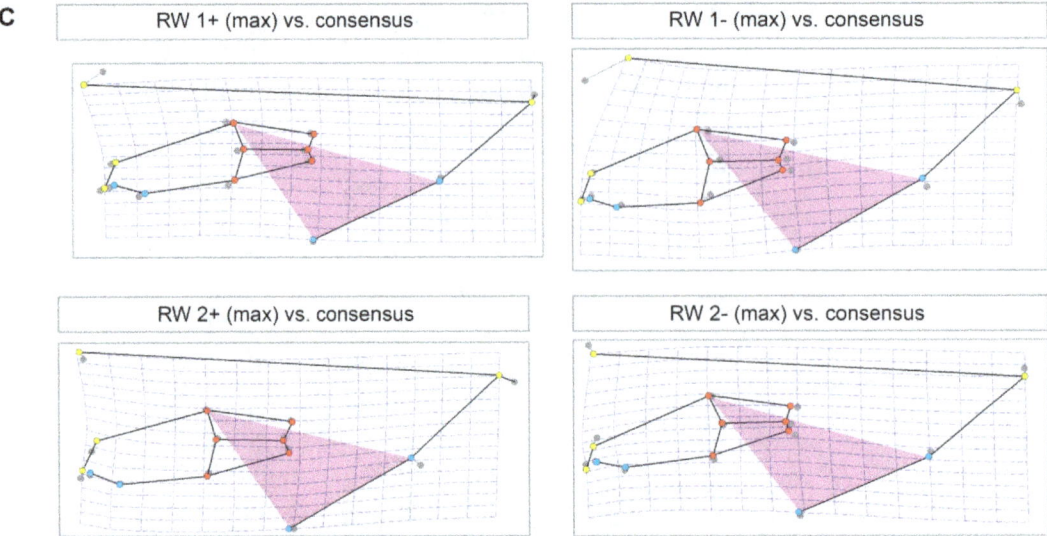

Figure 2. Relative warp (RW) analysis results. (**A**) The plot shows the morphological diversification of domestic and wild rabbits along RW 1 and 2. M = group mean configuration; (**B**) Scatterplot of all landmark configurations (black dots) and consensus shape (colored dots) as reference form after Procrustes superimposition. The purple area depicts the superficial masseter muscle (**C**) Thin-plate splines visualize the variation. The landmark configuration in grey represents the consensus shape (zero point in (**A**); equals mean shape of the sample as reference). The landmark configuration in color linked with black lines gives the shape information of the target shape associated with maximum and minimum RW scores, respectively.

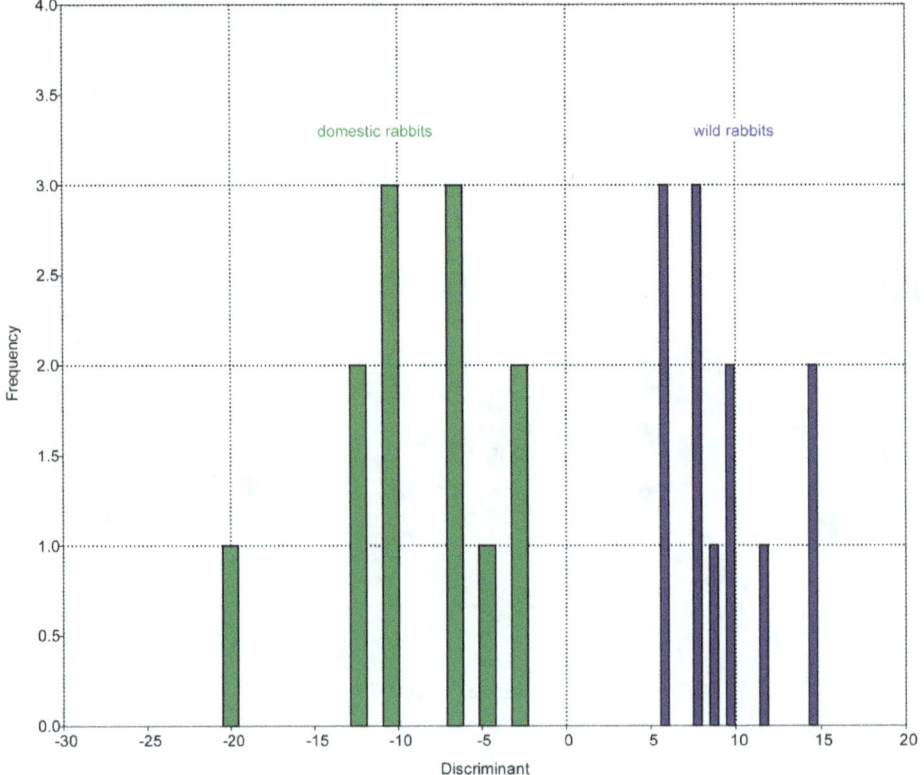

Figure 3. Discrimination analysis results. The histogram displays distinct separation between both groups of rabbits on basis of the morphological analysis.

Table 3. Multivariate regression of log centroid size against the first nine relative warps (RW), with coefficient of determination (r²) and significance value (p-value) for the null hypothesis. Asterisk (*) marks significant p-value.

	Log Centroid Size	
	r^2	p-Value
RW 1	0.035066	0.38092
RW 2	0.168757	0.046143 *
RW 3	0.010572	0.63258
RW 4	0.510982	8.67×10^{-5} *
RW 5	0.023031	0.47901
RW 6	0.017082	0.54269
RW 7	0.046522	0.31144
RW 8	0.001987	0.83617
RW 9	0.004693	0.75044

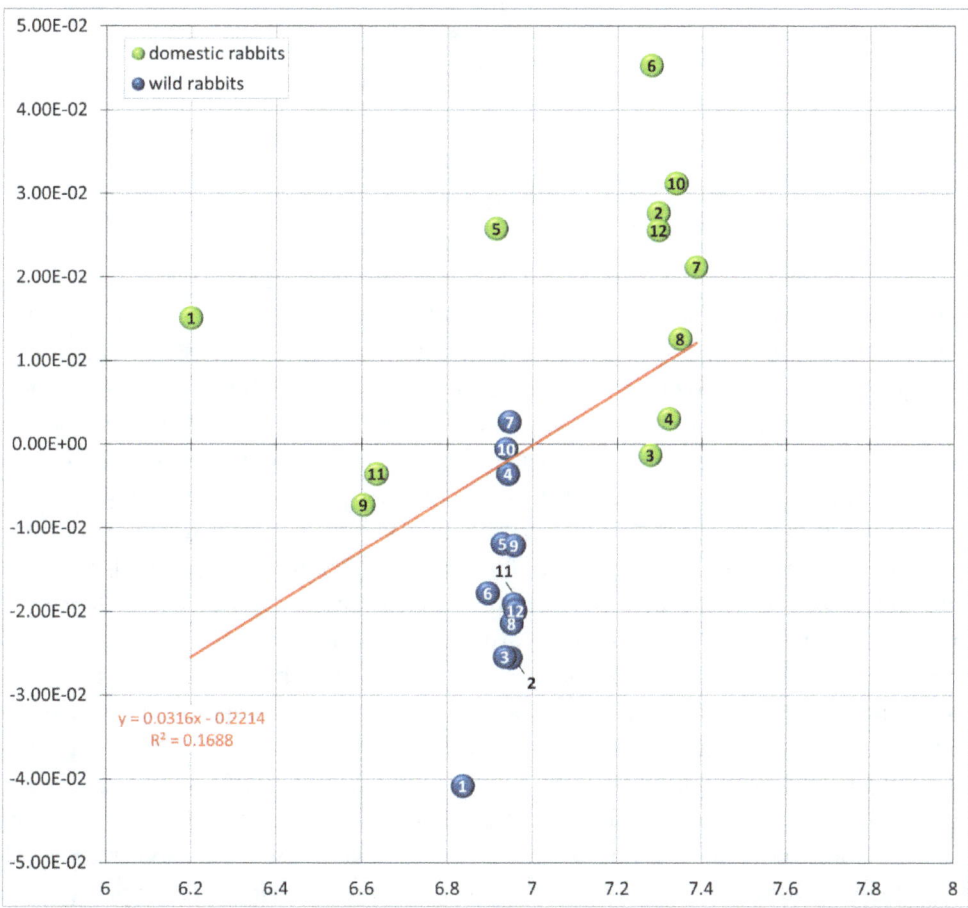

Figure 4. Regression of log centroid size (a measure of size) against the relative warp (RW) 2 (a measure of shape).

3.3. Landmark Variance

Comparing the consensus shape (mean shape of the sample) with all landmark configurations after Procrustes superimposition visualizes the shape variation within the sample (Figure 2B). It indicates the difference in location of corresponding landmarks. LM 1 (tip of nasal bone) reveals the highest variance by far (Table 4). Although by a magnitude smaller, LM 14 (tip of occipital protuberance) displays the second highest variance. The least variable homologous point is LM 3 (tip of incisor). LM 8 and 10 that characterize the last molar (m3), reveal a relatively low variance as well (Table 4).

Table 4. Variance (s^2) at applied landmarks (LM) (sorted in descending order).

LM	Variance (s^2)
1	1.6041×10^{-3}
14	0.32197×10^{-3}
12	0.23093×10^{-3}
6	0.20758×10^{-3}
13	0.1961×10^{-3}
2	0.1612×10^{-3}
11	0.13185×10^{-3}
4	0.12278×10^{-3}
5	0.10884×10^{-3}
7	0.10744×10^{-3}
9	0.10476×10^{-3}
10	0.09878×10^{-3}
8	0.08468×10^{-3}
3	0.07512×10^{-3}

3.4. Skull Shape Variation (Thin-Plate Splines)

RW 2 and to a lesser extent RW 1 separate wild and domestic rabbits. RW 1 and RW 2 primarily contrast anteroposteriorly elongated and dorsoventrally compressed skulls (positive RW 1 values, negative RW 2 values) against those that are anteroposteriorly compressed and dorsoventrally expanded (negative RW 1 values, positive RW 2 values) (Figure 2C). This pattern is driven in general by an overall change of the skull, but in particular combined by a change in the area of the nasal bone. Positive RW 1 and negative RW 2 scores are largely occupied by wild rabbits indicating that they tend to have a relatively long skull with the nasal bone projecting anteriorly over the incisors (Figure 2A,C). In contrast, negative RW 1 and positive RW 2 scores tend to characterize domestic rabbits displaying a relatively short skull and the tip of the nasal bone posterior to the incisors (Figure 2A,C). Other significant differences between both groups include the spatial displacement of important muscle unit attachment points, such as the relative position of the occipital protuberance and the angular process. In lateral view, the antegonial notch of the mandible lies on a vertical line with the last molars in wild rabbits (positive RW 1 values), whereas it is positioned posteriorly relative to the last molars in domestic rabbits (negative RW 1 values).

Focusing on RW 2, skull shape changes associated with positive RW 2 values include a shortening of the occipital region in anterior direction and a slight shift of the anterior cranial region (nasal bone and maxillary incisors) in dorsal direction (Figure 2C). Negative RW 2 values account for a shortening of the molar region in anterior direction and a slight shift of the anterior cranial region (nasal bone and maxillary incisors) in ventral direction. This pattern opposes domestic rabbits (positive RW 2 scores) against wild rabbits (negative RW 2 scores). In lateral view, the occiput is almost at the same level with the nasal bone in wild rabbits (negative RW 2 values), whereas it lies distinctly ventral to the tip of the nose in domestic rabbits (positive RW 2 values) (Figure 2C). Associated with positive RW 2 scores, the angular process is more or less at the same level with the tip of the lower incisors in wild rabbits. In contrast, associated with negative RW 2 scores, the angular process lies distinctly dorsal to the tip of the lower incisors in domestic rabbits. The oral cavity in the area of the diastema is also affected by skull shape changes. In dorsoventral direction, it is compressed in wild rabbits (negative RW 2 scores), whereas it is expanded in domestic rabbits (positive RW 2 scores) (Figure 2C).

3.5. Covariance

PLS 1 explains between 60% and 90% of the covariance between the three modules (Table 5). Testing the associations between two blocks of variables reveals a strong covariance between module 1 (cranium) and module 2 (mandible) for wild rabbits, whereas no correlation is detected for domestic rabbits (Figure 5A, Table 6). For both groups, the relationship between module 1 (cranium) and module 3 (cheek teeth) is significant (Figure 5B, Table 6). There is a weak covariance between module 2 (mandible) and module 3 (cheek teeth) in wild rabbits, and no correlation was detected for domestic rabbits (Figure 5C, Table 6).

Table 5. Covariance and cumulative covariance percentages per partial least squares axis (PLS).

PLS	Covariance (%)	Cumulative Covariance (%)
module 1 vs. 2		
PLS 1	82.08	82.08
PLS 2	12.35	94.43
module 1 vs. 3		
PLS 1	90.53	90.53
PLS 2	8.51	99.04
module 2 vs. 3		
PLS 1	59.55	59.55
PLS 2	22.60	82.15

Table 6. Linear regression of partial least square axis (PLS) 1 of module 1 (cranium) vs. 2 (mandible), 1 vs. 3 (cheek teeth) and 2 vs. 3, with coefficient of determination (r^2) and significance value (p-value) for the null hypothesis. Asterisk (*) marks significant p-value.

Module	Log Centroid Size	
	r^2	p-Value
module 1 vs. 2 (wild rabbits)	0.66167	0.0012895 *
module 1 vs. 2 (domestic rabbits)	0.27903	0.077491 *
module 1 vs. 3 (wild rabbits)	0.85269	1.82×10^{-5} *
module 1 vs. 3 (domestic rabbits)	0.64699	0.0016086 *
module 2 vs. 3 (wild rabbits)	0.46661	0.014344 *
module 2 vs. 3 (domestic rabbits)	0.034312	0.56437

4. Discussion

4.1. Morphological Diversification and Allometry

Evolution of craniomandibular shape in rabbits has been governed by ecological adaptation [56] including locomotion [57] and dietary habits [58,59]. Our analyses show that there are consistent differences in skull shape between wild and domestic rabbits. We find little overlap of the groups in the RWA (Figure 2A) and complete separation as revealed by the discriminant analysis (Figure 3). These results indicate that the craniomandibular system in wild and domestic rabbits was subjected to different constraints generating phenotypic divergence. The shape variation between both groups is partly coupled with skull size, and morphological differences are therefore partially the result of allometry. A future study including a greater variety of domestic rabbits (larger and smaller specimens, different breeds) may help to clarify the influence of morphological variation with changing size. Allometry is a major factor in the diversification of many domestic mammal breeds and, thus, may also be important in pet rabbits. Nevertheless, our study quantifies the observation that human-imposed artificial selection has led to non-adaptive variation in skull morphology in domestic rabbits [12].

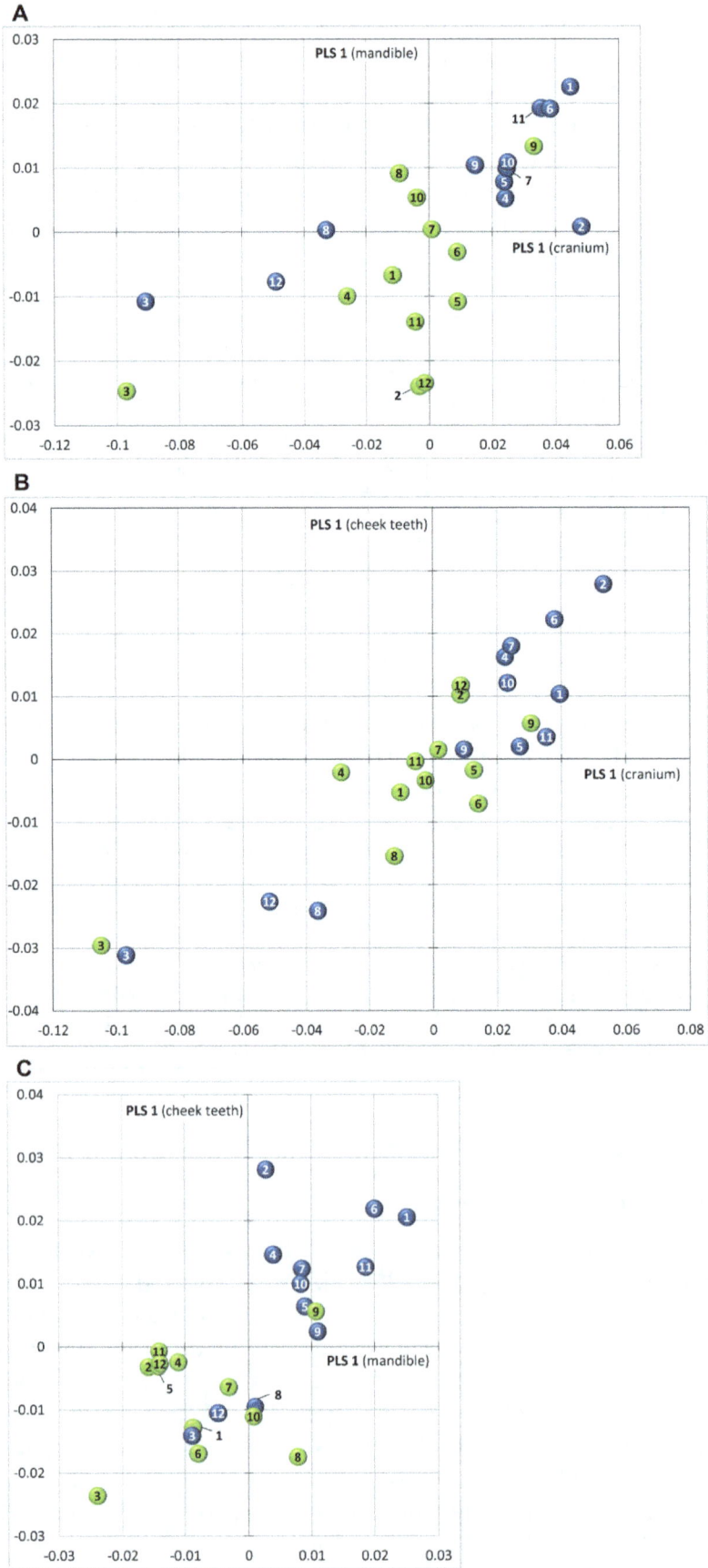

Figure 5. Two-block partial least squares (2-block PLS) analysis testing modular covariation between (**A**) cranium and mandible; (**B**) cranium and cheek teeth; (**C**) mandible and cheek teeth. Color coding as in Figures 2 and 4.

4.2. Variance and Covariance in Skull Shape: Implications for Diagnostic Analysis (Clinical Relevance)

In accordance with the breeding for "cuteness" (concept of baby schema, "Kindchenschema"), the present analysis reveals that the skull shape is generally more quadratic in domestic rabbits, whereas wild rabbits tend to have a long and flat skull. In particular, the relative length of the nasal bone (represented by LM 1) and the occiput (represented by LM 14) characterize this difference. In domestic rabbits, the reference line that marks the dorsal limitation of the maxillary tooth apices in lateral view of the skull is defined to connect the most anterior point of the nasal bone with the most posterior point of the occipital protuberance (white line in Figure 6) [4]. However, the application of this reference line in most wild rabbits might mistakenly indicate retrograde apical elongation of the maxillary cheek teeth—depending on the individual skull shape. Therefore, it is recommended that the non-modified application of this line is primarily restricted to pet rabbits.

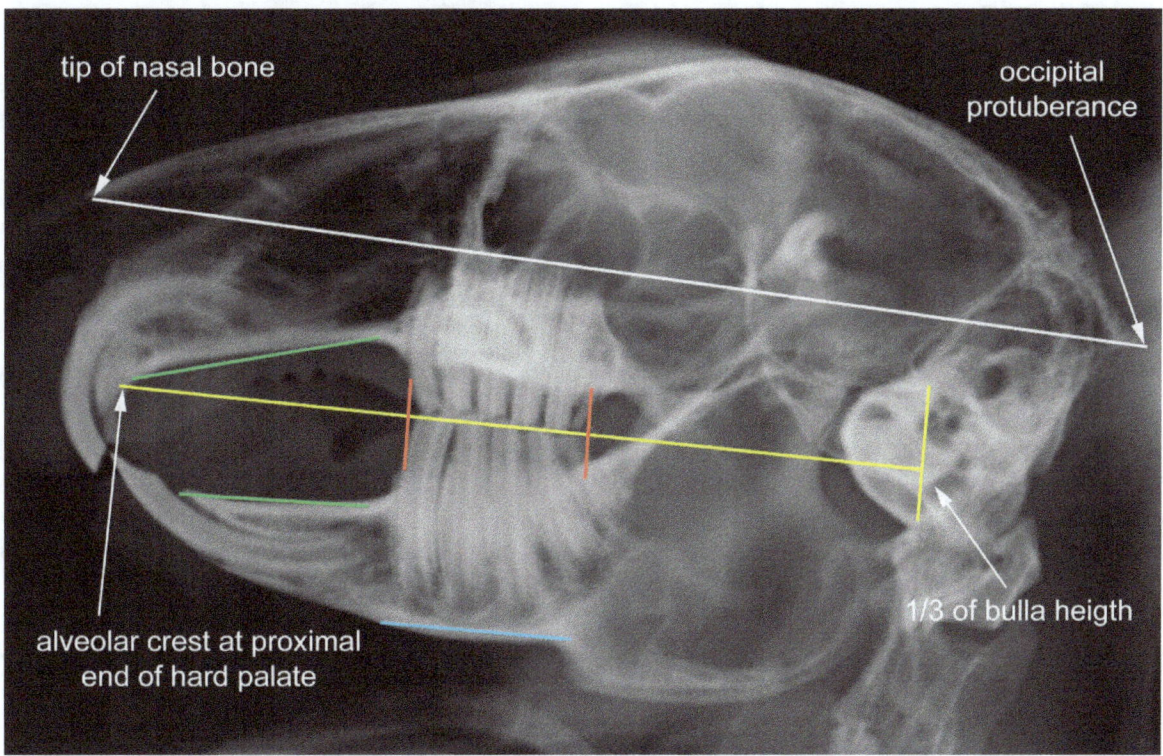

Figure 6. Species-specific reference lines superimposed on the radiograph of a clinically healthy pet rabbit in laterolateral view (according to [4]). The radiographic anatomic reference lines enable objective interpretation of malocclusion in domestic rabbits.

4.3. Effect of Variation in Incisor Region

Interestingly, the dentition itself forms a relatively unalterable unit that appears not to be essentially affected by the breeding for a shorter skull ("cuteness") or the evolution towards a shorter skull. This is based on the fact that despite the significant difference in the shape of the cranium between wild and domestic rabbits, the morphological configuration of the teeth themselves (represented by LM 2–11) is very similar across all samples. However, a closer look at the three sub-units of the dentition (incisors, diastema and molars) reveals that the tip of the maxillary incisors tends to project more ventrally in relation to the tip of the mandibular incisors in wild rabbits. This indicates slightly longer clinical crowns of the maxillary incisors. In contrast, the maxillary and mandibular incisors in domestic rabbits tend to occlude more bluntly with a slightly less chisel-shaped tooth tip. This may increase predisposition to incisor malocclusions with subsequent cheek tooth overgrowth.

Normally, incisors and cheek teeth are kept in shape by the continual processes of attrition and abrasion, respectively, which are compensated by continuous growth of the teeth (hypselodont teeth). Accordingly, in rabbits with a healthy dentition, an eruption rate of approximately 2.0 mm per week was recorded in the maxillary incisors and 2.4 mm per week in the mandibular incisors [60,61]. The persistent wear of the hypselodont teeth is basically induced by the natural fibrous diet of rabbits which is very abrasive due to the presence of lignin, cellulose and hard silicate phytoliths in grasses and other plants. Free living rabbits also strip bark off trees with their incisors and chew it just as they ribble at delicate roots. In addition to that, animals with a healthy dentition grind their incisors and cheek teeth periodically which is called "thegosis" or "bruxism". These planning jaw movements occur in the absence of food and help to maintain a physiological length and shape of the teeth. Thegosis is seen predominantly when rabbits are at rest [62]. Rabbits with a malocclusion, however, often avoid these special jaw movements due to dental pain. Elongated clinical crowns of both the incisors and cheek teeth are a consequence of this.

In rabbits with a healthy dentition, the incisors are continuously worn down during the biting and chewing of each masticatory cycle [63]. While rabbits graze longer grasses, the relatively resistant stems are taken into the mouth and cut near the ground between the incisors [64,65]. Hereby, the incisors meet edge to edge and then the mandibular incisors slide along the caudal surface of the maxillary first incisor, in a predominantly sagittal direction [63]. This reduces the food to manageable pieces that are transported by the tongue to the cheek teeth for further reduction. Pet rabbits fed predominantly on pelleted diets and chopped hay miss this action which might promote a blunter shape and a greater length of the clinical crowns as indicated by the present study.

In addition to that, incisors are worn down continuously while pieces of food are ground between the cheek teeth, provided the food is suitable for physiological jaw movements with a rostrolingually oriented shearing power stroke. This kind of jaw movement is most pronounced in hay mastication and causes that the tips of the mandibular incisors move forward till they touch the dorsal edge of the wear facet of the maxillary incisors (circular upward motion). Furthermore, they are swept transversely across the caudal aspect of the second maxillary incisors [64]. However, when the cheek teeth are crushing (carrot mastication), the mandibular incisors move merely upwards, in a predominantly vertical direction while their tips remain just caudal to the wear facets of the maxillary incisors [64,66]. This might be an additional explanation for the blunter occlusal plane of the maxillary incisors in the pet rabbit group in contrast to the more pointed incisor tip in the wild rabbit group.

4.4. Constraints in Molar Region

The present landmark analysis shows that the area lying between the maxillary and mandibular diastema (represented by LM 2, 4–7 and 11) is relatively long and flat in wild rabbits, whereas it is distinctly shorter and higher in domestic rabbits. In pet rabbits with a healthy dentition, the reference lines that mark the inclination of the palatine and mandibular bone plate slightly converge rostrally (green lines in Figure 6) [4]. This is also true for wild rabbits, but the amount of convergence is in general lower than in pet rabbits due to their slightly shorter cheek teeth and longer skulls. This is based on the fact that the clinical crowns of the cheek teeth (represented by LM 6–11) are moderately shorter in wild rabbits compared to those in domestic rabbits with their higher skulls (Figure 2C). This coincides with a study on chinchillas that showed the cheek teeth in pet animals being generally longer in axial direction compared to their wild counterparts [67]. However, the present work demonstrates that the molar sub-unit of the dentition reveals almost no variance in its morphological configuration to other skull structures, both in wild and domestic rabbits. This suggests that the morphofunctionality of the cheek teeth as a unit seems not to be essentially influenced by the domestication process. Yet, analyzed more in detail, RW 2 reveals a tendency of the cheek teeth to shift caudally in domestic rabbits, whereas in the longer skulls of wild rabbits a more rostral shift seems to dominate (Figure 2C).

4.5. Implications of Craniomandibular Shape Variation for Masticatory Performance

Another difference between domestic and wild rabbits concerns the position of the most posterior dorsal point of the angular process (represented by LM 13). The area which is defined by the antegonial notch of the mandibular ramus, the angular process and the posterior intersection between mandible and last mandibular molar (m3) (represented by LM 12, 13 and 9) forms a nearly right-angled triangle both in wild and domestic rabbits. In the latter, however, the mandibular ramus is posteriorly higher according to the relative position of the angular process which is gently shifted dorsally (Figure 2C). This results in a decrease of the distance between the jaw articulation and the muscle insertion near the angular process in pet rabbits compared to their wild counterparts. The difference in this distance may have an effect on important jaw closers, such as the posterior deep masseter and the medial pterygoid [66]. The force producing capacity of these muscles (in particular the medial pterygoid) is very high [59] and, thus, differences in the anatomical arrangement of the muscles potentially could be expected to influence bite force. However, future studies measuring the bite force and investigating the muscular differences between domestic rabbits and wild rabbits are necessary.

In this context, it is interesting to note that the part of the mandible that lies ventrocaudal to the antegonial notch (reaching up to the most posterior dorsal point of the angular process) is more pronounced in domestic rabbits than in their wild counterparts (Figure 1A). This may be a normal consequence of the progressive increase in skull height or it indicates the presence of stronger jaw muscles since this part of the mandible represents the major attachment area for the superficial and anterior deep part of the masseter muscle both acting as jaw closer. The latter statement seems more realistic since the muscle attachment areas seem to be more salient in pet rabbits (Figure 1A). In addition to that, the present landmark analysis reveals that the area depicting the superficial masseter (represented by LM 11–13) is noticeably larger in pet rabbits compared to data found in wild rabbits (Figure 2C). On one hand, the muscle needs space for its attachment onto the bone, but on the other hand it may also influence the shape of the mandible due to the forces it exerts [68]. Further studies focusing on muscular anatomy in more detail are needed to verify if the masseter muscle fibers are more vertically aligned in pet rabbits due to the relative shortness of the skull. In positive terms, it might be possible to assume that on basis of the correlation between bone shape and muscle properties, both facts probably influence the bite force at the cheek teeth area which then should be larger in domestic rabbits compared to the wild animals with their longer skulls.

It is generally assumed that in rabbits, dietary habits seem to be a major factor in developing acquired malocclusions (reviewed in [1]). Although the dentitions of the wild and domesticated rabbit seem to be in principle identical (confirmed by the present study), their diet definitely differs. Wild animals commonly eat lush green grasses, young tree shoots and delicate roots, while pet rabbits mostly consume a primarily pellet-type diet with additionally offered hay (freely available) which is more resistant than grass. This basic diet is especially popular among most rabbit breeders. Pet owners like to complement or replace this diet in part with a certain amount of daily offered fresh leafy and root vegetables. Furthermore, small pieces of fruits are given as treats. Since diet is known to largely influence skull morphology of different vertebrates [69] (Table 7), it is important to look first at the basic jaw movements in chewing rabbits which considerably differ dependent on the food resistance and are accompanied by a varying degree of strain on the incisors and cheek teeth.

Each masticatory cycle consists of a biting (see above) and chewing sequence [63]. Chewing starts with a jaw opening phase that is followed by a fast closing of the jaw. Subsequently, food is ground or crushed between the cheek teeth unilaterally during the slow closing phase of the masticatory cycle [66]. While the basic chewing rhythm is not affected by the food texture [65], the jaw movement, however, strongly depends on the type of food that is ingested (shearing or crushing power stroke) [63,66]. In addition to that, the force that is applied by the cheek teeth during crushing increases in proportion to the hardness of the food [63].

During the shearing stroke which is primarily used in hay mastication the working side condyle moves forward from a strongly retracted position while the balancing condyle shifts slightly backward.

Consequently, the mandibular cheek teeth on the working side are moved lingually (3–4 mm) and slightly rostrally (1 mm) with minimum vertical and maximum transverse jaw excursion [66]. Thus, they perform a buccolingually directed power stroke where a considerable shearing force is applied between the interlocked transverse ridges of the upper and lower (pre-) molars.

This jaw movement sometimes occurs in pellet mastication, but is never seen in carrot mastication. Carrots are always chewed with the aid of a crushing stroke where the position of the working condyle is initially more anterior. The forward movement of this condyle is less pronounced while the backward movement of the balancing condyle is enhanced. The mandibular cheek teeth of the working side move purely lingually without a rostromedial shearing action, just swinging slightly upward in the buccal and swinging slightly downward in the lingual phase. There is a maximum vertical gape and the result is primarily a crushing action that can also be observed in rabbits eating pellets. However, this type of chewing is never seen in hay mastication.

In summary, this suggests that in grazing wild rabbits cheek teeth are strained primarily in a laterorostral direction while shear forces on the interlocked enamel crests dominate and there is only a small amount of axial load on the cheek teeth. In this context, it is reasonable that the first mandibular cheek tooth is the largest of the rabbit dentition. Thus, the teeth lying behind it can firmly prop up against this stronger premolar. In contrast to wild animals, most pet and breeding rabbits predominantly crush "unnatural" food between their teeth (pellets, carrots and other root vegetables) which is accompanied with a much higher axial strain on the (pre-)molars and an insufficient tooth wear (higher clinical crowns) combined with a tendency to retrograde tooth elongation [1]. This fact appears also to explain why longitudinal splits of the first mandibular premolar (P3) are so common in pet rabbits. They are assumed to be the consequence of a load-related apical irritation that results in an abnormal tooth tissue formation (hypoplasia). Thus, the altered cement fails to connect both tooth bodies firmly together (bilophodont cheek teeth) resulting in a longitudinally "split" tooth [1].

Considering additionally that hay is more resistant than fresh grasses, it seems logical to develop further the hypothesis that pet and breeding rabbits had to develop stronger jaw muscles and secondarily larger axial bite forces than their wild counterparts to be able to crush their unnatural food more effectively. This might be supported by a shorter skull and more vertically oriented muscle fibers whereas a longer skull with a more anteriorly positioned masseter muscle (as seen in wild rabbits) reduces the vertical bite force due to a greater distribution of bite forces on all cheek teeth. As teeth at the rear of the dentition generally exert higher bite forces than the more rostrally positioned teeth, this might be an explanation for the found tendency of the cheek teeth to shift caudally in the group of the domestic rabbits. Furthermore, the presence of stronger muscles may explain the more salient appearance of the caudoventral part of the masseteric fossa (mandibular angle) in pet rabbits, as in different mammals (re-)modeling of the mandibular cortical bone has proven to be associated with oral processing of tough food (reviewed in [70]). This research has shown that especially a postnatal variation in diet-related jaw-loading patterns had a marked influence on the masticatory bone formation, leading to morphological variations between sister taxa in the long term [70]. With age, however, plasticity decreases. Based on this, rabbit breeders feeding predominantly pellets and hay seem to promote malocclusions in adult rabbits unknowingly as the masticatory apparatus of the weanlings is exposed to unphysiological strains that may result in changes of the skull morphology.

4.6. Phenotypic Plasticity in the Mammalian Feeding Apparatus

A series of studies have supported the hypothesis that an increase in jaw robustness is an evolutionary or plastic response (phenotypic plasticity) to generating higher-magnitude loads. They all found load-related morphometric variations and phenotypic changes in jaw and skull morphology in many different mammals (rabbits, chinchillas, rats, mice, ferrets, minipigs, lions, tigers, primates) being fed diets of different mechanical properties [12,67,69–99] (Table 7).

Table 7. Influence of food on skull morphology, muscle anatomy and tooth length (phenotypic plasticity). Abbreviations: TMJ = temporomandibular joint, ref. = reference.

Species	Ref.	Diet Fed	Feeding Period	Background	Results (Morphology, Anatomy)
laboratory mice (3 weeks old)	[88]	rodent pellets vs. ground pellets mixed with jelly	about 5 months	food consistency significantly influenced bone remodeling (shape of the mandible) as hard food generates greater stress in the jaw (bone remodeling)	mice fed on hard food displayed mandibles functionally more efficient for hard-food processing (higher mechanical advantage values), extended coronoid and angular processes, ventrally expanded incisor and molar zones; all functional modules except the molar zone showed shape differences. Mice fed on soft food showed jaw elongations (reduced mechanical advantage values)
mice (after weaning), healthy animals and mice with muscle dystrophy (pathological muscular defect)	[87]	hard pellets vs. pellets under the form of jelly	30 weeks	remodeling of the mandible as response to food consistency and muscular dystrophy	significant changes in mandible size whereby some parts of the mandible were more prone to remodeling (such as the angular process which is less robust when fed soft diet)
rats	[83]	hard diet vs. soft diet	about 4 months	in particular, the mandible depends on muscular function to grow to its normal size, maxillary growth seems to be under closer genetic programming	soft-diet animals had smaller jaw muscles and smaller jaws
farm-reared long-tailed chinchillas vs. museum skulls	[73]	granular feed (pellets) vs. natural diet	life-long	under natural habitat conditions, fiber constitutes almost 66% of the chinchilla diet, whereas under conditions of farm and domestic keeping granular feed with the fiber ranging from 12% to 18% is the main food; this does not require such hard work of the masticatory apparatus	crania and mandibles of farm-reared chinchillas were significantly larger than the museum specimens; only the frontal length did not show any significant differences between both groups; the length of the maxillary cheek-tooth row was larger in the museum crania

Table 7. *Cont.*

Species	Ref.	Diet Fed	Feeding Period	Background	Results (Morphology, Anatomy)
domestic (captive-bred) long-tailed chinchillas vs. wild-caught chinchillas and zoo specimens	[67]	granular feed (pellets) vs. natural diet	lifelong	captive bred animals with a normoclusion had longer cheek teeth (7.4 mm) than wild-caught chinchillas (5.9 mm) due to prolonged chewing of the naturally abrasive diet, zoo specimens lay in between (6.6 mm)	skulls of captive-bred chinchillas were on average 16% longer and slightly higher than the others (assumed to unrestricted food intake)
suckling rabbits	[100]	small food particles vs. milk	about 4 weeks	postnatal development of the masticatory apparatus due to change in function from suckling to chewing (shift of muscle activity)	the facial skull becomes higher and longer, increase in mandibular height and development of an angular process, anterior part of the superficial masseter attains a more vertical position, displacement of the mandibular angle in a ventroposterior direction, stronger jaw closing muscles and increased bite-force
juvenile rabbits	[99]	hard pellets vs. soft pellets (soaked in water)	87 days	influence of food consistency on the rabbit masseter muscle fibers (plasticity)	rabbits adjusted to altered foods within days resulting in changes in the masseter muscle; hard-diet animals increased the occlusal forces (larger fiber cross-sectional area); soft-diet animals decreased the occlusal forces (small fiber cross-sectional area)
rabbits (weanlings)	[74]	soft and hard/tough diet	15 weeks	influence of masticatory stresses on the development and structure of the hard palate (phenotypic plasticity)	rabbits subjected to elevated masticatory loading developed hard palates with significantly greater bone area, greater cortical bone thickness and thicker anterior plates
rabbits (weanlings)	[89]	ground rabbit pellets vs. intact pellets and hay blocks	105 days	phenotypic plasticity of the superficial masseter fiber architecture as dietary consistency influences its fiber type composition	tough diet causes an increase in physiological cross-sectional areas of the masseter muscle (increased muscle mass)

Table 7. *Cont.*

Species	Ref.	Diet Fed	Feeding Period	Background	Results (Morphology, Anatomy)
New Zealand rabbits (weanlings)	[101]	powdered pellets, intact pellets, intact pellets and hay blocks	26 weeks	diet-induced variations in masticatory stresses influence postorbital soft tissues (fibrocartilage)	more degraded organization of collagen fibers in the postorbital region due to increased masticatory forces (pellets and hay)
New Zealand white rabbits (4-week-old weanlings)	[82]	ground pellets vs. intact pellets with hay blocks	15 weeks	diet-related variation in masticatory stress affects structural properties and extracellular matrix composition of the TMJ and the symphysis (histology and immunohistochemistry of articular cartilage revealed a diminished articular cartilage viscoelasticity)	elevated masticatory loads result in an increase of the masseter muscle mass and a partial skull bone enlargement (mandibular corpus, condyle, symphysis) with a greater local bone density
ferrets (5 weeks old)	[84]	hard pellets vs. soft pellets (soaked in water)	6 months	effect of masticatory muscle function on craniofacial morphology	less tension on the periosteal membrane of the cranial bones, resulting in less periosteal bone apposition in the inserting areas

All studies showed a positive correlation between dietary properties and peak masticatory loads that caused the adjacent cortical bony tissue to change its structure and morphology whereby it normally became thicker and more mineralized. Therefore, rabbits and primates that routinely ingested stiff and tough food exhibited relatively larger jaws to counter elevated peak masticatory stresses (peak bite force) (reviewed in [70]). In rabbits, hay and pellets resulted in greater jaw-muscle activity and higher mandibular strain, compared to the ingestion of carrots [80]. Hay seems to be the most mechanically challenging food as it is tougher and stiffer than pellets and carrots [70]. It requires more chews per gram to be processed which results in longer chewing bouts compared to pellets and carrots. This means that over a longer period of time the teeth are predominantly axially loaded due to the elevated bite force. If we take into consideration that hay with a lot of hard stems has reduced nutritive properties and potential limits on digestibility, then rabbits eating predominantly hay need to consume large quantities to meet basic metabolic and nutritional demands [70]. All of this promotes retrograde tooth elongation and incursion of the apices into the adjacent bone (most common finding in malocclusions) [1]. Furthermore, hay also promotes periodontal diseases (impacted food) and, therefore is not the best nutrition for rabbits [31]. Grasses and other fresh plants, however, are abrasive, but relatively soft and, thus, can be ground down with relatively low axial load of the cheek teeth as the primary strain on the (pre-) molars occurs in a more physiological laterorostral direction with the aid of the shearing power stroke.

5. Conclusions

The present study is an intriguing example that highlights the importance of integrating evolution and veterinary science in order to improve the knowledge base. Evolutionary Veterinary Science is key to gain a comprehensive understanding of pathologies and, thus, opens up new avenues of research in veterinary medicine.

In summary, the landmark-based geometric morphometric analysis indicates that the craniomandibular shape of rabbits changed at different rates in the course of domestication since cranial morphometry strongly differs between domestic and wild rabbits although the dentition itself does not seem to differ significantly. This leads to a functional imbalance of the masticatory apparatus because the regions that are associated with the generation of masticatory forces (i.e., cranium and mandible) change independently from the regions that are associated with the resistance of masticatory forces (i.e., hypselodont teeth). Finally, this disequilibrium seems to result in a predisposition to dental problems in domestic rabbits. What caused shorter skulls in the course of the domestication? On the one hand, selective breeding for extremely short crania in dwarf rabbits is sometimes accompanied with the occurrence of extremely short skulls (brachygnathic rabbits with a shorter maxillary diastema and secondary congenital incisor malocclusion). On the other hand, it has been proven that diet has a significant influence on skull morphology as well (phenotypic plasticity) (Figure 7).

The present analysis comparing wild and domestic rabbits shows that in pet animals an increased skull height with a concurrently greater muscle insertion area (ventrocaudal enlargement of the mandibular ramus) and more vertically oriented jaw muscle fibers exhibit higher muscle strength and, thus, a larger bite force compared to wild rabbits. Previous studies confirm that the shorter skull morphology seems to be a long-term adaptation to the increased stress on the dentition due to feeding a diet consisting predominantly of harder particles than that found in the wild (pellets, hay, carrots) [70]. Instead of performing lateral gliding jaw movements which grind the hypselodont cheek teeth optimally in the long term, the more resistant food particles (stiff hay, pellets and carrots) are predominantly crushed between the teeth which requires stronger hinge movements (raising and lowering the jaw) [102]. Consequently, the cheek teeth have to withstand a higher masticatory pressure which also causes abnormal stress to the nearby bone with all its consequences (retrograde tooth elongation which is the most common finding in pet rabbits with a beginning or far advanced malocclusion [1]. Based on this knowledge, the diet of pet rabbits has to be strictly reconsidered as this has been already recommended by Böhmer [31]. A more natural nutrition of domestic rabbits appears to be all the more important because the present results show that, even in rabbits with a primarily healthy dentition, all cheek teeth already show an elongated clinical crown which makes the teeth much more susceptible to an abnormal axial load with secondary bending or shifting forces. All these facts strengthen the importance to offer pet rabbits an adequate close-to-nature nutrition throughout the whole life and especially beginning early parallel to weaning (phase of increased phenotypic plasticity) that ensures a normal strain on the teeth by promoting physiological lateral gliding movements and avoiding direct axial load [31].

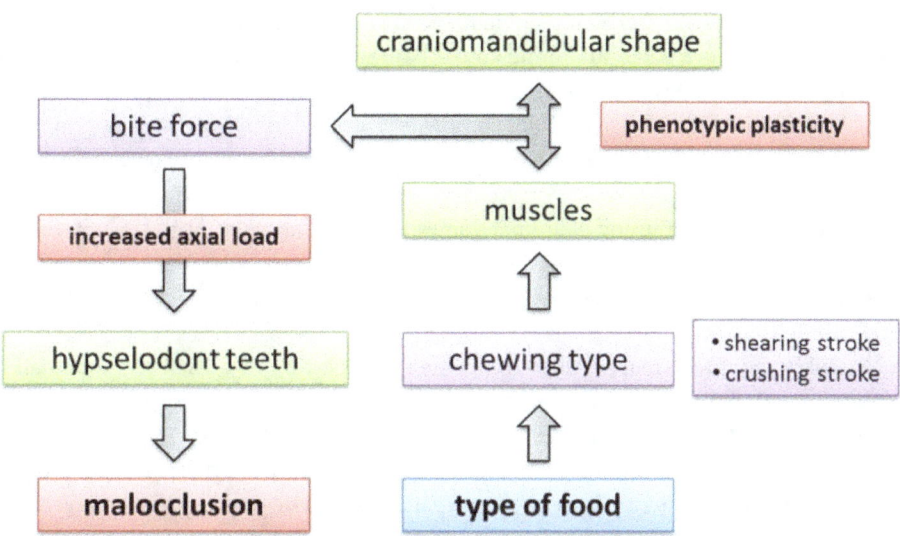

Figure 7. Flowchart summarizing the mechanisms involved in food-masticatory apparatus interactions as indicated by the present study. Type of food is the critical factor because it determines the performed chewing mechanism in rabbits. The chewing mechanism constrains the muscle performance, which has considerable impact on the craniomandibular shape via phenotypic plasticity. The musculoskeletal arrangement influences the bite force that acts on the teeth. The higher the bite force, the greater the axial load increasing the risk of malocclusions.

Acknowledgments: The research received no financial support from any funding agency.

Author Contributions: Both authors substantially contributed to the study concept and design. Estella Böhmer collected the data. Christine Böhmer conducted the analyses. Christine Böhmer and Estella Böhmer interpreted the data and wrote the manuscript.

References

1. Böhmer, E. *Dentistry in Rabbits and Rodents*; Wiley Blackwell: Chichester, UK, 2015; p. 288.
2. Jekl, V.; Hauptman, K.; Knotek, Z. Quantitative and qualitative assessments of intraoral lesions in 180 small herbivorous mammals. *Vet. Rec.* **2008**, *162*, 442–449. [CrossRef] [PubMed]
3. Crossley, D.A.; Penman, S. (Eds.) *Manual of Small Animal Dentistry*, 2nd ed.; British Small Animal Veterinary Association (BSAVA): Cheltenham, UK, 1995; p. 245.
4. Böhmer, E.; Crossley, D. Objective interpretation of dental disease in rabbits, guinea pigs and chinchillas. *Eur. J. Comp. Anim. Pract.* **2011**, *21*, 47–56.
5. Rooney, N.J.; Mullan, S.M.; Baker, P.E.; Hill, J.M.; Sealey, C.E.; Turner, M.J.; Held, S.D.E.; Blackwell, E.J.; Saunders, R. The current state of welfare, housing and husbandry of the English pet rabbit population. *BMC Res. Notes* **2014**, *7*, 942–954. [CrossRef] [PubMed]

6.   Mullan, S.M.; Main, D.C. Survey of the husbandry, health and welfare of 102 pet rabbits. *Vet. Rec.* **2006**, *159*, 103–109. [CrossRef] [PubMed]

7.   Harcourt-Brown, F.M. Diagnosis, treatment and prognosis of dental disease in pet rabbits. *In Pract.* **1997**, *19*, 407–427. [CrossRef]

8.   Crossley, D.A. Rodent and rabbit radiology. In *An Atlas of Veterinary Dental Radiology*; DeForge, D.H., Colmery, B.H., Eds.; Iowa State University Press: Ames, IA, USA, 2000; pp. 247–259.

9.   Gracis, M. Clinical technique: Normal dental radiography of rabbits, guinea pigs, and chinchillas. *J. Exot. Pet. Med.* **2008**, *17*, 78–86. [CrossRef]

10.   Crossley, D.A. Clinical aspects of rodent dental anatomy. *J. Vet. Dent.* **1995**, *12*, 131–135. [PubMed]

11.   Böhmer, E. Röntgendiagnostik bei Zahn-sowie Kiefererkrankungen der Hasenartigen und Nager. Teil 1: Tierartspezifische Zahn-und Kieferanatomie sowie Pathologie, Indikationen für die Röntgendiagnostik. *Tierarzliche Praxis Kleintiere* **2001**, *29*, 316–327.

12.   Darwin, C. *The Variation of Animals and Plants under Domestication*; John Murray: London, UK, 1868; p. 411.

13.   Clutton-Brock, J. *A Natural History of Domesticated Mammals*; Cambridge University Press: Cambridge, UK, 1999; p. 248.

14.   Larson, G.; Fuller, D.Q. The evolution of animal domestication. *Annu. Rev. Ecol. Evol. Syst.* **2014**, *45*, 115–136. [CrossRef]

15.   Zeder, M.A. Core questions in domestication research. *Proc. Natl. Acad. Sci. USA* **2015**, *112*, 3191–3198. [CrossRef] [PubMed]

16.   Carneiro, M.; Rubin, C.J.; Di Palma, F.; Albert, F.W.; Alfoldi, J.; Barrio, A.M.; Pielberg, G.; Rafati, N.; Sayyab, S.; Turner-Maier, J.; et al. Rabbit genome analysis reveals a polygenic basis for phenotypic change during domestication. *Science* **2014**, *345*, 1074–1079. [CrossRef] [PubMed]

17.   Albert, F.W.; Somel, M.; Carneiro, M.; Aximu-Petri, A.; Halbwax, M.; Thalmann, O.; Blanco-Aguiar, J.A.; Plyusnina, I.Z.; Trut, L.; Villafuerte, R.; et al. A comparison of brain gene expression levels in domesticated and wild animals. *PLoS Genet.* **2012**, *8*. [CrossRef] [PubMed]

18.   Trut, L.; Oskina, I.; Kharlamova, A. Animal evolution during domestication: The domesticated fox as a model. *Bioessays* **2009**, *31*, 349–360. [CrossRef] [PubMed]

19.   Frantz, L.A.; Schraiber, J.G.; Madsen, O.; Megens, H.J.; Cagan, A.; Bosse, M.; Paudel, Y.; Crooijmans, R.P.; Larson, G.; Groenen, M.A. Evidence of long-term gene flow and selection during domestication from analyses of Eurasian wild and domestic pig genomes. *Nat. Genet.* **2015**, *47*, 1141–1148. [CrossRef] [PubMed]

20.   Larson, G.; Piperno, D.R.; Allaby, R.G.; Purugganan, M.D.; Andersson, L.; Arroyo-Kalin, M.; Barton, L.; Vigueira, C.C.; Denham, T.; Dobney, K.; et al. Current perspectives and the future of domestication studies. *Proc. Natl. Acad. Sci. USA* **2014**, *111*, 6139–6146. [CrossRef] [PubMed]

21.   Wiener, P.; Wilkinson, S. Deciphering the genetic basis of animal domestication. *Proc. Biol. Sci.* **2011**, *278*, 3161–3170. [CrossRef] [PubMed]

22.   Wright, D. The genetic architecture of domestication in animals. *Bioinform. Biol. Insights* **2015**, *9*, 11–20. [CrossRef] [PubMed]

23.   Wayne, R.K. Cranial morphology of domestic and wild canids: The influence of development on morphological change. *Evolution* **1986**, *40*, 243–261. [CrossRef]

24.   Morey, D.F. Size, shape, and development in the evolution of the domestic dog. *J. Archaeol. Sci.* **1992**, *19*, 181–204. [CrossRef]

25.   Evin, A.; Dobney, K.; Schafberg, R.; Owen, J.; Vidarsdottir, U.S.; Larson, G.; Cucchi, T. Phenotype and animal domestication: A study of dental variation between domestic, wild, captive, hybrid and insular Sus scrofa. *BMC Evol. Biol.* **2015**, *15*. [CrossRef] [PubMed]

26.   Young, A.; Bannasch, D. Morphological variation in the dog. In *The Dog and Its Genome*; Ostrander, E.A., Giger, U., Lindblad-Toh, K., Eds.; Cold Spring Harbor Laboratory Press: New York, NY, USA, 2006; pp. 47–65.

27.   Drake, A.G.; Klingenberg, C.P. Large-scale diversification of skull shape in domestic dogs: Disparity and modularity. *Am. Nat.* **2010**, *175*, 289–301. [CrossRef] [PubMed]

28.   Owen, J.; Dobney, K.; Evin, A.; Cucchi, T.; Larson, G.; Vidarsdottir, U.S. The zooarchaeological application of quantifying cranial shape differences in wild boar and domestic pigs (*Sus scrofa*) using 3D geometric morphometrics. *J. Archaeol. Sci.* **2014**, *43*, 159–167. [CrossRef]

29. Künzel, W.; Breit, S.; Oppel, M. Morphometric investigations of breed-specific features in feline skulls and considerations on their functional implications. *Anat. Histol. Embryol.* **2003**, *32*, 218–223. [CrossRef] [PubMed]

30. Nussbaumer, M. Über die Variabilität der dorso-basalen Schädelknickungen bei Haushunden. *Zool. Anz.* **1982**, *209*, 1–32.

31. Böhmer, E. *Warum Leiden Hauskaninchen so Häufig an Gebiss-und Verdauungsproblemen? Ein Ratgeber für die Ernährung von Kaninchen*; Curoxray: München, Germany, 2014; p. 248.

32. Okuda, A.; Hori, Y.; Ichihara, N.; Asari, M.; Wiggs, R.B. Comparative observation of skeletal-dental abnormalities in wild, domestic, and laboratory rabbits. *J. Vet. Dent.* **2007**, *24*, 224–229. [CrossRef] [PubMed]

33. Ungar, P.S. *Mammal. Teeth: Origin, Evolution, and Diversity*; The Johns Hopkins University Press: Baltimore, MD, USA, 2010; p. 304.

34. Koenigswald, W.V. Diversity of hypsodont teeth in mammalian dentitions—Construction and classification. *Palaeontogr. Abt. A* **2011**, *294*, 63–94.

35. Damuth, J.; Janis, C.M. On the relationship between hypsodonty and feeding ecology in ungulate mammals, and its utility in palaeoecology. *Biol. Rev. Camb. Philos. Soc.* **2011**, *86*, 733–758. [CrossRef] [PubMed]

36. Williams, S.H.; Kay, R.F. A comparative test of adaptive explanations for hypsodonty in ungulates and rodents. *J. Mamm. Evol.* **2001**, *8*, 207–229. [CrossRef]

37. Rose, K.D.; DeLeon, V.B.; Missiaen, P.; Rana, R.S.; Sahni, A.; Singh, L.; Smith, T. Early Eocene lagomorph (Mammalia) from Western India and the early diversification of Lagomorpha. *Proc. Biol. Sci.* **2008**, *275*, 1203–1208. [CrossRef] [PubMed]

38. Ge, D.; Wen, Z.; Xia, L.; Zhang, Z.; Erbajeva, M.; Huang, C.; Yang, Q. Evolutionary history of lagomorphs in response to global environmental change. *PLoS ONE* **2013**, *8*. [CrossRef] [PubMed]

39. Sun, J.; Ni, X.; Bi, S.; Wu, W.; Ye, J.; Meng, J.; Windley, B.F. Synchronous turnover of flora, fauna, and climate at the Eocene-Oligocene Boundary in Asia. *Sci. Rep.* **2014**, *4*. [CrossRef] [PubMed]

40. Alves, P.C.; Ferrand, N.; Hackländer, K. (Eds.) *Lagomorph Biology. Evolution, Ecology, and Conservation*; Springer: Berlin, Germany, 2008; p. 413.

41. Herre, W.; Röhrs, M. *Haustiere—Zoologisch Gesehen*; Springer: Berlin, Germany, 2013; p. 412.

42. Carneiro, M.; Afonso, S.; Geraldes, A.; Garreau, H.; Bolet, G.; Boucher, S.; Ferrand, N. The genetic structure of domestic rabbits. *Mol. Biol. Evol.* **2011**, *28*, 1801–1816. [CrossRef] [PubMed]

43. Logan, M.; Sanson, G. The association of tooth wear with sociality of free-ranging male koalas (*Phascolarctos cinereus* Goldfuss). *Aust. J. Zool.* **2002**, *50*, 621–626. [CrossRef]

44. Cox, P.G.; Hautier, L. *Evolution of the Rodents: Advances in Phylogeny, Functional Morphology and Development*; Cambridge University Press: Cambridge, UK, 2015; p. 624.

45. Schmidt-Kittler, N. Feeding specializations in rodents. *Senckenberg. Lethaea* **2002**, *82*, 141–152. [CrossRef]

46. Müller, J.; Clauss, M.; Codron, D.; Schulz, E.; Hummel, J.; Fortelius, M.; Hatt, J.M. Growth and wear of incisor and cheek teeth in domestic rabbits (*Oryctolagus cuniculus*) fed diets of different abrasiveness. *J. Exp. Zool. A Ecol. Genet. Physiol.* **2014**, *321*, 283–298. [CrossRef] [PubMed]

47. Wolf, P.; Kamphues, J. Probleme der art-und bedarfsgerechten Ernährung kleiner Nager als Heimtiere. *Prakt Tierarzt* **1995**, *88*, 1088–1092.

48. Wolf, P.; Kamphues, J. Untersuchungen zu Fütterungseinflüssen auf die Entwicklung der Incisivi bei Kaninchen, Chinchilla und Ratte. *Kleintierpraxis* **1996**, *10*, 723–732.

49. Rohlf, F.J. tpsDig2. 2.17. Stony Brook, New York: Department of Ecology and Evolution, State University of New York at Stony Brook, 2013. Available online: http://life.bio.sunysb.ed/morph/ (accessed on 4 October 2012).

50. Bookstein, F.L. *Morphometric Tools for Landmark Data: Geometry and Biology*; Cambridge University Press: Cambridge, UK, 1991; p. 435.

51. O'Higgins, P.; Jones, N. Morphologika^2. 2.5: Hull York Medical School, 2006. Available online: http://sites.google.com/site/hymsfme/downloadmorphologica (accessed on 13 October 2012).

52. Hammer, Ø.; Harper, D.A.T.; Ryan, P.D. PAST: Palaeontological Statistics software package for education and data analysis. *Palaeontol. Electron.* **2001**, *4*, 1–9.

53. Zelditch, M.L.; Swiderski, D.L.; Sheets, H.D.; Fink, W.L. *Geometric Morphometrics for Biologists: A Primer*; Elsevier Academic Press: New York, NY, USA, 2004; p. 443.

54. Foote, M. Contributions of individual taxa to overall morphological disparity. *Paleobiology* **1993**, *19*, 403–419. [CrossRef]

55. Rohlf, F.J.; Corti, M. Use of two-block partial least-squares to study covariation in shape. *Syst. Biol.* **2000**, *49*, 740–753. [PubMed]

56. Ge, D.; Yao, L.; Xia, L.; Zhang, Z.; Yang, Q. Geometric morphometric analysis of skull morphology reveals loss of phylogenetic signal at the generic level in extant lagomorphs (Mammalia: Lagomorpha). *Contrib. Zool.* **2015**, *84*, 267–284.

57. Kraatz, B.P.; Sherratt, E.; Bumacod, N.; Wedel, M.J. Ecological correlates to cranial morphology in Leporids (Mammalia, Lagomorpha). *PeerJ* **2015**, *3*. [CrossRef] [PubMed]

58. Koenigswald, W.v.; Anders, U.; Engels, S.; Schultz, J.A.; Ruf, I. Tooth morphology in fossil and extant Lagomorpha (Mammalia) reflects different mastication patterns. *J. Mamm. Evol.* **2010**, *17*, 275–299. [CrossRef]

59. Watson, P.J.; Groning, F.; Curtis, N.; Fitton, L.C.; Herrel, A.; McCormack, S.W.; Fagan, M.J. Masticatory biomechanics in the rabbit: A multi-body dynamics analysis. *J. R. Soc. Interface* **2014**, *11*. [CrossRef] [PubMed]

60. Shadle, A.R. The attrition and extrusive growth of the four major incisor teeth of domestic rabbits. *J. Mammal.* **1936**, *17*, 15–21. [CrossRef]

61. Hamidur Rahman, A.S.M.; Al-Mahmud, K.A.; Nashiru-Islam, K.M. Dental malocclusion in New Zealand white rabbit. *Bangladesh Vet. J.* **1983**, *16*, 85–88.

62. Keil, A. Über die Frage des natürlichen Vorkommens und der experimentellen Erzeugung echter Karies bei Tieren (Discussion of the natural occurrence of dental caries and it sexperimental production of true caries in animals. *Deutsche Zahnärztl. Ztschr.* **1949**, *4*, 694–704.

63. Harcourt-Brown, F.M. Metabolic Bone Disease as a Possible Cause of Dental Disease in Pet Rabbits. Postgraduate Fellowship Thesis, The Royal College of Veterinary Surgeons (RCVS), London, UK, 2006.

64. Ardran, G.M.; Kemp, F.H. A radiographic analysis of mastication and swallowing in the domestic rabbit: *Oryctolagus cuniculus*. *Proc. Zool. Soc. Lond.* **1958**, *130*, 257–274. [CrossRef]

65. Yamada, Y.; Yamamura, K. Possible factors which may affect phase durations in the natural chewing rhythm. *Brain Res.* **1996**, *706*, 237–242. [CrossRef]

66. Weijs, W.A.; Dantuma, R. Functional anatomy of the masticatory apparatus in the rabbit (*Oryctolagus cuniculus* L.). *Neth. J. Zool.* **1981**, *31*, 99–147. [CrossRef]

67. Crossley, D.A.; Miguelez, M.M. Skull size and cheek-tooth length in wild-caught and captive-bred chinchillas. *Arch. Oral Biol.* **2001**, *46*, 919–928. [CrossRef]

68. Cornette, R.; Tresset, A.; Herrel, A. The shrew tamed by Wolff's law: Do functional constraints shape the skull through muscle and bone covariation? *J. Morphol.* **2015**, *276*, 301–309. [CrossRef] [PubMed]

69. Smuts, G.L. Age determination of the African lion (*Panthera leo*). *J. Zool.* **1978**, *185*, 365–373. [CrossRef]

70. Ravosa, M.J.; Scott, J.E.; McAbee, K.R.; Veit, A.J.; Fling, A.L. Chewed out: An experimental link between food material properties and repetitive loading of the masticatory apparatus in mammals. *PeerJ* **2015**, *3*. [CrossRef] [PubMed]

71. Hartstone-Rose, A.; Selvey, H.; Villari, J.R.; Atwell, M.; Schmidt, T. The three-dimensional morphological effects of captivity. *PLoS ONE* **2014**, *9*. [CrossRef] [PubMed]

72. Saragusty, J.; Shavit-Meyrav, A.; Yamaguchi, N.; Nadler, R.; Bdolah-Abram, T.; Gibeon, L.; Shamir, M.H. Comparative skull analysis suggests species-specific captivity-related malformation in lions (*Panthera leo*). *PLoS ONE* **2014**, *9*. [CrossRef] [PubMed]

73. Baranowski, P.; Wróblewska, M.; Nowak, P.; Pezinska, K. Biometry of the skull of wild and farm long-tailed Chinchilla (*Chinchilla laniger*, Molina, 1782). *Int. J. Morphol.* **2013**, *31*, 1003–1011. [CrossRef]

74. Menegaz, R.A.; Sublett, S.V.; Figueroa, S.D.; Hoffman, T.J.; Ravosa, M.J. Phenotypic plasticity and function of the hard palate in growing rabbits. *Anat. Rec.* **2009**, *292*, 277–284. [CrossRef] [PubMed]

75. Menegaz, R.A.; Sublett, S.V.; Figueroa, S.D.; Hoffman, T.J.; Ravosa, M.J.; Aldridge, K. Evidence for the influence of diet on cranial form and robusticity. *Anat. Rec.* **2010**, *293*, 630–641. [CrossRef] [PubMed]

76. Hylander, W.L. The functional significance of primate mandibular form. *J. Morphol.* **1979**, *160*, 223–240. [CrossRef] [PubMed]

77. Hylander, W.L. Mandibular function in Galago crassicaudatus and Macaca fascicularis: An in vivo approach to stress analysis of the mandible. *J. Morphol.* **1979**, *159*, 253–296. [CrossRef] [PubMed]

78. Zuccarelli, M.D. Comparative morphometric analysis of captive vs. wild African lion (*Panthera leo*) skulls. *Bios* **2004**, *75*, 131–138. [CrossRef]

79. O'Regan, H.J.; Kitchener, A.C. The effects of captivity on the morphology of captive, domesticated and feral mammals. *Mammal. Rev.* **2005**, *35*, 215–230. [CrossRef]

80. Weijs, W.A.; Brugman, P.; Grimbergen, C.A. Jaw movements and muscle activity during mastication in growing rabbits. *Anat. Rec.* **1989**, *224*, 407–416. [CrossRef] [PubMed]

81. Block, M.S.; Unhold, G.; Bouvier, M. The effect of diet texture on healing following temporomandibular joint discectomy in rabbits. *J. Oral Maxillofac. Surg.* **1988**, *46*, 580–588. [CrossRef]

82. Ravosa, M.J.; Kunwar, R.; Stock, S.R.; Stack, M.S. Pushing the limit: Masticatory stress and adaptive plasticity in mammalian craniomandibular joints. *J. Exp. Biol.* **2007**, *210*, 628–641. [CrossRef] [PubMed]

83. Beecher, R.M.; Corruccini, R.S. Effects of dietary consistency on craniofacial and occlusal development in the rat. *Angle Orthod.* **1981**, *51*, 61–69. [PubMed]

84. He, T.; Kiliaridis, S. Effects of masticatory muscle function on craniofacial morphology in growing ferrets (*Mustela putorius furo*). *Eur. J. Oral Sci.* **2003**, *111*, 510–517. [CrossRef] [PubMed]

85. Avis, V. The significance of the angle of the mandible: An experimental and comparative study. *Am. J. Phys. Anthropol.* **1961**, *19*, 55–61. [CrossRef] [PubMed]

86. Herring, S.W. The ontogeny of mammalian mastication. *Am. Zool.* **1985**, *25*, 339–349. [CrossRef]

87. Renaud, S.; Auffray, J.C.; de la Porte, S. Epigenetic effects on the mouse mandible: Common features and discrepancies in remodeling due to muscular dystrophy and response to food consistency. *BMC Evol. Biol.* **2010**, *10*. [CrossRef] [PubMed]

88. Anderson, P.S.; Renaud, S.; Rayfield, E.J. Adaptive plasticity in the mouse mandible. *BMC Evol. Biol.* **2014**, *14*. [CrossRef] [PubMed]

89. Taylor, A.B.; Jones, K.E.; Kunwar, R.; Ravosa, M.J. Dietary consistency and plasticity of masseter fiber architecture in postweaning rabbits. *Anat. Rec. A Discov. Mol. Cell. Evol. Biol.* **2006**, *288*, 1105–1111. [CrossRef] [PubMed]

90. Bouvier, M.; Zimny, M.L. Effects of mechanical loads on surface morphology of the condylar cartilage of the mandible in rats. *Acta Anat.* **1987**, *129*, 293–300. [CrossRef] [PubMed]

91. Ciochon, R.L.; Nisbett, R.A.; Corruccini, R.S. Dietary consistency and craniofacial development related to masticatory function in minipigs. *J. Craniofac. Genet. Dev. Biol.* **1997**, *17*, 96–102. [PubMed]

92. Gotthard, K.; Nylin, S. Adaptive plasticity and plasticity as an adaptation: A selective review of plasticity in animal morphology and life history. *Oikos* **1995**, *74*, 3–17. [CrossRef]

93. Katsaros, C.; Berg, R.; Kiliaridis, S. Influence of masticatory muscle function on transverse skull dimensions in the growing rat. *J. Orofac. Orthop.* **2002**, *63*, 5–13. [CrossRef] [PubMed]

94. Kiliaridis, S.; Engstrom, C.; Thilander, B. The relationship between masticatory function and craniofacial morphology. I. A cephalometric longitudinal analysis in the growing rat fed a soft diet. *Eur. J. Orthod.* **1985**, *7*, 273–283. [CrossRef] [PubMed]

95. Kim, S.G.; Park, J.C.; Kang, D.W.; Kim, B.O.; Yoon, J.H.; Cho, S.I.; Bae, C.S. Correlation of immunohistochemical characteristics of the craniomandibular joint with the degree of mandibular lengthening in rabbits. *J. Oral Maxillofac. Surg.* **2003**, *61*, 1189–1197. [CrossRef]

96. Mavropoulos, A.; Bresin, A.; Kiliaridis, S. Morphometric analysis of the mandible in growing rats with different masticatory functional demands: Adaptation to an upper posterior bite block. *Eur. J. Oral Sci.* **2004**, *112*, 259–266. [CrossRef] [PubMed]

97. Mavropoulos, A.; Ammann, P.; Bresin, A.; Kiliaridis, S. Masticatory demands induce region-specific changes in mandibular bone density in growing rats. *Angle Orthod.* **2005**, *75*, 625–630. [PubMed]

98. Bouvier, M.; Hylander, W.L. The effect of dietary consistency on gross and histologic morphology in the craniofacial region of young rats. *Am. J. Anat.* **1984**, *170*, 117–126. [CrossRef] [PubMed]

99. Langenbach, G.; van de Pavert, S.; Savalle, W.; Korfage, H.; van Eijden, T. Influence of food consistency on the rabbit masseter muscle fibres. *Eur. J. Oral. Sci.* **2003**, *111*, 81–84. [CrossRef] [PubMed]

100. Langenbach, G.E.; Weijs, W.A.; Koolstra, J.H. Biomechanical changes in the rabbit masticatory system during postnatal development. *Anat. Rec.* **1991**, *230*, 406–416. [CrossRef] [PubMed]

101. Jasarevic, E.; Ning, J.; Daniel, A.N.; Menegaz, R.A.; Johnson, J.J.; Stack, M.S.; Ravosa, M.J. Masticatory loading, function, and plasticity: A microanatomical analysis of mammalian circumorbital soft-tissue structures. *Anat. Rec.* **2010**, *293*, 642–650. [CrossRef] [PubMed]

102. Greaves, W.S. *Mammalian Jaw. A Mechanical Analysis*; Cambridge University Press: Cambridge, UK, 2012; p. 114.

3

Review on Usage of Vancomycin in Livestock and Humans: Maintaining Its Efficacy, Prevention of Resistance and Alternative Therapy

Panditharathnalage Nishantha Kumara Wijesekara [1], Wikum Widuranga Kumbukgolla [2], Jayaweera Arachchige Asela Sampath Jayaweera [3,*] and Diwan Rawat [4]

[1] Human Recourse Department, University Grants Commission, 20, Ward Place, Colombo 07 10000, Sri Lanka; nkwijesekara@gmail.com

[2] Department of Biochemistry, Faculty of Medicine and Allied Sciences, Rajarata University Mihintale, Mihintale 50008, Sri Lanka; kumbukgolla@yahoo.com

[3] Department of Microbiology, Faculty of Medicine and Allied Sciences, Rajarata University Mihintale, Mihintale 50008, Sri Lanka

[4] Department of Chemistry, University of Delhi, Delhi 110007, India; dsrawat@chemistry.du.ac.in

* Correspondence: jaasjayaweera@med.rjt.ac.lk

Academic Editor: Patrick Butaye

Abstract: Vancomycin is one of the "last-line" classes of antibiotics used in the treatment of life-threatening infections caused by Gram-positive bacteria. Even though vancomycin was discovered in the 1950s, it was widely used after the 1980s for the treatment of infections caused by methicillin-resistant *Staphylococci*, as the prevalence of these strains were increased. However, it is currently evident that vancomycin-resistant *Staphylococcus aureus* and vancomycin-resistant *Enterococci* have developed for various reasons, including the use of avaparcin—an analog of vancomycin—as a feed additive in livestock. Therefore, prophylactic and empiric use of antibiotics and their analogues need to be minimized. Herein we discuss the rational use of vancomycin in treating humans, horses, farm animals, and pet animals such as dogs, cats, and rabbits. In present day context, more attention should be paid to the prevention of the emergence of resistance to antibiotics in order to maintain their efficacy. In order to prevent emergence of resistance, proper guidance for the responsible use of antimicrobials is indispensable. Therefore, almost all stakeholders who use antibiotics should have an in-depth understanding of the antibiotic that they use. As such, it is imperative to be aware of the important aspects of vancomycin. In the present review, efforts have been made to discuss the pharmacokinetics and pharmacodynamics, indications, emergence of resistance, control of resistance, adverse effects, and alternative therapy for vancomycin.

Keywords: vancomycin; broad view; veterinary use at a glance; rational use; alternatives

1. Introduction

Vancomycin was first discovered from a soil sample in the interior jungle of Borneo in the 1950s, and its usage was very limited due to the presence of impurities that caused toxicities in the earlier preparations. However, the use of vancomycin was reconsidered after the emergence of methicillin-resistant *Staphylococci* in the 1970s, and its usage increased from the 1980s after purer preparations were made in late 1970s [1]. Now, vancomycin has become the most common injectable drug of choice to treat methicillin-resistant *Staphylococci* species and drug resistant *Enterococcus* species [2].

Vancomycin exhibits bactericidal activity by inhibiting the cell wall synthesis against aerobic and anaerobic Gram-positive bacteria [3]. Vancomycin is active against most strains of Clostridia, almost all strains of *Staphylococcus aureus* (including those that produce β-lactamases and methicillin resistant strains), coagulase-negative Staphylococci, and Viridans group Staphylococci and Enterococci. Vancomycin is not effective against Gram-negative bacteria [4]. Vancomycin is one of the antibiotics of last resort, used only after treatment with other antibiotics has failed in the treatment of life-threatening infections by Gram-positive bacteria. Even though vancomycin has great potential in treating infections in animals, the use of vancomycin in veterinary medicine is limited because it is expensive and requires continuous intravenous infusion [5].

Available dosage forms of vancomycin are 500 mg, 1 g, 5 g, and 10 g vials for injections. Powdered vancomycin is reconstituted in sterile water, which results in a dark-colored solution, and it is further diluted in 5% dextrose or saline when it is administered. The reconstituted solution is stable for 14 days either at room temperature or in a refrigerator. Additionally, 125 mg and 250 mg vancomycin tablets are available for oral administration [6].

Improper use of antibiotics is largely responsible for the microbial drug resistance problems. Therefore, the people who use antibiotics in animals and humans must be vigilant about the adverse effects and the proper doses—especially in case of last-line antibiotics such as vancomycin. In this review, efforts have been made to illustrate the usage of vancomycin in animals and humans; however, the review shows areas that need more clinical trials on animal models, as little information is available for its use in animals. The limited use of vancomycin in animals is due to various reasons, such as it is a last line of antibiotic in humans, it is inconvenient to administer in animals, the emergence of vancomycin-resistant *Enterococci*, and the threat of spread of vancomycin-resistant genes to other gram-positive organisms. However, vancomycin is a valuable drug of choice for the treatment of infections of animals that are caused by multi drug resistant *Enterococci* and *Staphylococci* species [7].

2. Pharmacokinetics and Pharmacodynamics of Vancomycin

Vancomycin is a large glycopeptide compound with a molecular weight of 1448 Da which inhibits a late stage in bacterial cell wall peptidoglycan synthesis [8,9]. Amino acids present in vancomycin are synthesized, joined together, and cross-linked to assemble vancomycin [10]. The chemical structure of vancomycin is displayed in Figure 1. The three-dimensional structure of vancomycin contains a cleft that fits by hydrogen bonding with the peptides of a highly specific configuration of L-alanyl-D-alanyl-D-alanyl which is found only in bacterial cell walls; therefore, vancomycin is selectively toxic by forming stable complexes [11].

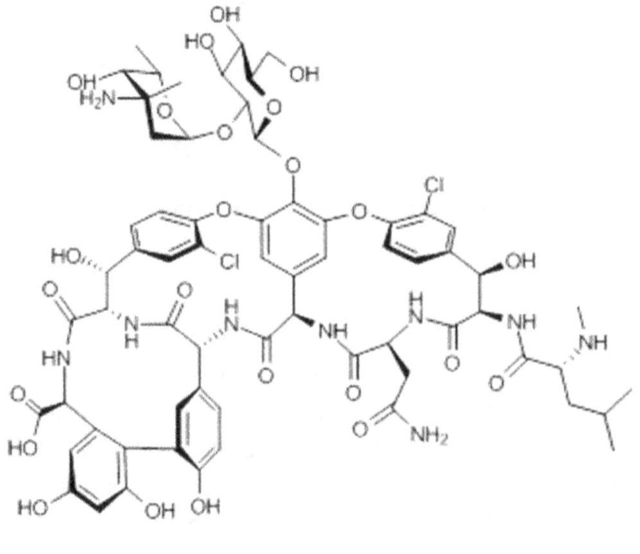

Figure 1. Chemical structure of vancomycin [12].

The factors that affect the activity of vancomycin are its tissue distribution, its protein-binding, inoculum size, and resistant organisms. The volume of distribution in humans is 0.4–1 L/kg; in dogs, 0.4–5.5 L/kg [13]. The binding of vancomycin to protein has a range from 10% to 50%. A 1–8-fold increase in the minimum inhibitory concentration (MIC) has been shown in several in vitro assessments as a result of the presence of albumin, whereas the presence of serum has had a more variable effect [14,15]. It is evident in an in vitro pharmacodynamic model that the time taken to kill is longer when the inoculum size is high (9.5 $\log_{10}$ CFU/g) compared to a moderate inoculum (5.5 $\log_{10}$ CFU/g): 48 versus 72 h, respectively, for both the methicillin sensitive *Staphylococci* and methicillin-resistant *Staphylococci* organisms isolated from human patients [16,17].

Vancomycin penetrates into most body spaces, and the penetrability is dependent on the degree of inflammation present. The concentration of vancomycin in different body spaces is different [18]. The inflamed meninges improve the penetration of vancomycin into the cerebral spinal fluid, with reported concentrations of 6.4–11.1 mg/L, whereas uninflamed meninges have resulted in low concentrations of 0–3.45 mg/L in humans [19]. Furthermore, it has been shown in a rabbit model that a high concentration of vancomycin is present in the cerebral spinal fluid of inflamed meninges [20]. Therapeutic concentrations of vancomycin in ascitic, pericardial, pleural, and synovial fluids are greater than 2.5 mg/L in humans [21].

More than 80% and 50% of a vancomycin dose is excreted unchanged in the urine (mostly by way of glomerular filtration) within 24 h after administration in humans and dogs, respectively, and the concentration of vancomycin in liver tissue and bile is below detectable levels. Vancomycin has a distribution phase of 30 min to 1 h. The half-life of vancomycin in patients with normal creatinine clearance in humans is about 6 h; dogs, 2 h; horses, 3 h [22,23].

3. Therapeutic Indications of Vancomycin

As vancomycin is a last resort antibiotic in humans, its use in humans and animals is limited. That may be the reason for the scarcity of available reference materials on the use of vancomycin in livestock. However, vancomycin would be a compulsory drug of choice in valuable animals such as breeding animals in similar indications as humans. Even though the reference material for following indications mainly deal with human medical conditions, vancomycin can be used in those conditions in animals, as vancomycin has been tested in lab animals and it is suggested for clinical trials in animals so as to establish proper guidelines for veterinary clinical practice.

A significant reduction of the number of colony forming units of *Staphylococcus aureus* in mouse blood was observed following vancomycin therapy [11]. It was shown that 165 *Enterococcus* strains isolated from dogs were sensitive to vancomycin, despite the fact that they show a high frequency of resistance to erythromycin, tetracycline, rifampicin, and enrofloxacin [24].

Vancomycin is given to humans by the intravenous route in prophylaxis when there is a high risk of methicillin-resistant staphylococci, and for treatment of endocarditis, osteomyelitis, acute bacterial prostatitis, and other serious infections caused by Gram-positive cocci [25]. Human patients with normal renal function should receive a loading dosage of 25–30 mg of vancomycin per kg intravenously over 1 h, followed by a regular dose every 12 h [26,27]. However, the practical dosing intervals can be 8, 12, 24, and 48 h based on the creatinine clearance of the patient [28].

Currently, dosages of vancomycin for administration in animals are highly empirical. In general, intravenous administration of vancomycin (diluted in 200 mL of 5% dextrose) for animals is at a dose rate of 20 mg/kg over a 1-h period at 12 h intervals [29]. More specifically, the vancomycin dosage for horses is 4.3–7.5 mg/kg in 8 h intervals, and for dogs it is 15 mg/kg in 6 h intervals, intravenously over a 1-h period. For dogs, a loading dose of 3.5 mg/kg and constant rate infusion of 1.5 mg/kg/h can be administered [2,30,31]. Vancomycin can be used to treat infections caused by erythromycin- and rifampin-resistant *Rhodococcus equi* in young horses [32,33]. In view of the above, it is apparent that the intravenous dose rate of vancomycin for horses falls within the range of dose recommended for humans. In healthy horses, a therapeutic concentration of vancomycin can be reached and maintained in synovial fluid after IV administration [34]. Vancomycin is a good therapeutic option in children having hematogenous osteomyelitis caused by methicillin-resistant *Staphylococcus aureus* (MRSA). In contrast, a case series pointed out that the potential drawback of vancomycin therapy in foals in severe osseous or physeal lesions (multiple physeal abscesses) or severe joint disease (fibrinous septic arthritis) may have a limited drug delivery to the site(s) of infection [35]. However, it is necessary to execute clinical trials to establish exact dose rates for animals, and it is desirable to measure creatinine clearance in animals to decide upon practical dosing intervals.

Vancomycin is administered locally to treat localized joint or bone infection in horses by regional limb perfusion of 300 mg diluted in a 0.5% solution [2,36]. Vancomycin is given to lobsters suffering from gaffkaemia due to Gram-positive bacteria, by way of giving injection in to abdominal sinus at a dose rate of 25 mg/kg [37].

Vancomycin is used in humans by mouth, at a dosage of 125 mg every 6 h for 7 to 10 days in the treatment of pseudomembranous colitis caused by overgrowth of *Clostridium difficile*. *Clostridium difficile* also causes *Clostridium difficile*-associated diseases in swine, calf, and horses [38,39]. The empirical dose rate for oral administration in animals is 5–10 mg/kg every 12 h. Vancomycin can be used orally for *Clostridium perfringens* enteritis and *Clostridium spiroforme* enteritis in rabbits, or *Clostridium difficile* in hamsters [40] and other species, including horses. It has been clinically proven that vancomycin can be used to treat for cholangio-hepatitis caused by a beta-lactam-resistant *Enterococcus* in cats at a dose rate of 12–15 mg/kg/h intravenously [41]. Thus, the exact dosage for those indications also should be established with proper dosage intervals. For the treatment of peritonitis in humans, vancomycin is added to dialysis fluid [42].

Vancomycin can be more effective in combination with other antibiotics for cases in which vancomycin alone is ineffective. The synergistic action of vancomycin either with gentamicin or streptomycin helps to kill susceptible strains of enterococci [43]. It has been demonstrated in humans that vancomycin is better than trimethoprim-sulfamethoxazole in efficacy and safety in treating staphylococcal infections [44]. As such, it is necessary to conduct animal clinical trials investigating the synergistic action of vancomycin with other drugs. This phenomenon has been demonstrated in vitro using a modified disk diffusion test to elucidate the synergistic action of vancomycin with ceftriaxone, ceftazidime, cefpodoxime, and amoxicillin-clavulanate against methicillin-resistant staphylococci. It was shown using a rabbit model that the combination of vancomycin with nafcillin has greater efficacy against vancomycin intermediate-susceptible *S. aureus* in aortic valvular vegetation and renal abscesses than by either treatment alone [45].

4. Emergence of Resistance to Vancomycin

Antibiotic use either as therapy, in the prevention of bacterial diseases, or as performance enhancers has resulted in antibiotic-resistant micro-organisms in pathogens and among bacteria of the endogenous microflora of animals. Antibiotic-resistant bacteria present in animals can be transmitted to humans via contact or via the food chain. Furthermore, resistance genes of animal bacteria can be transferred to human pathogens in the intestinal flora of humans [37].

The development of intermediate and high levels of resistance to vancomycin for *Staphylococcus aureus* was reported for the first time in Japan in 1997 [46]. According to guidelines of the Clinical Laboratory Standards Institute, susceptibility break points of vancomycin are ≤4 mcg/mL for *Enterococcus*, ≤1 mcg/mL for *Streptococcus*, and ≤4 mcg/mL for *Staphylococcus*. However, in 2006, the vancomycin MIC breakpoints for *S. aureus* were lowered to 2 μg/mL for "susceptible", 4–8 μg/mL for "intermediate", and 16 μg/mL for "resistant" [47]. Enterococci should be regularly tested in vitro for susceptibility to vancomycin for determination of MIC. Enterococci are deemed susceptible to vancomycin if MICs are ≤4 μg/mL; they are considered as intermediate level resistance to vancomycin if MICs are 8 to 16 μg/mL; and as complete resistance to vancomycin if MICs are >16 μg/mL [23].

Mortality of people increases when the MRSA bacteremia was caused by strains with a high vancomycin resistance (MIC > 1 μg/mL) and when it was treated empirically either with inappropriate antibiotic or vancomycin [48–50]. Avoparcin (a vancomycin analog) is a glycopeptide antibiotic that can suppress the growth of Gram-positive bacteria, and it has been used in livestock feed for growth promotion in broiler chickens, growing pigs, calves, and beef cattle. Avoparcin has also been used for preventing necrotic enteritis in poultry. In countries where avoparcin was used for the above purposes, it was evident that vancomycin-resistant enterococci (VRE) are commonly found in the commensal microbiota of food animals and in the meat from these animals. The presence of VRE in the commensal microbiota of healthy humans has been observed despite the very low usage of vancomycin in hospitals [37].

The harmless commensal of enterococci have evolved over the years to opportunistic pathogens mainly causing nosocomial infections (hospital acquired infections). The development of VRE is one of the consequences of this phenomenon. The most clinically important bacterial species with a resistance gene is *Enterococcus faecium* with vanA type vancomycin resistance, which is the most common VRE variant among farm animals, where avoparcin is widely used for growth promotion. When the use of avoparcin was discontinued, the prevalence of VRE among farm animals reduced [51–54].

5. Control of Resistance for Vancomycin

The development of preventive strategies to limit existing resistance and to avoid the emergence of resistant bacteria is of paramount importance in maintaining the efficacy of antibiotics in both human medicine and veterinary medicine. Therefore, understanding the epidemiology of antibacterial resistance will enable us to develop preventive strategies to limit existing resistance and to avoid the emergence of new strains of resistant bacteria [55,56].

In order to control emergence of resistance, hygienic measures to prevent cross contamination and a decrease in the usage of antibiotics are desirable. The reduction of the need for antibiotics is the best possible way of controlling resistance in large groups of animals. This can be accomplished by proper vaccination against infectious diseases, the adoption of good hygienic practice in animal husbandry, stopping the use of antibiotics as feed additives for growth promotion in animals bred as a food source, the appropriate use of antibiotics for food animals, and the development of guidelines, codes of practice, and policies on the appropriate use of antibiotics. Farm workers and owners of pets being treated with antibiotics need to pay attention to hygiene during and after handling treated animals [37].

In an infection caused by MRSA strains with elevated vancomycin MIC ($2~\mu g/mL$) needs elevated vancomycin dosing to achieve a serum concentration of vancomycin greater than $15~\mu g/mL$. To get such concentrations, it is required to increase the recommended dosage, which may cause toxicities. Hence, a combination or alternative therapy should be considered for such infections [57,58]. The calculation of doses of vancomycin based on MIC values relevant to the infected bacterial strain and physiological condition of the animal is important [59]. Vancomycin usage in animals should be restricted to infections which respond only to vancomycin and for which there are no other reasonable alternatives; when it is used in animals, it should be given at proper dosage, proper dosage interval, and proper duration of treatment [32].

6. Adverse Effect of Vancomycin

Although there is a little information on toxicity in animals, there is a high possibility in animals for the following adverse effects, which are evident in human clinical trials [5]. It is reported that vancomycin administration may lead to fatal enterotoxaemia in guinea pigs [42].

Prolonged intravenous use of vancomycin may cause neutropenia, thrombophlebitis, rash, fever, anemia, thrombocytopenia, and ototoxic reactions in humans and animals. Vancomycin should be administered intravenously in diluted form, because it is highly irritable for the tissues. It may cause local phlebitis at the site of injection in animals [6,8]. Vancomycin should be infused for ≥ 1 h to reduce the risk of the histamine release-associated "red man" syndrome in humans. It is advised not to administer intravenous rapidly, so as to avoid acute adverse reaction in animals [2]. The major drawback of vancomycin usage is auditory damage in humans; however, tinnitus and deafness might improve once the treatment is ceased. In addition to that, nausea, chills, phlebitis, severe hypotension, wheezing, dyspnoea, urticaria, and pruritus have been observed with the treatment of vancomycin in humans [60–63]. In some instances, neutropenia was detected with prolonged therapy [64].

There is a potential for nephrotoxicity and ototoxicity with vancomycin in animals [65]. Toxicities are minimal in vancomycin monotherapy at conventional dosages of 1 g (15 mg/kg) every 12 h in humans [66]. However, increased incidence of nephrotoxicity has been established with doses of 4 g/day or higher. As a result of elevated dosage, serum concentrations may increase, which may lead to toxicity [67–70]. Vancomycin increases the risk of nephrotoxicity in humans with drugs such as amphotericin, capreomycin, cyclosporine, cisplatin, colistimethate, polymyxins, and tacrolimus [42]. There are veterinary indications for the above drugs, such as amphotericin used in systemic fungal infections; cyclosporine used in atopy; cisplatin used in osteosarcoma; polymyxins used in gut infections; and tacrolimus used in keratoconjunctivitis sicca in small animals. Depending on the circumstances such as concurrent malignancy or fungal infection in association with MRSA infection, veterinarians would combine such drugs with vancomycin [30,31,71,72]. Therefore, it is desirable to investigate the adverse effects when the above drugs are administered concurrently with vancomycin in animals.

7. Alternative Therapy for Vancomycin

Alternative therapies should be considered for humans with *S. aureus* infections that show a vancomycin MIC of 2 mg/L or greater [49]. Lysostaphin (an endopeptidase) is more effective than vancomycin in treating methicillin-resistant *Staphylococcus aureus* in a neonatal pup model [15,24].

Oral bacitracin can be considered as an alternative to vancomycin in the treatment of antibiotic-associated pseudomembranous colitis caused by *Clostridium difficile* cytotoxin in animals. Bacitracin is used for bacitracin-sensitive infections in pigs, chicken, and turkeys [65].

Linezolid—an oxazolidinone active against Gram-positive bacteria—is one of the options for vancomycin in the treatment of infections that are caused by antibacterials including methicillin-resistant *Staphylococcus aureus* and vancomycin-resistant enterococci infections in humans. It has been shown in a murine model that linezolid can be used to control *Mycobacterium tuberculosis* infection. Linezolid such as Zyvox is also used in dogs [73]. Moreover, linezolid is used in animals for the treatment of nocardiosis. Therefore, it is necessary to establish efficacy and dose rates for linezolid in animals [74,75]. Prolonged usage and dose less than that recommended may lead to the development of resistance to linezolid. As linezolid is not active against Gram-negative organisms, it must be coupled with another antibacterial agent if the infection involves both Gram-positive and Gram-negative organisms, and this combination should be used for infections only when other treatments are not available [72]. It has been demonstrated in a rat model that linezolid with rifampin or vancomycin with rifampin is effective in an animal model of MRSA foreign body osteomyelitis [76]. Teicoplanin has a similar activity on MRSA with minimal renal toxicity. Further, red man syndrome is less frequent [77]. The therapeutic drug monitoring of vancomycin suggests that an area under the curve to Minimal inhibitory concentration (AUC/MIC) ratio of ≥ 400 µg·h/mL AUC/MIC ratio of ≥ 400 is the pharmacodynamic and pharmacokinetic (PK/PD) parameter associated with clinical and bacteriological responses to vancomycin therapy. In contrast in teicoplanin, an AUC_{24}/MIC ratio of ≥ 900 µg·h/mL is required [35].

Other therapeutic options for vancomycin are trimethoprim-sulfamethoxazole, doxycycline, or minocycline either with or without rifampin. Although vancomycin is superior to trimethoprim-sulfamethoxazole in efficacy and safety, trimethoprim-sulfamethoxazole can be given in selected cases of MRSA infection where there is a treatment failure with vancomycin treatment [45]. All of the above drugs are used in animals [65]. Rifampin can be used to treat pneumonic condition in foals caused by *Rhodcoccusequi* at a dose rate of 5 to 10 mg/kg orally at 12 h intervals. Rifampin has been suggested for use in the treatment of atypical bacterial infection in cats [5,65]. Further, the novel anti-MRSA cephalosporin ceftobiprole is in the pipeline. Its efficacy in veterinary medicine needs to be elucidated.

It has been shown in chicks that dietary cell-wall preparation of *Enterococcus faecalis* strain EC-12 can be used to stimulate the gut immune system and to reinforce the immune reaction against the vancomycin-resistant enterococci [78].

8. Conclusions

As vancomycin is a last resort antibiotic where other antibiotics cannot be used, it is essential to maintain efficacy of vancomycin for treating humans, pet animals and livestock species. In order to achieve the above-mentioned objective, vancomycin should be used only in instances where it is necessary to use the proper dosing, dosing interval, and appropriate duration of treatment based on MIC values of the disease-causing agent, physiological condition of the animal, and combination of antibiotics (where appropriate). There is scant research on the use of vancomycin in animals. According to the facts discussed in this review, it is necessary to establish novel parameters for the clinical usage of vancomycin in treating animals, by conducting animal clinical trials in order to minimize the emerging antibiotic resistance of micro-organisms against vancomycin in animals and transferring those organisms to humans. Some countries have prohibited the use of vancomycin analogues in animal food additives, which seems to be a late decision because vancomycin-resistant genes were already evolved before the bans were instituted. Therefore, vigilance in monitoring antibiotic resistance is useful to prevent such incidents in the future.

Author Contributions: All four authors contributed equally for this work.

References

1. Moellering, R.C., Jr. Vancomycin: A 50-year reassessment. *Clin. Infect. Dis.* **2006**, *42*, S3–S4. [CrossRef] [PubMed]
2. Mark, G.P. *Saunders Handbook of Veterinary Drugs Small and Large Animal*, 3rd ed.; Saunders: Philadelphia, PA, USA, 2011.
3. Bassetti, M.; Temperoni, C.; Astilean, A. Review: New antibiotics for bad bugs: Where are we? *Ann. Clin. Microbiol. Antimicrob.* **2013**, *12*, 1–15. [CrossRef] [PubMed]
4. Bennett, P.N.; Brown, M.J. *Vancomycin, Clinical Pharmacology*, 9th ed.; Churchill Livingstone: London, UK, 2000.
5. John, F.P.; Baggot, J.D.; Walker, R.D. *Glycopeptides: Vancomycin, Teicoplanin, and Avoparcin, Antimicrobial Therapy in Veterinary Medicine*, 3rd ed.; Blackwell Publishing Professional: Ames, IA, USA, 2000.
6. Dana, G.A.; Dowling, M.; Smith, D.A. Vancomycin. In *Handbook of Veterinary Drugs*, 3rd ed.; Lippincott Williams & Wilkins: Philadelphia, PA, USA, 2005.
7. Cetinkaya, Y.; Falk, P.; Mayhall, C.G. Vancomycin-Resistant Enterococci. *Clin. Microbiol. Rev.* **2000**, *13*, 686–707. [CrossRef] [PubMed]
8. Cynthia, M.K. Vancomycin. In *Merck Veterinary Manual*, 10th ed.; Merck Sharp & Dohme Corp.: Kenilworth, NJ, USA, 2010; Available online: http://www.merckvetmanual.com/mvm/index.jsp?cfile=htm/bc/191279.htm (accessed on 3 August 2016).
9. Gungor, S.; Charro, M.B.D.; Perez, B.R.; Schubert, W.; Isom, P.; Moslemy, P.; Patane, M.A.; Guy, R.H. Trans-scleral iontophoretic delivery of low molecular weight therapeutics. *J. Control. Release* **2010**, *147*, 225–231. [CrossRef] [PubMed]
10. Hubbard, B.K.; Walsh, C.T. Vancomycin Assembly: Nature's Way. *Angew. Chem.* **2003**, *42*, 730–765. [CrossRef] [PubMed]
11. Reynolds, P.E. Structure, biochemistry and mechanism of action of glycopeptide antibiotics. *Eur. J. Clin. Microbiol. Infect. Dis.* **1989**, *8*, 943–950. [CrossRef] [PubMed]
12. Nitanai, Y.; Kikuchi, T.; Kakoi, K.; Hanamaki, S.; Fujisawa, I.; Aoki, K. Crystal structures of the complexes between vancomycin and cell-wall precursor analogs. *J. Mol. Biol.* **2009**, *385*, 1422–1432. [CrossRef] [PubMed]
13. Zaghlol, H.A.; Brown, S.A. Single- and multiple-dose pharmacokinetics of intravenously administered vancomycin in dogs. *Am. J. Vet. Res.* **1988**, *49*, 1637–1640. [PubMed]

14. LaPlante, K.L.; Rybak, M.J. Impact of high-inoculum *Staphylococcus aureus* on the activities of nafcillin, vancomycin, linezolid, and daptomycin, alone and in combination with gentamicin, in an in vitro pharmacodynamic model. *Antimicrob. Agents Chemother.* **2004**, *48*, 4665–4672. [CrossRef] [PubMed]

15. Levison, M.E.; Levison, J.H. Pharmacokinetics and Pharmacodynamics of Antibacterial Agents. *Infect. Dis. Clin. N. Am.* **2009**, *23*, 791–815. [CrossRef] [PubMed]

16. Cantu, T.G.; Dick, J.D.; Elliott, D.E.; Humphrey, R.L.; Kornhauser, D.M. Protein binding of vancomycin in a patient with immunoglobulin A myeloma. *Antimicrob. Agents Chemother.* **1990**, *34*, 1459–1461. [CrossRef] [PubMed]

17. Micek, S.T. Alternatives to vancomycin for the treatment of methicillin-resistant Staphylococcus aureus infections. *Clin. Infect. Dis.* **2007**, *45*, S184–S190. [CrossRef] [PubMed]

18. Koteva, K.; Hong, H.L.; Wang, X.D.; Nazi, I.; Hughes, D.; Naldrett, M.J.; Buttner, M.J.; Wright, G.D. A vancomycin photoprobe identifies the histidine kinase VanSsc as a vancomycin receptor. *Nat. Chem. Biol.* **2010**, *6*, 327–329. [CrossRef] [PubMed]

19. Albanese, J.; Leone, M.; Bruguerolle, B.; Ayem, M.L.; Lacarelle, B.; Martin, C. Cerebrospinal fluid penetration and pharmacokinetics of vancomycin administered by continuous infusion to mechanically ventilated patients in an intensive care unit. *Antimicrob. Agents Chemother.* **2000**, *44*, 1356–1358. [CrossRef] [PubMed]

20. Nau, R.; Sörgel, F.; Eiffert, H. Penetration of Drugs through the Blood-Cerebrospinal Fluid/Blood-Brain Barrier for Treatment of Central Nervous System Infections. *Clin. Microbiol. Rev.* **2010**, *23*, 858–883. [CrossRef] [PubMed]

21. Matzneller, P.; Burian, A.; Zeitlinger, M.; Sauermann, R. Understanding the Activity of Antibiotics in Cerebrospinal Fluid in vitro. *Pharmacology* **2016**, *97*, 233–244. [CrossRef] [PubMed]

22. Forouzesh, A.; Moise, P.A.; Sakoulas, G. Vancomycin ototoxicity: A reevaluation in an era of increasing doses. *Antimicrob. Agents Chemother.* **2009**, *53*, 2483–2486. [CrossRef] [PubMed]

23. Chavers, L.S.; Moser, S.A.; Benjamin, W.H.; Banks, S.E.; Steinhauer, J.R.; Smith, A.M.; Johnson, C.N.; Funkhouser, E.; Chavers, L.P.; Stamm, A.M.; et al. Vancomycin-resistant enterococci: 15 years and counting. *J. Hosp. Infect.* **2003**, *53*, 159–171. [CrossRef] [PubMed]

24. Anuradha, G.; Scot, D.E.; Ludek, Z. Dogs Leaving the ICU Carry a Very Large Multi-Drug Resistant Enterococcal Population with Capacity for Biofilm Formation and Horizontal Gene Transfer. *PLoS ONE* **2011**, *6*. Available online: http://journals.plos.org/plosone/article/file (accessed on 1 January 2017).

25. Leekha, S.; Terrell, C.L.; Edson, R.S. General Principles of Antimicrobial Therapy. *Mayo. Clin. Proc.* **2011**, *86*, 156–167. [CrossRef] [PubMed]

26. Cheong, J.Y.; Bakry, M.M.; Lau, C.L.; Rahman, R.A. The relationship between trough concentration of vancomycin and effect on methicillin-resistant Staphylococcus aureus in critically ill patients. *S. Afr. Med. J.* **2012**, *102*, 616–619. [CrossRef] [PubMed]

27. Wu, C.; Shen, L.; Hsu, L.; Ko, W.; Wu, F.L. Pharmacokinetics of vancomycin in adults receiving extracorporeal membrane oxygenation. *J. Formos. Med. Assoc.* **2016**, *115*, 560–570. [CrossRef] [PubMed]

28. Cisek, A.A.; Rzewuska, M.; Witkowski, W.; Binek, M. Antimicrobial resistance in Rhodococcus equi. *Acta Biochim. Pol.* **2014**, *61*, 633–638. [PubMed]

29. Steer, A.C.; Carapetis, J.R. Acute hematogenous osteomyelitis in children: Recognition and management. *Paediatr. Drugs* **2004**, *6*, 333–346. [CrossRef] [PubMed]

30. Mevius, D.J.; Koene, M.G.J.; Wit, B.; van Pelt, W.; Bondt, N. Monitoring of Antimicrobial Resistance and Antibiotic Usage in Animals in the Netherlands. 2012. Available online: http://www.uu.nl/SiteCollection Images (accessed on 1 January 2017).

31. Diesal, A.; Moriello, K.A. A busy clinician's review of cyclosporine. *Vet. Med.* **2008**, *103*, 266. Available online: http://veterinarymedicine.dvm360.com/busy-clinicians-review-cyclosporine (accessed on 2 January 2017).

32. Nath, S.R.; Mathew, A.P.; Mohan, A.; Anila, K.R. Rhodococcusequi granulomatous mastitis in an immuno-competent patient—A case report. *J. Med. Microbiol.* **2013**, *62*, 1253–1255. [CrossRef] [PubMed]

33. Orsini, J.A.; Parsons, C.S.; Stine, L.; Haddock, M.; Ramberg, C.F.; Benson, C.E.; Nunamaker, D.M. Vancomycin for the treatment of methicillin-resistant staphylococcal and enterococcal infections in 15 horses. *Can. J. Vet. Res.* **2005**, *69*, 278–286. [PubMed]

34. Matsumoto, K.; Watanabe, E.; Kanazawa, N.; Fukamizu, T.; Shiemi, A.; Yokoyama, Y.; Ikawa, K.; Morikawa, N.; Takeda, Y. Pharmacokinetic/pharmacodynamic analysis of teicoplanin in patients with MRSA infections. *Clin. Pharmacol.* **2016**, *8*, 15–18. [PubMed]

35. Svetitsky, S.; Leibovici, L.; Paul, M. Comparative efficacy and safety of vancomycin versus teicoplanin: Systematic review and meta-analysis. *Antimicrob. Agents Chemother.* **2009**, *53*, 4069–4079. [CrossRef] [PubMed]

36. Martinez, L.M.; Sanroman, J.L.; Cruz, A.M.; Tendillo, F.; Rioja, E.; Roman, F. Evaluation of safety and pharmacokinetics of vancomycin after intraosseous regional limb perfusion and comparison of results with those obtained after intravenous regional limb perfusion in horses. *Am. J. Vet. Res.* **2006**, *67*, 1701–1707. [CrossRef] [PubMed]

37. Slovis, N.M.; Elam, J.; Estrada, M.; Leutenegger, C.M. Infectious agents associated with diarrhoea in neonatal foals in central Kentucky: A comprehensive molecular study. *Equine. Vet. J.* **2014**, *46*, 311–316. [CrossRef] [PubMed]

38. Bandelj, P.; Briski, F.; Frlic, O.; Rataj, A.V.; Rupnik, M.; Ocepek, M.; Vengust, M. Identification of risk factors influencing *Clostridium difficile* prevalence in middle-size dairy farms. *BMC Vet. Res.* **2016**, *47*, 41. [CrossRef] [PubMed]

39. Keel, K.; Brazier, J.S.; Post, K.W.; Weese, S.; Songer, G. Prevalence of PCR Ribotypes among *Clostridium difficile* Isolates from Pigs, Calves, and Other Species. *J. Clin. Microbiol.* **2007**, *45*, 1963–1964. [CrossRef] [PubMed]

40. Boss, S.M.; Gries, C.L.; Kirchner, B.K.; Smith, G.D.; Francis, P.C. Use of vancomycin hydrochloride for treatment of *Clostridium difficile* enteritis in Syrian hamsters. *J. Am. Assoc. Lab. Anim. Sci.* **1994**, *44*, 31–37.

41. Fish, R.; Nipah, R.; Jones, C.; Finney, H.; Fan, S.L. Intraperitoneal Vancomycin Concentrations during Peritoneal Dialysis–Associated Peritonitis: Correlation with Serum Levels. *Perit. Dial. Int.* **2012**, *32*, 332–338. [CrossRef] [PubMed]

42. British Medical Association. Vancomycin. In *British National Formulary*, 68th ed.; British National Formulary Publications, Royal Pharmaceutical Society of Great Britain: London, UK, 2015; Available online: http://www.bnf.org/bnf/index.htm (accessed on 8 October 2016).

43. Arias, C.A.; Singh, K.V.; Panesso, D.; Murray, B.E. Time-Kill and Synergism Studies of Ceftobiprole against *Enterococcus faecalis*, Including β-Lactamase-Producing and Vancomycin-Resistant Isolates. *Antimicrob. Agents Chemother.* **2007**, *51*, 2043–2047. [CrossRef] [PubMed]

44. Azimian, A.; Havaei, S.A.; Fazeli, H.; Naderi, M.; Ghazvini, K.; Samiee, S.M.; Soleimani, M.; Peerayeh, S.N. Genetic Characterization of a Vancomycin-Resistant *Staphylococcus aureus* Isolate from the Respiratory Tract of a Patient in a University Hospital in Northeastern Iran. *J. Clin. Microbiol.* **2012**, *50*, 3581–3585. [CrossRef] [PubMed]

45. Climo, M.W.; Patron, R.L.; Archer, G. Combinations of Vancomycin and β-Lactams are synergistic against Staphylococci with reduced susceptibilities to Vancomycin. *Antimicrob. Agents Chemother.* **1999**, *43*, 1747–1753. [PubMed]

46. Chen, C.Y.; Huang, Y.C. Review: New epidemiology of *Staphylococcus aureus* infection in Asia. *Clin. Microbiol. Infect.* **2014**, *20*, 605–623. [CrossRef] [PubMed]

47. Tenover, F.C., Jr.; Moellering, R.C. The rationale for revising the Clinical and Laboratory Standards Institute vancomycin minimal inhibitory concentration interpretive criteria for *Staphylococcus aureus*. *Clin. Infect. Dis.* **2007**, *44*, 1208–1215. [CrossRef] [PubMed]

48. Lodise, T.P.; Miller, C.D.; Graves, J.; Evans, A.; Graffunder, E.; Helmecke, M.; Stellrecht, K. Predictors of high vancomycin MIC values among patients with methicillin-resistant *Staphylococcus aureus* bacteremia. *J. Antimicrob. Chemother.* **2008**, *62*, 1138–1141. [CrossRef] [PubMed]

49. Rybak, M.; Lomaestro, B., Jr.; Moellering, R.; Craig, W.; Billeter, M.; Dalovisio, J.R.; Dalovisio, J.R.; Levine, D.P. Therapeutic Monitoring of Vancomycin in Adults. *Am. J. Health Syst. Pharm.* **2009**, *66*, 82–98. [CrossRef] [PubMed]

50. Soriano, A.; Marco, F.; Martínez, J.A.; Pisos, E.; Almela, M.; Dimova, V.P.; Alamo, D.; Ortega, M.; Lopez, J.; Mensa, J. Influence of vancomycin minimum inhibitory concentration on the treatment of methicillin-resistant *Staphylococcus aureus* bacteremia. *Clin. Infect. Dis.* **2008**, *46*, 193–200. [CrossRef] [PubMed]

51. Bogaard, A.E.V.D.; Stobberingh, E.E. Epidemiology of resistance to antibiotics links between animals and humans. *Int. J. Antimicrob. Agents* **2000**, *14*, 327–335. [CrossRef]

52. Devriese, L.A.; Ieven, M.; Goossens, H.; Vandamme, P.; Pot, B.; Hommez, J.; Haesebrouck, F. Presence of vancomycin-resistant enterococci in farm and pet animals. *Antimicrob. Agents Chemother.* **1996**, *40*, 2285–2287. [PubMed]

53. Nilsson, O. Vancomycin resistant enterococci in farm animals—Occurrence and importance. *Infect. Ecol. Epidermiol.* **2012**, *2*. [CrossRef] [PubMed]

54. Bogaard, A.E.V.D.; Bruinsma, N.; Stobberingh, E.E. The effect of banning avoparcin on VRE carriage in The Netherlands. *J. Antimicrob. Chemother.* **2000**, *46*, 146–148. [CrossRef] [PubMed]

55. Guillemot, D. Antibiotic use in humans and bacterial resistance. *Curr. Opin. Microbiol.* **1999**, *2*, 494–498. [CrossRef]

56. Lathers, C.M. Role of veterinary medicine in public health: Antibiotic use in food animals and humans and the effect on evolution of antibacterial resistance. *J. Clin. Pharmacol.* **2001**, *41*, 595–599. [CrossRef] [PubMed]

57. Hidayat, L.K.; Hsu, D.I.; Quist, R.; Shriner, K.A.; Beringer, W. High-dose vancomycin therapy for methicillin-resistant Staphylococcus aureus infections: Efficacy and toxicity. *Arch. Intern. Med.* **2006**, *166*, 2138–2144. [CrossRef] [PubMed]

58. Jones, R.N. Microbiological Features of Vancomycin in the 21st Century: Minimum Inhibitory Concentration Creep, Bactericidal/Static Activity, and Applied Breakpoints to Predict Clinical Outcomes or Detect Resistant Strains. *Clin. Infect. Dis.* **2006**, *42* (Suppl. 1), S13–S24. [CrossRef] [PubMed]

59. Giuliano, C.; Haase, K.K.; Hall, R. Use of vancomycin pharmacokinetic—Pharmacodynamic properties in the treatment of MRSA infections. *Expert Rev. Anti-Infect. Ther.* **2010**, *8*, 95–106. [CrossRef] [PubMed]

60. Brummett, R.E.; Fox, K.E. Vancomycin- and erythromycin-induced hearing loss in humans. *Antimicrob. Agents Chemother.* **1989**, *33*, 791–796. [CrossRef] [PubMed]

61. Elting, L.S.; Rubenstein, E.B.; Kurtin, D.; Rolston, K.V.; Fangtang, J.; Martin, C.G.; Raad, I.I.; Whimbey, E.E.; Manzullo, E.; Bodey, G.P. Mississippi mud in the 1990s: Risks and outcomes of vancomycin-associated toxicity in general oncology practice. *Cancer* **1998**, *83*, 2597–2607. [PubMed]

62. Stanley, D.; McGrath, B.J.; Lamp, K.C.; Rybak, M.J. Effect of human serum on killing activity of vancomycin and teicoplanin against *Staphylococcus aureus*. *Pharmacotherapy* **1994**, *14*, 35–39.

63. Tange, R.A.; Kieviet, H.L.; Marle, J.V.; Sjoback, D.B.; Ring, W. An experimental study of vancomycin-induced cochlear damage. *Arch. Otorhinolaryngol.* **1989**, *246*, 67–70. [CrossRef] [PubMed]

64. Pai, M.P.; Mercier, R.C.; Koster, S.A. Epidemiology of vancomycin-induced neutropenia in patients receiving home intravenous infusion therapy. *Ann. Pharmacother.* **2006**, *40*, 224–228. [CrossRef] [PubMed]

65. Bishop, T. Vancomycin. In *The Veterinary Formulary*, 6th ed.; Pharmaceutical Press: London, UK, 2005.

66. Ray, A.S.; Haikal, A.; Hammoud, K.A.; Yu, S.L. Vancomycin and the Risk of AKI: A Systematic Review and Meta-Analysis. *CJASN* **2016**, *11*, 2132–2140.

67. Bailie, G.R.; Neal, D. Vancomycin ototoxicity and nephrotoxicity. *Med. Toxicol. Advers. Drug Exp.* **1988**, *3*, 376–386. [CrossRef]

68. Drygalski, A.V.; Curtis, B.R.; Bougie, D.W.; McFarland, J.G.; Ahl, S.; Limbu, I.; Baker, K.R.; Aster, R.H. Vancomycin-induced immune thrombocytopenia. *N. Engl. J. Med.* **2007**, *356*, 904–910. [CrossRef] [PubMed]

69. Healy, D.P.; Sahai, J.V.; Fuller, S.H.; Polk, R.E. Vancomycin-induced histamine release and "red man syndrome": Comparison of 1-and 2-hour infusions. *Antimicrob. Agents Chemother.* **1990**, *34*, 550–554. [CrossRef] [PubMed]

70. Michael, J.R. The Pharmacokinetic and Pharmacodynamic Properties of Vancomycin. *Clin. Infect. Dis.* **2006**, *42*, S35–S39.

71. Glycopetides. Available online: http://www.merckmanuals.com/vet/search.html (accessed on 3 November 2016).

72. Radostits, O.M.; Gay, C.C.; Blood, D.C.; Hinchcliff, K.W. *Veterinary Medicine: A Textbook of the Diseases of Cattle, Horses, Sheep, Pigs and Goats*, 9th ed.; W B Saunders: Philadelphia, PA, USA, 2000.

73. Ruben, D. Cisplatin for Dogs. 2015. Available online: http://www.petplace.com/article/drug-library/library (accessed on 1 January 2017).

74. Cynamon, M.H.; Klemens, S.P.; Sharpe, C.A.; Chase, S. Activities of several novel oxazolidinones against *Mycobacterium tuberculosis* in a murine model. *Antimicrob. Agents Chemother.* **1999**, *43*, 1189–1191. [PubMed]

75. Slatter, J.G.; Adams, L.A.; Bush, C.E.; Chiba, K.; Yates, P.T.D.; Feenstra, K.L.; Koike, S.; Ozawa, N.; Peng, G.W.; Sams, J.P.; et al. Pharmacokinetics, toxicokinetics, distribution, metabolism and excretion of linezolid in mouse, rat and dog. *Xenobiotica* **2002**, *32*, 907–924. [CrossRef] [PubMed]

76. Vergidis, P.; Rouse, M.S.; Euba, G.; Karau, M.J.; Schmidt, S.M.; Mandrekar, J.N.; Steckelberg, J.M.; Patel, R. Treatment with Linezolid or Vancomycin in Combination with Rifampin Is Effective in an Animal Model of Methicillin-Resistant *Staphylococcus aureus* Foreign Body Osteomyelitis. *Antimicrob. Agents Chemother.* **2011**, *55*, 1182–1186. [CrossRef] [PubMed]

77.   Rodriguez, A.B.; Pedrera, M.I.; Barriga, C. In vivo effect of teicoplanin and vancomycin upon haemolytic and bactericidal activity of serum against *Staphylococcus aureus*. *Comp. Immunol. Microbiol. Infect. Dis.* **1996**, *19*, 283–288. [CrossRef]

78.   Sakai, Y.; Tsukahara, T.; Bukawa, W.; Matsubara, N.; Ushida, K. Cell Preparation of *Enterococcus faecalis* Strain EC-12 Prevents Vancomycin-Resistant Enterococci Colonization in the Cecum of Newly Hatched Chicks. *Poultry. Sci. J.* **2006**, *85*, 273–277. [CrossRef]

4

Feline Immunodeficiency Virus Neuropathogenesis: A Model for HIV-Induced CNS Inflammation and Neurodegeneration

Rick B. Meeker [1,*] and Lola Hudson [2]

[1] Department of Neurology, University of North Carolina, Chapel Hill, NC 27599, USA
[2] Department of Molecular Biomedical Sciences, College of Veterinary Medicine,
     North Carolina State University, Raleigh, NC 27607, USA; lola_hudson@ncsu.edu
*   Correspondence: meekerr@neurology.unc.edu

Academic Editor: Patrick Butaye

Abstract: Feline Immunodeficiency virus (FIV), similar to its human analog human immunodeficiency virus (HIV), enters the central nervous system (CNS) soon after infection and establishes a protected viral reservoir. The ensuing inflammation and damage give rise to varying degrees of cognitive decline collectively known as HIV-associated neurocognitive disorders (HAND). Because of the similarities to HIV infection and disease, FIV has provided a useful model for both in vitro and in vivo studies of CNS infection, inflammation and pathology. This mini review summarizes insights gained from studies of early infection, immune cell trafficking, inflammation and the mechanisms of neuropathogenesis. Advances in our understanding of these processes have contributed to the development of therapeutic interventions designed to protect neurons and regulate inflammatory activity.

Keywords: AIDS; human immunodeficiency virus; dementia; neurons; microglia; macrophages

1. Introduction

FIV, similar to HIV, is a lentivirus that infects and replicates in T cells and cells of monocyte lineage including perivascular macrophages and microglia [1–11]. Soon after initial systemic infection with HIV or FIV, the virus enters the central nervous system (CNS). During infection, the virus inserts its RNA core into the host cell, which is then reverse transcribed into DNA and integrated into the host cell genome. Since both T cell and monocytoid cells can be long lived, they can maintain a virus reservoir within infected tissues including the CNS. Antiretroviral therapy targeted to various steps in the virus lifecycle can now suppress systemic viral burden to low or undetectable levels and has greatly increased survival in infected individuals. However, because antiretroviral drugs penetrate the blood-brain barrier poorly and are substrates for active efflux transporters, the virus persists in the brain and has led to an increasing prevalence of cognitive dysfunction as the infected population ages [12–15], even with suppression of both the systemic and cerebrospinal fluid (CSF) viral load [16]. Substantial effort is focused on the development of strategies that will eliminate virus from cellular reservoirs. In the CNS the self-sustaining nature of the microglial population [17,18] and the ability of monocytic cells to sustain viral replication in the absence of T cells [19] make eradication of virus a daunting task. To reduce or eliminate CNS effects of lentiviral infection, we need a better understanding of viral replication in the CNS and the mechanisms that underlie neuronal damage. Because of the difficulty of exploring these processes in humans, animal models have played an essential role in this endeavor.

2. FIV Infection of the Nervous System

2.1. General Background

FIV was isolated from naturally infected domestic cats soon after the identification of HIV [20] and was subsequently shown to be genetically and functionally similar to HIV including similar cell tropism and the ability to produce a severe acquired immune deficiency syndrome (AIDS) [21]. Many investigators have explored the virology, immunology and pathogenesis of FIV to gain insights into treatment strategies for both veterinary and human medicine. Among the many achievements, these efforts led to approval of an effective FIV vaccine in 2002. Recent studies have addressed important issues such as mechanisms of FIV transmission, replication and evolution [22–27], FIV vaccine efficacy [28,29], the role of neutralizing antibodies in disease progression [28,30,31], virus assembly and release [32,33], viral latency and eradication strategies [34–36], development of adjunctive therapies [37–40], immunology [41–45], interactions with the microbiome [46,47], development of antiretroviral compounds [48–50] and development of protocols for assessing feline cognitive function [51–54]. Many of these efforts are summarized in this volume and in a review by Bienzle [55]. In the following sections, we summarize in vitro and in vivo studies of FIV that have provided insights into infection and pathogenesis in the central nervous system (CNS).

In contrast to HIV-1, FIV uses CD134 as a primary receptor instead of CD4 [56,57]. Similar to HIV-1, FIV uses the alpha chemokine receptor, CXCR4, as a co-receptor [58–62]. Although most primary isolates of FIV will infect both T-lymphocytes and monocytes, productive replication in vivo is predominantly within FIV-infected T-lymphocytes [2,63–65].

FIV and HIV are thought to gain initial access to the CNS via trafficking of infected monocytes although other mechanisms may contribute such as trafficking of T cells, penetration of free virus across a damaged blood–brain barrier and trafficking across the blood-cerebrospinal fluid (CSF) barrier. Once the virus gains access to the CNS, infection spreads to microglia and astrocytes but not neurons. Virus production in the CNS is typically low and may be controlled in part by CD8+ T cells [66–69]. Early studies of FIV tropism demonstrated that virus could be recovered from brain and CSF of infected cats [70–73]. In vitro studies of CNS cell tropism showed that FIV can infect feline astrocytes [70,74–76], microglia [6,70,75], choroid plexus macrophages [77] and perhaps brain microvascular endothelial cells [78]. In vivo studies indicated that most virus production in the CNS is maintained by macrophages and microglia [2,6]. However, although microglia and macrophages are primary targets of FIV in the brain and choroid plexus, they support a relatively low level of productive infection [6,77,79] and show negligible cell death. This slow virus production in viable microglia or macrophages can infect peripheral blood mononuclear cells (PBMCs) with high efficiency, rapidly leading to a robust productive infection [6,77]. This can be a source of peripheral infection when antiretroviral therapy is non-compliant or discontinued even when systemic virus levels are undetectable.

One of the questions of interest has been whether virus in the CNS represents uniquely adapted quasispecies that may account for both neurotropism and neurovirulence. Studies of FIV envelope diversity during the early stages of infection have shown that the virus that first appears in the CSF is similar to plasma [80]. Over time there can be significant divergence in the pattern of variants in the CSF versus plasma including the rare appearance of unique variants. However, similar to humans, the profile of FIV quasispecies in the CSF in long-term infection is largely composed of variants in plasma with minor contributions from unique variants indicating that the contribution from virus production within the CNS is quite low. Brain-specific FIV sequences have been isolated from the CSF [71,81] that exhibit greater neurovirulence but evidence for consistent selection of specific FIV variants within the CNS is lacking. Thus, infection of the feline CNS closely parallels HIV infection of the human CNS but evidence for unique strains that are responsible for CNS dysfunction is limited. How viral infection is sustained in the nervous system has been an important but elusive question. With the discovery that microglia are a self-sustaining population of cells within the brain [17,18] and monocytic cell infection can be maintained in the absence of T cells [19] it is expected that microglia will have the capacity to maintain the HIV/FIV reservoir indefinitely. Exploration of the mechanisms that control CNS viral replication remains an important area of research essential to the development of strategies to eradicate virus and the FIV model provides a versatile system for the investigation of these processes through all stages of pathogenesis.

2.2. FIV Trafficking across the Blood-Brain Barrier

In vitro studies using fetal feline brain microvascular endothelial cells grown on transwell insert membranes containing 5 μm pores have been used to investigate trafficking of immune cells across the feline blood-brain barrier [82]. These studies used various combinations of astrocytes and/or microglia on the opposite side of the membrane to evaluate the role of parenchymal cells in the trafficking of PBMCs [83,84]. Monocytes, CD4+ T cells, CD8+ T cells and B cells were all observed to cross the endothelium. The transmigration was facilitated by the presence of astrocytes suggesting that although these cells contribute to the blood-brain barrier they also provide signals that support transmigration. The inflammatory cytokine, tumor necrosis factor alpha (TNFα) may provide one such signal as it promotes the transmigration of virus and both infected and uninfected lymphocytes [84]. Exposure of the endothelial/astrocyte cultures to FIV did not induce any preferential trafficking of monocytes, in agreement with previous trafficking studies of human monocytes infected with HIV-1 [85]. Of all the major PBMC subsets, only CD8+ T cells were subject to positive regulation when the feline cultures were exposed to FIV. This observation was consistent with the role of CD8 T cells in the control of CNS infection [66–69]. When microglia were added to the endothelial/astrocyte cultures the trafficking of T cells, B cells and monocytes was suppressed [83]. The suppression of monocyte trafficking by the microglia was partially reversed when the cultures were inoculated with FIV indicating a largely unexplored role of microglia in the control of immune cell trafficking. The range of trafficking cells seen in vitro was consistent with in vivo trafficking studies that showed early invasion of T cells and B cells within the brain of cats 8–10 weeks after infection with FIV_{GL8} [86]. FIV provirus was measured in the brain as early as two to four weeks post-inoculation indicating that the early immune cell trafficking carries virus into the CNS [87,88]. FIV replication was confirmed by the presence of FIV RNA at 10 weeks when the infiltration of mononuclear cells was at a peak [88]. However, the tissue viral loads and pathology decreased over time indicating significant recovery from this acute phase of infection. Although the ability of FIV or HIV to establish a latent infection in the CNS is controversial, several studies have reported a sustained proviral burden in FIV-infected cats in the brain [72,89] even in the absence of significant viral RNA.

2.3. FIV Trafficking across the Blood–CSF Barrier

In addition to penetration across the blood-brain barrier, virus may also penetrate into the brain via the blood-CSF barrier. This barrier differs from the blood–brain barrier as there are no tight junctions at the vascular endothelium. This allows easier penetration of virus and immune cells into the choroid plexus stroma which contains a large population of macrophages and dendritic cells, excellent targets for infection by FIV. The blood-CSF barrier is formed by tight junctions between the cuboidal epithelial cells of the choroid plexus [82]. Trafficking of choroid plexus macrophages across the epithelial barrier can be quite robust and is positively modulated by FIV [90]. In studies of mouse choroid plexus, the epithelium has been shown to constitutively express intracellular adhesion molecule-1 (ICAM-1) and vascular cell adhesion molecule-1 (VCAM-1) which increase in response to inflammatory stimuli [91]. These molecules support the trafficking of cells into the cerebral ventricles and CSF. In both HIV and FIV infection, a relatively robust infiltration of mononuclear cells was seen in the choroid plexus, meninges and subarachnoid space as early as four weeks post-infection [86,92–94]. This influx is consistent with studies of envelope sequence diversity described above which showed that most FIV/HIV in the CSF is likely to be of systemic origin [80,95–97].

Interactions between macrophages and T cells could be particularly prominent within perivascular regions and within the choroid plexus where infected macrophages are commonly seen in HIV, simian immunodeficiency virus (SIV) and FIV infections. In addition, many studies have documented an admixture of systemic and CNS lentiviral transcripts within the choroid plexus of infected hosts [98–101] suggesting the potential interaction of infected perivascular macrophages and trafficking T cells. Thus, the choroid plexus is an important interface between the systemic immune system and the brain but the functional role of the choroid plexus in immune cell trafficking and the fate of trafficking cells are still poorly understood. One study suggests that trafficking through the choroid plexus may confer a unique phenotype during recovery of the nervous system after injury [102]. In unpublished studies we have demonstrated the potency of trafficking macrophages after infusion of cultured, FIV-infected feline choroid plexus macrophages into the lateral ventricle of naïve cats. These experiments were designed to evaluate the role of infected macrophage trafficking across the blood-CSF barrier in the early establishment of CNS infection. Although we saw no evidence for CNS infection via this route a high dose of macrophages (3.6×10^5 macrophages/200 μL into the lateral ventricle) induced a massive influx of neutrophils throughout the brain in the absence of local infusion damage or bleeding. The effect was subsequently confirmed in rats using macrophages tagged with fluorescent polystyrene 1 μm spheres. The macrophages were tracked to the cervical lymph nodes but were not seen in the brain parenchyma. This observation, although limited, is an indication of the profound effect ventricular macrophages can have on immune cell trafficking into the brain. It is also a caution that the ventricular environment is an immunologically active environment. This should be taken into consideration in experiments employing intracranial infusions. Important questions remain concerning the sentinel functions of ventricular macrophages and their specific role in the regulation of the CNS immune environment.

3. FIV and Neuropathogenesis

3.1. Neurological Signs

Because the course of FIV-induced disease, including CNS infection, parallels HIV infection, FIV has been used as a model to investigate the processes that lead to neural damage. One of the difficulties associated with the use of FIV as a model for HIV-associated neurodegenerative disease is the very gradual decline in CNS function with few overt signs until after about 5–8 years, often overlapping with the development of acquired immune deficiency syndrome (AIDS). In addition, as in HIV-infected humans, only a small subset of infected cats show readily apparent neurological signs as they become immune deficient. A question often raised is whether cats naturally infected with FIV have neurological disease since there is little indication of clinically relevant neurological deficits. The brains of random source FIV infected cats examined post mortem show clear signs of degeneration. Less is known about well maintained domestic cats and several factors complicate the assessment of these cats. The deficits seen in HIV infected patients are cognitive-motor processing deficits with no primary motor deficits. In patients maintained on antiretroviral therapy cognitive decline reflects frontal cortex deficits such as attention and executive functions [14,15]. These deficits would not easily be picked up in routine neurological exams of cats (similar for humans where neuropsychological tests are often required to document deficits). It is also likely that such deficits would impact the lives of cats far less than humans. Behavioral deficits seen in immune deficient cats may also be overlooked in the context of opportunistic infections. As cats age the impact of FIV infection is likely to become greater but this remains to be tested.

In contrast to the clinical setting, neural and behavioral dysfunction are commonly seen in experimentally infected cats using sensitive physiological and behavioral methods. Because these methods are complex and/or expensive they are not practical in the clinic. In addition, because of the slow course and low natural prevalence of neural deficits, experimental studies of FIV-associated neurological disease have adopted strategies to accelerate neuropathogenesis. These strategies have employed neonatal inoculation with FIV [81], the use of neurovirulent strains of FIV [73,81,103–107] and a combination of neurovirulent strains and direct intracranial inoculation [80]. An example of a typical infection following direct inoculation into the lateral ventricle is illustrated in Figure 1. A rapid and robust FIV production is seen in CSF that meets and often exceeds levels in plasma. Cats inoculated systemically typically show a delayed appearance of virus in CSF with much lower titers, even though the plasma FIV titers are similar to intracranial inoculation. FIV titers in the CSF can vary substantially and the correlation between plasma and CSF virus is relatively low. Spikes of FIV can appear in the CSF in the absence of changes in plasma FIV suggesting independent control of replication.

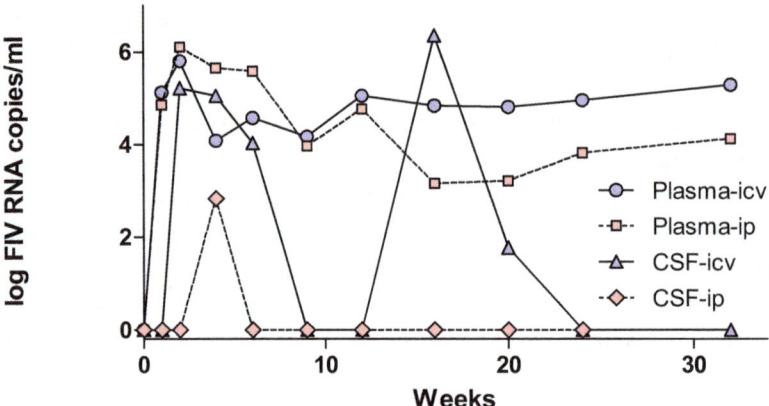

Figure 1. Example of the development of FIV titers in plasma and CSF after systemic (ip) or intracereroventricular (ICV) inoculation of specific pathogen free cats with 2×10^5 copies of FIV. In both cases plasma viremia develops rapidly, peaking at 1–2 weeks post-inoculation. The sustained plasma viral load is maintained at higher levels after ICV inoculation (blue circles). CSF viral titers (blue triangles) closely parallel the acute plasma virus and occasionally exceeds plasma titers indicating a CNS origin. Chronic CSF FIV titers may show independent spikes of activity and generally average about 10^3–10^4 copies/mL. Following systemic inoculation, FIV titers in CSF show a modest delayed peak followed by relative recovery to low levels.

In studies of experimentally infected specific pathogen free cats, designed to mimic HIV infection in humans, neurological signs can be detected as early as 12 months post infection. The signs include abnormal, stereotypic motor behaviors, anisocoria, increased aggression, increased cortical slow wave activity in quantitative electroencephalograms, prolonged latencies in brainstem evoked potentials, delayed righting and pupillary reflexes, decreased nerve conduction velocities, changes in sleep architecture and deficits in cognitive-motor functions [52,54,104–110]. Proton magnetic resonance spectroscopy (MRS) demonstrated reductions in the concentrations of the neuronal marker, N-acetyl-aspartate (NAA) and the NAA/choline or NAA/creatine ratio within the brains of FIV-infected cats [81,106]. Neurotoxic activity in the CSF of FIV-infected cats could be detected as early as 4 months after intracranial inoculation [111] prior to any observable deficits. These observations highlight the early and progressive nature of the disease and the importance of early therapeutic intervention to suppress neurodegeneration, particularly in HIV-infected patients. The feline model continues to make important contributions to the development and testing of such interventions. As discussed below, there is an expectation that FIV infection will contribute to the development of age-associated CNS disease including the development of Alzheimer-like pathologies. A valuable contribution to our understanding of the interaction between infection and aging could be made through the development of simple behavioral and/or physiological tests that could routinely be used in veterinary clinics. Information on age-associated cognitive decline in the large domestic cat population has the potential to contribute substantially to our understanding of neurodegeneration relevant to an aging population of HIV-infected patients.

3.2. FIV Neuropathology

The CNS pathology that develops in cats experimentally infected with FIV reflects the low grade inflammation seen in pre-AIDS/encephalitis patients and current patients on antiretroviral therapy. Findings include infiltration of perivascular macrophages, microglial activation, astrogliosis, myelin pallor, diffusely distributed signs of neural damage in the form of beaded and/or fragmented dendrites [112–116] (Figure 2A,B). Other studies have shown increased immunoreactivity for neurofilament protein in cortical pyramidal neurons [117] and decreased expression of microtubule associated protein-2 (MAP-2) and glutamic acid decarboxylase (GAD) [118]. In addition, a significant 32% loss of large pyramidal cells within layers two, three and five of the frontal/parietal cortex and large cells within the striatum has been seen in asymptomatic cats approximately three years after infection with a FIV isolated from a naturally infected cat (FIV$_{NCSU1}$) [119]. The loss of neurons correlated with decreases in the CD4:CD8 ratio suggesting a close relationship to systemic immune dysfunction. However, it is worth noting that, although a significant decrease was seen in these specific neuron populations, other neurons were minimally affected (as with HIV) such that the net neuron loss in the cortex was 2.3%. Because the overall loss is modest it is not surprising that these cats typically have deficits that would not be apparent in routine clinical neurologic evaluations. This again parallels HIV infection where sensitive neuropsychological testing is often required to demonstrate underlying cognitive deficits.

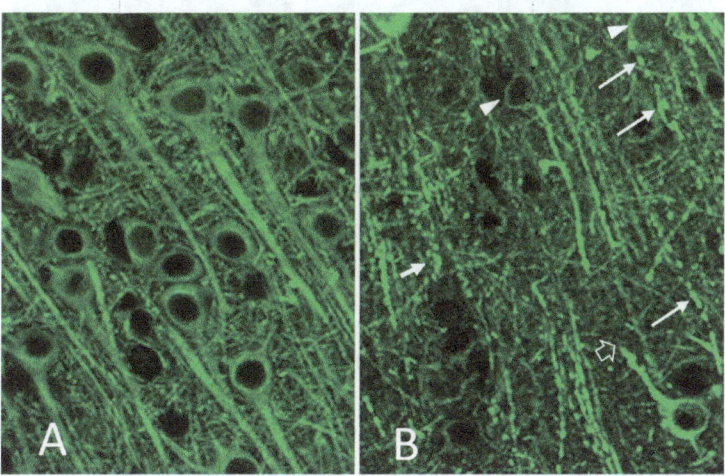

Figure 2. Stain for MAP-2 (green) in the cortex of an FIV-infected cat: (**A**) example of normal cortical pyramidal cells; and (**B**) adjacent areas often show early signs of damage indicated by a fragmented appearance of the MAP-2 stained dendrites and signs of focal swelling.

With the exception of advanced stages of disease progression where neuron loss becomes evident, the pathology largely reflects ongoing inflammation which is potentially reversible. Figure 3 illustrates inflammatory changes seen in the brain of FIV infected cats at approximately three years post-infection. Iba1 immunoreactive microglia are abundant in white matter (Figure 3A). A subset of neurons stained with MAP-2 show signs of dendritic beading (Figure 3B, arrows) and in subcortical white matter-gray matter boundaries neurons are often seen wrapped by microglia (Figure 3C, MAP-2 stained neurons, green; Iba1 stained microglia, red). Increased numbers of macrophages are seen in the choroid plexus, particularly adjacent to penetrating blood vessels (Figure 3D, Iba1 stained macrophages, red; cytokeratin stained epithelium, blue). Accumulations of Mac387 stained monocyte/macrophages are seen surrounding blood vessels in the basal ganglia (Figure 3E) and cortex. It is notable that, in addition to the inflammatory activity, signs of repair activities can also be seen as increased cortical synaptophysin immunoreactivity in the cortex [119] and increased Timms staining (sprouting) in the hippocampus of FIV-infected cats [120] during the asymptomatic stages of disease. Restorative processes may be mediated by the same cells responsible for inflammatory damage. Studies of human macrophages exposed to HIV have shown that various growth factors and anti-inflammatory cytokines are concurrently secreted with neurotoxic factors indicating a constant balance between toxic and repair processes. Treatments designed to precisely regulate these functions have significant therapeutic potential.

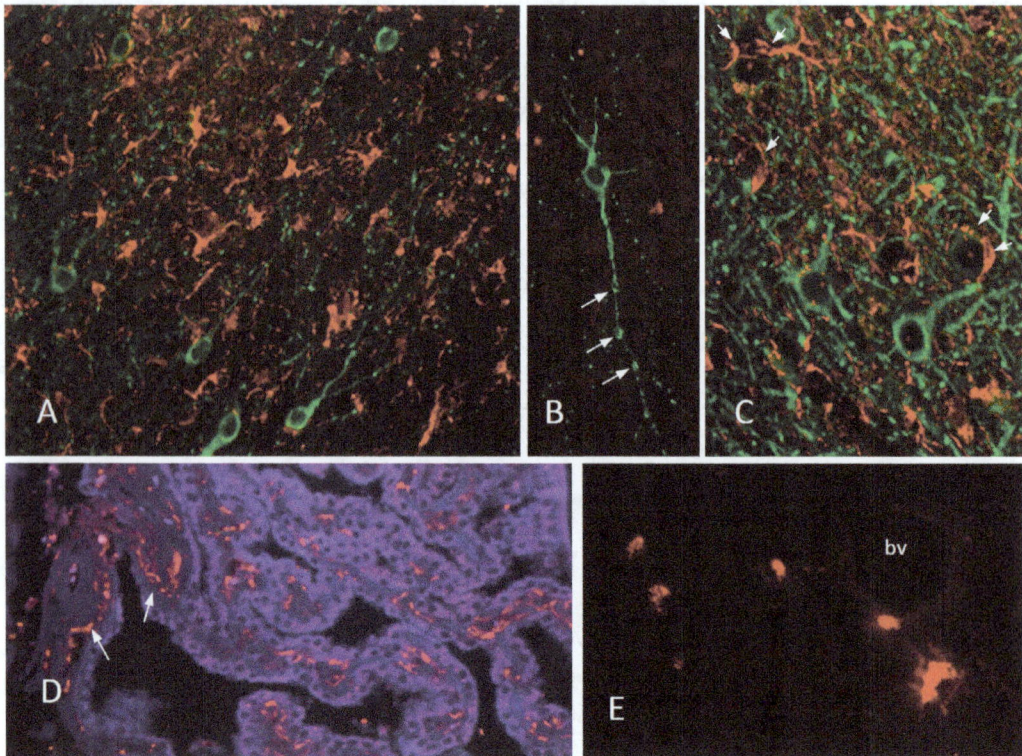

Figure 3. The CNS response to FIV infection. (**A**) Activated microglia stained with an antibody to Iba1 (red) are abundant in the subcortical white matter at the interface between the frontal cortex and basal ganglia. Neurons are stained for MAP-2 (green). (**B**) An example of a single MAP-2+ neuron (green) at the cortical-basal ganglia interface with varicosities in the dendrites indicative of early damage. (**C**) Iba1+ microglia (red) are often seen wrapping neurons in the FIV infected brain but are rare in normal brain. (**D**) An increased number of Iba1+ macrophages (red) populate the choroid plexus in an FIV infected cat. The cuboidal epithelium is stained for cytokeratin (blue). (**E**) Small clusters and scattered macrophages stained for Mac387 (red), a marker of newly migrated macrophages, are seen surrounding blood vessels (bv) in the basal ganglia and cortex (not shown).

An important observation that deserves greater attention is the development of Tau pathology in aged cats [120–122]. Two major efforts in the quest to combat neurodegenerative diseases are focused on understanding the development of Tau pathology and the ability of inflammatory diseases such as HIV infection to enhance age-associated neurodegenerative diseases including Alzheimer's disease (AD). Experimental models of the disease process are limited since few species other than humans have been shown to develop Tau pathology. The identification of pathological Tau in cats in early studies [121,122] and subsequently in a more detailed study of cats ranging in age from two weeks to 22 years [123] have indicated that aged cats, similar to humans, develop amyloid deposits and pathological changes in Tau. The expression of Tau tangles in the cats was rare indicating that the Tau pathology was still developing or was less severe than that seen in humans with dementia. The appearance of age-related pathology may be at least partially dependent on environmental influences. A study contrasting systemic amyloid deposition in naturally and experimentally infected cats identified deposits in 35% of the naturally infected cats [124] but no amyloid accumulation in experimentally infected specific pathogen free cats. This observation is an important reminder that factors such as immune activation/inflammation are likely to play a significant role in the development of pathology. It is recognized that a large percentage of domestic cats will develop feline cognitive dysfunction as they reach ages >10 years [125,126]. Identification of the early processes leading to age-dependent Tau pathology is critical to our understanding of the natural disease process and studies of cat aging may be a significant source of new insights.

4. Mechanisms of FIV Neurotoxicity

4.1. Studies Using Cultured Fetal Feline Cells

The availability of fetal tissue from cats provides the opportunity to perform in vitro experiments that explore the cellular processes that lead to pathology. Neurons are easily cultured from fetuses at approximately 35–40 days gestation (~6–7 cm fetus) [21,111,127–130]. In addition, microglia, choroid plexus epithelium and choroid plexus macrophages have been cultured from the fetal brain [77,90,131] and microvascular endothelial cells have been cultured from late gestation brain tissue [83,132,133]. Figure 4 illustrates various cultures prepared from fetal cat brain. Studies of FIV interactions with these cells have led to a number of important insights into the cellular processes associated with calcium dysregulation and neural dysfunction.

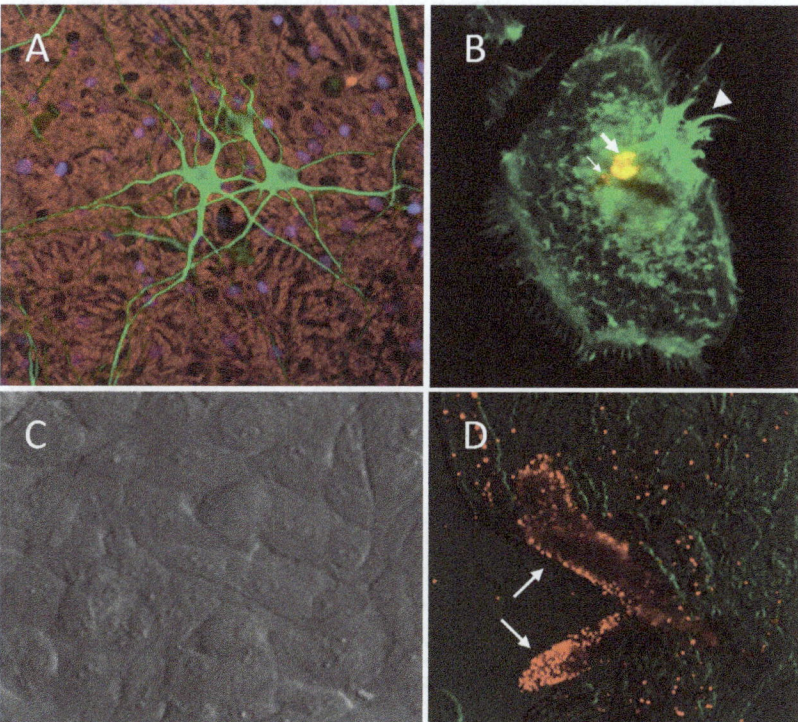

Figure 4. Examples of feline cells grown in culture for basic research on neuro-immune interactions and FIV neuropathogenesis. Excellent recognition of feline proteins is seen with a variety of antibodies to standard markers. (**A**) Neurons identified with MAP-2 immunocytochemistry (green) on a bed of GFAP immunoreactive astrocytes (red). (**B**) A cultured feline choroid plexus macrophage stained with an antibody to FIV (red) and counterstained with phalloidin (green) to show actin structure. FIV is compartmentalized within the cells (large arrow) and can be also seen in small endosome-like structures (small arrow). Ruffles are expressed on the surface of the cell and prominently on one side (arrowhead). (**C**) Cultured feline microvascular endothelial cells viewed with differential interference contrast. (**D**) Macrophages stained with DiI-acetylated-LDL (red) are prominent surrounding penetrating vessels in a whole mount preparation of choroid plexus illustrating the abundance of these cells at the blood-CSF interface.

In early studies of virus interactions with primary feline mixed neuronal cultures (e.g., Figure 4A), the addition of FIV produced minimal cell death but, instead, primed the neurons for damage in response to a normally subtoxic excitatory challenge with glutamate [129]. The concentration-effect curve for glutamate toxicity was shifted approximately three-fold to the left indicating an increase in the neuronal sensitivity to the glutamate. The effect of FIV developed gradually for up to seven days suggesting a cumulative release of soluble toxic factors, presumably from microglia. Subsequent studies using choroid plexus macrophages (Figure 4B) demonstrated that FIV induced the release of potent "toxins" that caused a dysregulation of calcium homeostasis in the neurons [127]. Although small amounts of FIV provirus were detected in some of these cultures at 17–24 days post-inoculation, no evidence of productive infection was observed during the period of toxin generation that peaked between approximately 3–6 days. A comparison of live virus, inactivated virus and viral envelope protein showed that each could induce the same secretion of neurotoxic factors from macrophages demonstrating that the inflammatory response leading to neuronal damage was independent of infection [128]. Other studies described above have used preparations of endothelial cells (Figure 4C) and choroid plexus (Figure 4D) for trafficking studies.

4.2. FIV and Intracellular Calcium Homeostasis

The identity of the soluble factors that impair neuronal function is still largely unknown. While a diverse range of HIV-associated, macrophage-derived factors have been proposed to be responsible for neurotoxicity [4,134–137], none have been shown to recapitulate the effects of the macrophage supernatant on neural calcium homeostasis and damage (which mimics pathology in vivo). Most investigators agree that accumulation of intracellular calcium is a pivotal neural response early in the pathological cascade. Thus, stabilization of intracellular calcium has been a focus of many efforts to prevent damage [138,139]. Studies with primary feline neurons showed that the accumulation of intracellular calcium was due to a gradual delayed increase that could be dissociated from acute increases in calcium [127,130]. An example of a typical response of feline neurons to conditioned medium from choroid plexus macrophages is shown in Figure 5.

When conditioned medium from FIV-treated choroid plexus macrophages was added to cultured feline neurons (1:5 dilution) an acute increase in intracellular calcium was seen (Figure 5B) followed by partial recovery (Figure 5C) and then a gradual delayed rise to high levels with structural damage in the form of beading (Figure 5D, arrows). The typical average calcium response in Figure 5E illustrates the acute rise, sustained plateau and the gradual delayed rise necessary for the development of cytoskeletal damage. Basal calcium in control cultures does not change over the same time course. The conditioned medium always provoked a much greater toxic response than cell-free FIV virions, consistent with the idea that macrophage activation is a primary cause of neurotoxicity. These early pathological changes are reversible but, if the exposure is sustained, the beading is followed by dendritic pruning and eventually cell death. The reason for the delayed rise is not completely understood. However, studies with HIV-infected human CSF have indicated that a loss of sodium-calcium exchanger (NCX) function contributes to the calcium destabilization [140] by reducing the ability to export excess intracellular calcium. This deficit would synergistically increase the magnitude of the intracellular calcium rise regardless of the source of calcium entry into the cytosol [127]. Evidence from these studies indicate that NMDA glutamate receptor activity makes the greatest contribution to pathology, consistent with numerous studies using different models of HIV neuropathogenesis [137,141–146]. Another mechanism hypothesized to lead to enhancement of glutamatergic activity is the inhibition of astrocyte glutamate transporters [147] resulting in prolonged exposure of neurons to glutamate. FIV infection of astrocytes in vitro resulted in a 50%–60% reduction in the ability to transport glutamate [76]. The extent of this effect in vivo is still unclear but increased concentrations of glutamate have been reported in extracts prepared from brains of FIV-infected cats [71].

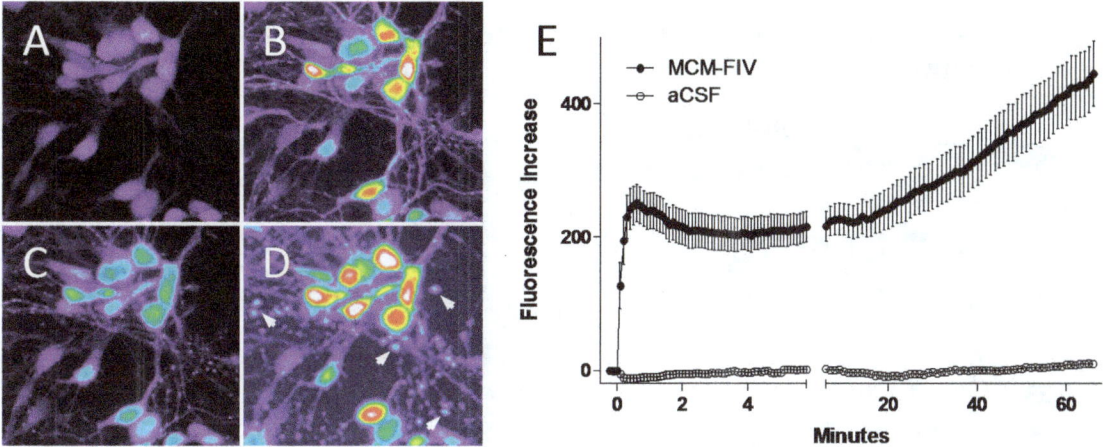

Figure 5. Exposure of cultured feline cortical neurons to soluble factors secreted by choroid plexus macrophages infected with FIV results in a dysregulation of calcium homeostasis followed by cytoskeletal damage. (**A**) Pseudocolored image showing resting calcium in feline cortical neurons. (**B**) Acute increase in calcium triggered by addition of conditioned medium from macrophages inoculated with FIV. (**C**) Partial recovery of calcium is typically seen over the first few minutes. (**D**) The acute increase is followed by a gradual, progressive increase in intracellular calcium. This delayed deregulation of calcium triggers the development of focal swellings in dendrites and axons (beading), a reversible hallmark of early pathogenesis. Similar results are seen with inactivated virions or FIV surface glycoprotein (envelope) indicating that infection is not necessary to provoke the secretion of neurotoxic factors. (**E**) Example of the average profile of calcium increase in response to macrophage conditioned medium (MCM) relative to normal basal calcium levels in cells treated with artificial cerebrospinal fluid (aCSF). Beading typical appears at approximately 20–30 min during the delayed rise and is independent of the acute increase.

Overall, these studies illustrate that inflammation sensitizes neurons in a fashion that encourages the development of more severe neurodegenerative pathologies. Therapeutic approaches that prevent the early neuronal dysfunction have the potential to interrupt the pathological cascade at a point where it is largely reversible. The FIV model offers many benefits for these efforts. Nevertheless, it is also important to recognize limitations of the model. Lack of species-specific reagents and assays can prevent detailed exploration of toxic factors and mechanisms. In spite of these limitations, the FIV model offers the ability to assess potential neuroprotective strategies both in vitro and in vivo.

5. Development of Neuroprotective Treatments

Insights from the above studies have supported a model of neuropathogenesis illustrated in Figure 6. FIV penetration into the nervous systems via infected monocytes establishes a viral reservoir with chronic activation of macrophages and microglia. The subsequent inflammatory response, triggered in part by putative FIV interactions with CXCR4, causes the release of soluble factors that act on neurons to provoke a dysregulation of calcium homeostasis. Progressive accumulation of calcium due to decreased export of calcium in conjunction with NMDA receptor activity drives pathological changes in the cytoskeleton through mechanisms that are not well understood but may include calcium-dependent activation of calpain, calcium-calmodulin protein kinase II (CamKII) or calcineurin. The net result is the loss of actin structure, inefficient transport and the development of focal swellings in the dendrites and axons (beading) where organelles, amyloid precursor protein and Tau accumulate.

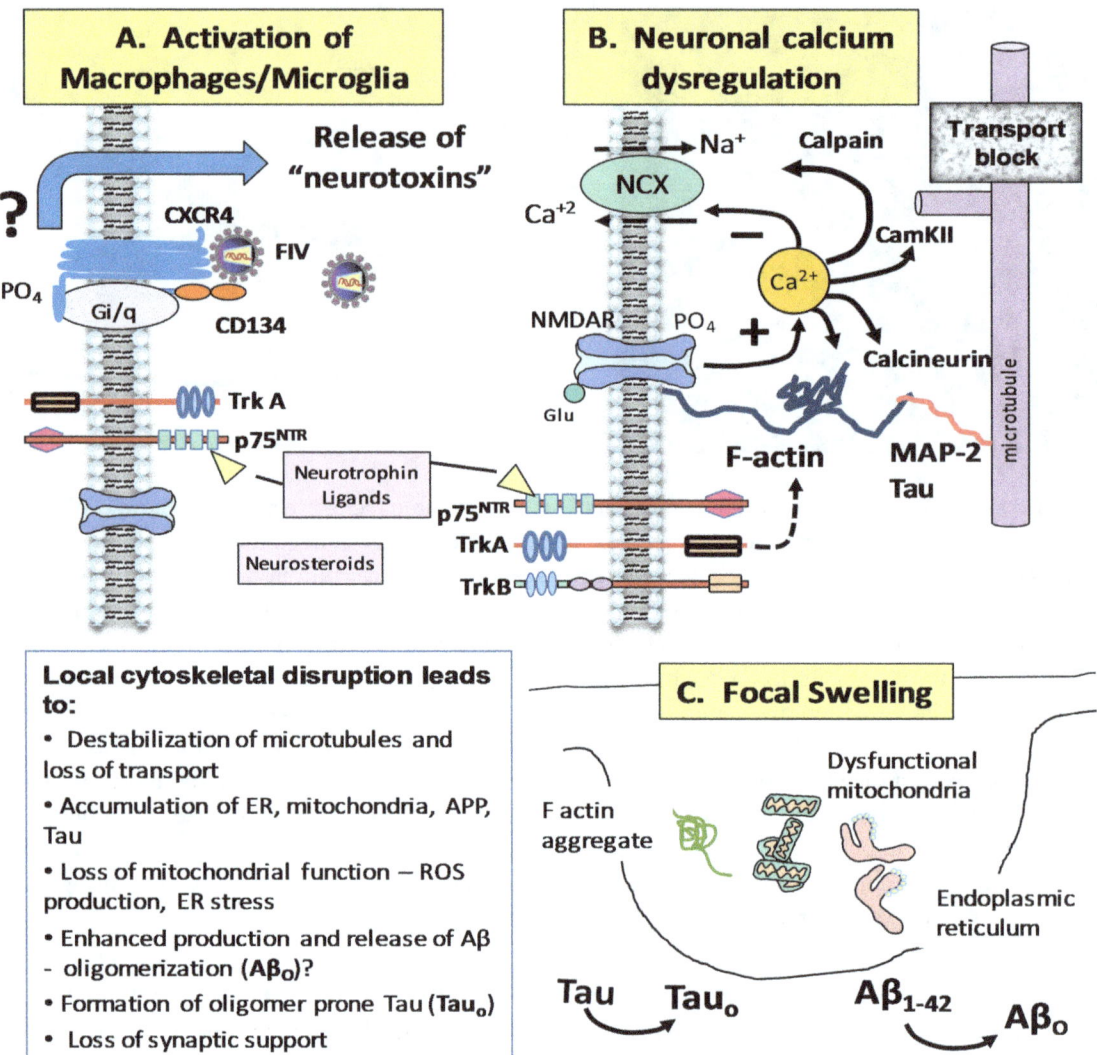

Figure 6. Summary of inflammation-associated neuropathogenesis in response to FIV. (**A**) FIV infects monocytes and macrophages through interactions with CD134 and CXCR4. The virus rapidly gains access to the brain via transmigration of infected monocytes at the blood brain barrier or macrophages at the blood-CSF barrier and establishes what is thought to be a self-sustaining reservoir within microglia. Activation by FIV results in the release of factors that have toxic effects on neurons. The processes that control toxin release are not well understood but appear to be regulated in part by neurotrophins. (**B**) Factors ("Neurotoxins") in the secretome of the mononuclear phagocytes enhance neuronal calcium signaling in response to glutamate and inhibit the ability of neurons to recover to resting calcium levels. The loss of recovery is thought to be due to a loss of sodium-calcium exchanger (NCX) function. The net result is a gradual, sustained accumulation of calcium that disrupts the cytoskeleton. Activation of calcium-dependent enzymes such as calpain, CamKII, and calcineurin may contribute to actin destabilization and loss of structure. (**C**) The loss of structure disrupts transport and results in focal swelling (beading) of axons and dendrites. The accumulation of mitochondria, endoplasmic reticulum, amyloid precursor protein (APP) and Tau in the swellings may set the stage for oxidative stress and potential cleavage of oligomerization prone Abeta and Tau. The p75 neurotrophin receptor ligand LM11A-31 reduces calcium accumulation and protects the cytoskeleton. Neurosteroids may offer protection by reducing inflammation.

Neurotrophin ligands may act at receptors on neurons or macrophages/microglia to prevent the calcium dysregulation and cytoskeletal disruption. Because FIV neuropathology and neurodegenerative mechanisms are highly similar to HIV it provides the opportunity to test potential therapies in FIV infected cats. Studies of cultured feline neurons have shown that a novel neurotrophin ligand which targets the p75 neurotrophin receptor (p75^{NTR}) has strong neuroprotective efficacy. At 10 nM, the ligand protected neurons from the long-term toxic effects of FIV in mixed neural cultures, suppressed the delayed accumulation of intracellular calcium (but not the acute increase) and greatly decreased dendritic damage [130]. The in vivo efficacy of the compound is currently being assessed in FIV infected cats.

In a separate series of studies Maingat et al. [53] demonstrated the potential for neurosteroids to prevent FIV associated degeneration. Treatment of experimentally infected cats with sulfated dehydroepiandrosterone (DHEA-S) reduced inflammation and prevented behavioral deficits and neuron loss indicating that neurosteroids could be useful for the treatment of inflammation-mediated neurodegeneration. Together, these studies [53,130] show that the FIV model parallels the development of neurodegenerative disease in humans and can be used to identify therapeutic strategies that protect the nervous system.

6. Conclusions

FIV infection of the nervous system shares many common features with HIV infection including usage of the co-receptor, CXCR4, similar cellular targets, rapid penetration and infection of the CNS, the generation of a diffuse CNS inflammatory response and gradual, progressive pathogenesis. Although there are differences between FIV and HIV virus structure, primary receptor usage and severity of CNS disease, the basic mechanisms that disable neurons appear to be almost identical providing the opportunity to investigate disease mechanisms. In vitro and in vivo studies of FIV have provided insights into: (1) the natural progression of CNS disease; (2) the role of astrocytes and microglia in immune cell trafficking across the blood-brain and blood-CSF barriers; (3) the mechanisms of early infection, viral diversification and disease progression in the CNS; (4) the potential importance of the choroid plexus blood-CSF barrier as a site of virus entry; (5) the potential mechanisms that lead to the loss of neuronal calcium homeostasis and neuronal pathology; and (6) have facilitated the identification and testing of novel treatments. The FIV model recapitulates many features of inflammation-associated neurodegeneration that are thought to promote various neurodegenerative diseases. The ability to investigate the pathogenesis of FIV in specific-pathogen free cats in parallel with in vitro studies of cultured feline cells provides the opportunity for translational studies that should facilitate the design and evaluation of new therapeutic strategies that prevent neurodegeneration.

Acknowledgments: Supported by NIH Grants R21 NS086426 and R01 MH085606. No funds were provided to publish in open access.

Author Contributions: Much of the work described in the review was performed jointly by Meeker and Hudson with Meeker performing the invitro studies and Hudson the in vivo studies. The review was written by Meeker with the assistance of Hudson.

References

1. Brinkmann, R.; Schwinn, A.; Narayan, O.; Zink, C.; Kreth, H.W.; Roggendorf, W.; Dorries, R.; Schwender, S.; Imrich, H.; Ter, M.V. Human immunodeficiency virus infection in microglia: Correlation between cells infected in the brain and cells cultured from infectious brain tissue. *Ann. Neurol.* **1992**, *31*, 361–365. [CrossRef] [PubMed]
2. Dow, S.W.; Mathiason, C.K.; Hoover, E.A. In vivo monocyte tropism of pathogenic feline immunodeficiency viruses. *J. Virol.* **1999**, *73*, 6852–6861. [PubMed]
3. Fischer-Smith, T.; Croul, S.; Sverstiuk, A.E.; Capini, C.; L'Heureux, D.; Regulier, E.G.; Richardson, M.W.; Amini, S.; Morgello, S.; Khalili, K.; et al. Cns invasion by cd14+/cd16+ peripheral blood-derived monocytes in hiv dementia: Perivascular accumulation and reservoir of hiv infection. *J. NeuroVirol.* **2001**, *7*, 528–541. [CrossRef] [PubMed]

4.   Gonzalez-Scarano, F.; Martin-Garcia, J. The neuropathogenesis of aids. *Nat. Rev. Immunol.* **2005**, *5*, 69–81. [CrossRef] [PubMed]

5.   Gorry, P.R.; Bristol, G.; Zack, J.A.; Ritola, K.; Swanstrom, R.; Birch, C.J.; Bell, J.E.; Bannert, N.; Crawford, K.; Wang, H.; et al. Macrophage tropism of human immunodeficiency virus type 1 isolates from brain and lymphoid tissues predicts neurotropism independent of coreceptor specificity. *J. Virol.* **2001**, *75*, 10073–10089. [CrossRef] [PubMed]

6.   Hein, A.; Martin, J.P.; Koehren, F.; Bingen, A.; Dorries, R. In vivo infection of ramified microglia from adult cat central nervous system by feline immunodeficiency virus. *Virology* **2000**, *268*, 420–429. [CrossRef] [PubMed]

7.   Koenig, S.; Gendelman, H.E.; Orenstein, J.M.; Dal Canto, M.C.; Pezeshkpour, G.H.; Yungbluth, M.; Janotta, F.; Aksamit, A.; Martin, M.A.; Fauci, A.S. Detection of aids virus in macrophages in brain tissue from aids patients with encephalopathy. *Science* **1986**, *233*, 1089–1093. [CrossRef] [PubMed]

8.   Lane, J.H.; Sasseville, V.G.; Smith, M.O.; Vogel, P.; Pauley, D.R.; Heyes, M.P.; Lackner, A.A. Neuroinvasion by simian immunodeficiency virus coincides with increased numbers of perivascular macrophages/microglia and intrathecal immune activation. *J. NeuroVirol.* **1996**, *2*, 423–432. [CrossRef] [PubMed]

9.   Petito, C.K. Human immunodeficiency virus type 1 compartmentalization in the central nervous system. *J. NeuroVirol.* **2004**, *10*, 21–24. [CrossRef] [PubMed]

10.   Williams, K.C.; Corey, S.; Westmoreland, S.V.; Pauley, D.; Knight, H.; deBakker, C.; Alvarez, X.; Lackner, A.A. Perivascular macrophages are the primary cell type productively infected by simian immunodeficiency virus in the brains of macaques: Implications for the neuropathogenesis of aids. *J. Exp. Med.* **2001**, *193*, 905–915. [CrossRef] [PubMed]

11.   Zenger, E.; Tiffany-Castiglioni, E.; Collisson, E.W. Cellular mechanisms of feline immunodeficiency virus (FIV)-induced neuropathogenesis. *Front. Biosci.* **1997**, *2*, d527–d537. [CrossRef] [PubMed]

12.   Anthony, I.C.; Ramage, S.N.; Carnie, F.W.; Simmonds, P.; Bell, J.E. Influence of haart on HIV-related CNS disease and neuroinflammation. *J. Neuropathol. Exp. Neurol.* **2005**, *64*, 529–536. [CrossRef] [PubMed]

13.   Neuenburg, J.K.; Brodt, H.R.; Herndier, B.G.; Bickel, M.; Bacchetti, P.; Price, R.W.; Grant, R.M.; Schlote, W. Hiv-related neuropathology, 1985 to 1999: Rising prevalence of hiv encephalopathy in the era of highly active antiretroviral therapy. *J. Acquir. Immune Defic. Syndr.* **2002**, *31*, 171–177. [CrossRef] [PubMed]

14.   Sacktor, N.; McDermott, M.P.; Marder, K.; Schifitto, G.; Selnes, O.A.; McArthur, J.C.; Stern, Y.; Albert, S.; Palumbo, D.; Kieburtz, K.; et al. Hiv-associated cognitive impairment before and after the advent of combination therapy. *J. NeuroVirol.* **2002**, *8*, 136–142. [CrossRef] [PubMed]

15.   Heaton, R.K.; Franklin, D.R.; Ellis, R.J.; McCutchan, J.A.; Letendre, S.L.; Leblanc, S.; Corkran, S.H.; Duarte, N.A.; Clifford, D.B.; Woods, S.P.; et al. HIV-associated neurocognitive disorders before and during the era of combination antiretroviral therapy: Differences in rates, nature, and predictors. *J. NeuroVirol.* **2011**, *17*, 3–16. [CrossRef] [PubMed]

16.   Cysique, L.A.; Brew, B.J.; Halman, M.; Catalan, J.; Sacktor, N.; Price, R.W.; Brown, S.; Atkinson, J.H.; Clifford, D.B.; Simpson, D.; et al. Undetectable cerebrospinal fluid hiv rna and beta-2 microglobulin do not indicate inactive aids dementia complex in highly active antiretroviral therapy-treated patients. *J. Acquir. Immune Defic. Syndr.* **2005**, *39*, 426–429. [CrossRef] [PubMed]

17.   Ginhoux, F.; Prinz, M. Origin of microglia: Current concepts and past controversies. *Cold Spring Harb. Perspect Biol.* **2015**, *7*, a020537. [CrossRef] [PubMed]

18.   Gomez Perdiguero, E.; Klapproth, K.; Schulz, C.; Busch, K.; Azzoni, E.; Crozet, L.; Garner, H.; Trouillet, C.; de Bruijn, M.F.; Geissmann, F.; et al. Tissue-resident macrophages originate from yolk-sac-derived erythro-myeloid progenitors. *Nature* **2015**, *518*, 547–551. [CrossRef] [PubMed]

19.   Honeycutt, J.B.; Wahl, A.; Baker, C.; Spagnuolo, R.A.; Foster, J.; Zakharova, O.; Wietgrefe, S.; Caro-Vegas, C.; Madden, V.; Sharpe, G.; et al. Macrophages sustain HIV replication in vivo independently of T cells. *J. Clin. Investig.* **2016**, *126*, 1353–1366. [CrossRef] [PubMed]

20.   Pedersen, N.C.; Ho, E.W.; Brown, M.L.; Yamamoto, J.K. Isolation of a t-lymphotropic virus from domestic cats with an immunodeficiency-like syndrome. *Science* **1987**, *235*, 790–793. [CrossRef] [PubMed]

21.   Meeker, R.B. Feline immunodeficiency virus neuropathogenesis: From cats to calcium. *J. Neuroimmune Pharmacol.* **2007**, *2*, 154–170. [CrossRef] [PubMed]

22.   Moench, T.R. Cell-associated transmission of HIV type 1 and other lentiviruses in small-animal models. *J. Infect. Dis.* **2014**, *210*, S654–S659. [CrossRef] [PubMed]

23. Willett, B.J.; Hosie, M.J. The virus-receptor interaction in the replication of feline immunodeficiency virus (FIV). *Curr. Opin. Virol.* **2013**, *3*, 670–675. [CrossRef] [PubMed]

24. Willett, B.J.; Kraase, M.; Logan, N.; McMonagle, E.; Varela, M.; Hosie, M.J. Selective expansion of viral variants following experimental transmission of a reconstituted feline immunodeficiency virus quasispecies. *PLoS One* **2013**, *8*, e54871.

25. Beczkowski, P.M.; Hughes, J.; Biek, R.; Litster, A.; Willett, B.J.; Hosie, M.J. Rapid evolution of the ENV gene leader sequence in cats naturally infected with feline immunodeficiency virus. *J. Gen. Virol.* **2015**, *96*, 893–903. [CrossRef] [PubMed]

26. Beczkowski, P.M.; Techakriengkrai, N.; Logan, N.; McMonagle, E.; Litster, A.; Willett, B.J.; Hosie, M.J. Emergence of cd134 cysteine-rich domain 2 (crd2)-independent strains of feline immunodeficiency virus (FIV) is associated with disease progression in naturally infected cats. *Retrovirology* **2014**, *11*, 95. [CrossRef] [PubMed]

27. Yoshikawa, R.; Izumi, T.; Yamada, E.; Nakano, Y.; Misawa, N.; Ren, F.; Carpenter, M.A.; Ikeda, T.; Munk, C.; Harris, R.S.; et al. A naturally occurring domestic cat apobec3 variant confers resistance to feline immunodeficiency virus infection. *J. Virol.* **2015**, *90*, 474–485. [CrossRef] [PubMed]

28. Beczkowski, P.M.; Logan, N.; McMonagle, E.; Litster, A.; Willett, B.J.; Hosie, M.J. An investigation of the breadth of neutralizing antibody response in cats naturally infected with feline immunodeficiency virus. *J. Gen. Virol.* **2015**, *96*, 671–680. [CrossRef] [PubMed]

29. Westman, M.E.; Malik, R.; Hall, E.; Harris, M.; Norris, J.M. The protective rate of the feline immunodeficiency virus vaccine: An Australian field study. *Vaccine* **2016**, *34*, 4752–4758. [CrossRef] [PubMed]

30. Beczkowski, P.M.; Harris, M.; Techakriengkrai, N.; Beatty, J.A.; Willett, B.J.; Hosie, M.J. Neutralising antibody response in domestic cats immunised with a commercial feline immunodeficiency virus (FIV) vaccine. *Vaccine* **2015**, *33*, 977–984. [CrossRef] [PubMed]

31. Coleman, J.K.; Pu, R.; Martin, M.M.; Noon-Song, E.N.; Zwijnenberg, R.; Yamamoto, J.K. Feline immunodeficiency virus (FIV) vaccine efficacy and FIV neutralizing antibodies. *Vaccine* **2014**, *32*, 746–754. [CrossRef] [PubMed]

32. Morrison, J.H.; Guevara, R.B.; Marcano, A.C.; Saenz, D.T.; Fadel, H.J.; Rogstad, D.K.; Poeschla, E.M. Feline immunodeficiency virus envelope glycoproteins antagonize tetherin through a distinctive mechanism that requires virion incorporation. *J. Virol.* **2014**, *88*, 3255–3272. [CrossRef] [PubMed]

33. Brown, L.A.; Cox, C.; Baptiste, J.; Summers, H.; Button, R.; Bahlow, K.; Spurrier, V.; Kyser, J.; Luttge, B.G.; Kuo, L.; et al. Nmr structure of the myristylated feline immunodeficiency virus matrix protein. *Viruses* **2015**, *7*, 2210–2229. [CrossRef] [PubMed]

34. McDonnel, S.J.; Sparger, E.E.; Luciw, P.A.; Murphy, B.G. Pharmacologic reactivation of latent feline immunodeficiency virus ex vivo in peripheral cd4+ t-lymphocytes. *Virus Res.* **2012**, *170*, 174–179. [CrossRef] [PubMed]

35. McDonnel, S.J.; Sparger, E.E.; Murphy, B.G. Feline immunodeficiency virus latency. *Retrovirology* **2013**, *10*, 69. [CrossRef] [PubMed]

36. Murphy, B.; Vapniarsky, N.; Hillman, C.; Castillo, D.; McDonnel, S.; Moore, P.; Luciw, P.A.; Sparger, E.E. FIV establishes a latent infection in feline peripheral blood cd4+ t lymphocytes in vivo during the asymptomatic phase of infection. *Retrovirology* **2012**, *9*, 12. [CrossRef] [PubMed]

37. Roberts, E.S.; VanLare, K.A.; Roycroft, L.M.; King, S. Effect of high-dose ciclosporin on the immune response to primary and booster vaccination in immunocompetent cats. *J. Feline Med. Surg.* **2015**, *17*, 101–109. [CrossRef] [PubMed]

38. Gil, S.; Leal, R.O.; McGahie, D.; Sepulveda, N.; Duarte, A.; Niza, M.M.; Tavares, L. Oral recombinant feline interferon-omega as an alternative immune modulation therapy in FIV positive cats: Clinical and laboratory evaluation. *Res. Vet. Sci.* **2014**, *96*, 79–85. [CrossRef] [PubMed]

39. Leal, R.O.; Gil, S.; Duarte, A.; McGahie, D.; Sepulveda, N.; Niza, M.M.; Tavares, L. Evaluation of viremia, proviral load and cytokine profile in naturally feline immunodeficiency virus infected cats treated with two different protocols of recombinant feline interferon omega. *Res. Vet. Sci.* **2015**, *99*, 87–95. [CrossRef] [PubMed]

40. Leal, R.O.; Gil, S.; Sepulveda, N.; McGahie, D.; Duarte, A.; Niza, M.M.; Tavares, L. Monitoring acute phase proteins in retrovirus infected cats undergoing feline interferon-omega therapy. *J. Small Anim. Pract.* **2014**, *55*, 39–45. [CrossRef] [PubMed]

41. Meng, L.; Tompkins, M.; Miller, M.; Fogle, J. Lentivirus-activated t regulatory cells suppress t helper cell interleukin-2 production by inhibiting nuclear factor of activated t cells 2 binding to the interleukin-2 promoter. *AIDS Res. Hum. Retrovir.* **2014**, *30*, 58–66. [CrossRef] [PubMed]

42. Miller, M.M.; Akaronu, N.; Thompson, E.M.; Hood, S.F.; Fogle, J.E. Modulating DNA methylation in activated cd8+ t cells inhibits regulatory t cell-induced binding of foxp3 to the cd8+ t cell il-2 promoter. *J. Immunol.* **2015**, *194*, 990–998. [CrossRef] [PubMed]

43. Miller, M.M.; Fogle, J.E.; Tompkins, M.B. Infection with feline immunodeficiency virus directly activates CD4+ CD25+ t regulatory cells. *J. Virol.* **2013**, *87*, 9373–9378. [CrossRef] [PubMed]

44. Miller, M.M.; Petty, C.S.; Tompkins, M.B.; Fogle, J.E. CD4+CD25+ t regulatory cells activated during feline immunodeficiency virus infection convert t helper cells into functional suppressors through a membrane-bound tgfbeta / garp-mediated mechanism. *Virol. J.* **2014**, *11*. [CrossRef] [PubMed]

45. Zhang, L.; Reckling, S.; Dean, G.A. Phenotypic and functional analysis of cd1a+ dendritic cells from cats chronically infected with feline immunodeficiency virus. *Comp. Immunol. Microbiol. Infect. Dis.* **2015**, *42*, 53–59. [CrossRef] [PubMed]

46. Weese, J.S.; Nichols, J.; Jalali, M.; Litster, A. The rectal microbiota of cats infected with feline immunodeficiency virus infection and uninfected controls. *Vet. Microbiol.* **2015**, *180*, 96–102. [CrossRef] [PubMed]

47. Branton, W.G.; Ellestad, K.K.; Maingat, F.; Wheatley, B.M.; Rud, E.; Warren, R.L.; Holt, R.A.; Surette, M.G.; Power, C. Brain microbial populations in hiv/aids: Alpha-proteobacteria predominate independent of host immune status. *PLoS ONE* **2013**, *8*. [CrossRef]

48. Asquith, C.R.; Meli, M.L.; Konstantinova, L.S.; Laitinen, T.; Perakyla, M.; Poso, A.; Rakitin, O.A.; Allenspach, K.; Hofmann-Lehmann, R.; Hilton, S.T. Evaluation of the antiviral efficacy of bis[1,2]dithiolo[1,4]thiazines and bis[1,2]dithiolopyrrole derivatives against the nucelocapsid protein of the feline immunodeficiency virus (FIV) as a model for HIV infection. *Bioorg. Med. Chem. Lett.* **2014**, *24*, 2640–2644. [CrossRef] [PubMed]

49. Asquith, C.R.; Meli, M.L.; Konstantinova, L.S.; Laitinen, T.; Poso, A.; Rakitin, O.A.; Hofmann-Lehmann, R.; Allenspach, K.; Hilton, S.T. Novel fused tetrathiocines as antivirals that target the nucleocapsid zinc finger containing protein of the feline immunodeficiency virus (FIV) as a model of hiv infection. *Bioorg. Med. Chem. Lett.* **2015**, *25*, 1352–1355. [CrossRef]

50. Taffin, E.; Paepe, D.; Goris, N.; Auwerx, J.; Debille, M.; Neyts, J.; Van de Maele, I.; Daminet, S. Antiviral treatment of feline immunodeficiency virus-infected cats with (r)-9-(2-phosphonylmethoxypropyl)-2,6-diaminopurine. *J. Feline Med. Surg.* **2015**, *17*, 79–86. [CrossRef] [PubMed]

51. Sherman, B.L.; Gruen, M.E.; Meeker, R.B.; Milgram, B.; DiRivera, C.; Thomson, A.; Clary, G.; Hudson, L. The use of a T-maze to measure cognitive-motor function in cats (*Felis catus*). *J. Vet. Behav.* **2013**, *8*, 32–39. [CrossRef] [PubMed]

52. Maingat, F.; Vivithanaporn, P.; Zhu, Y.; Taylor, A.; Baker, G.; Pearson, K.; Power, C. Neurobehavioral performance in feline immunodeficiency virus infection: Integrated analysis of viral burden, neuroinflammation, and neuronal injury in cortex. *J. Neurosci.* **2009**, *29*, 8429–8437. [CrossRef] [PubMed]

53. Maingat, F.G.; Polyak, M.J.; Paul, A.M.; Vivithanaporn, P.; Noorbakhsh, F.; Ahboucha, S.; Baker, G.B.; Pearson, K.; Power, C. Neurosteroid-mediated regulation of brain innate immunity in HIV/AIDs: Dhea-s suppresses neurovirulence. *FASEB J.* **2013**, *27*, 725–737. [CrossRef] [PubMed]

54. Steigerwald, E.S.; Sarter, M.; March, P.; Podell, M. Effects of feline immunodeficiency virus on cognition and behavioral function in cats. *J. Acquir. Immune Defic. Syndr. Hum. Retrovirol.* **1999**, *20*, 411–419. [CrossRef] [PubMed]

55. Bienzle, D. Fiv in cats—A useful model of HIV in people? *Vet. Immunol. Immunopathol.* **2014**, *159*, 171–179. [CrossRef] [PubMed]

56. De Parseval, A.; Chatterji, U.; Sun, P.; Elder, J.H. Feline immunodeficiency virus targets activated cd4+ t cells by using cd134 as a binding receptor. *Proc. Natl. Acad. Sci. USA* **2004**, *101*, 13044–13049. [CrossRef] [PubMed]

57. Shimojima, M.; Miyazawa, T.; Ikeda, Y.; McMonagle, E.L.; Haining, H.; Akashi, H.; Takeuchi, Y.; Hosie, M.J.; Willett, B.J. Use of cd134 as a primary receptor by the feline immunodeficiency virus. *Science* **2004**, *303*, 1192–1195. [CrossRef] [PubMed]

58. Egberink, H.F.; De Clercq, E.; van Vliet, A.L.; Balzarini, J.; Bridger, G.J.; Henson, G.; Horzinek, M.C.; Schols, D. Bicyclams, selective antagonists of the human chemokine receptor cxcr4, potently inhibit feline immunodeficiency virus replication. *J. Virol.* **1999**, *73*, 6346–6352. [PubMed]

59. Hosie, M.J.; Broere, N.; Hesselgesser, J.; Turner, J.D.; Hoxie, J.A.; Neil, J.C.; Willett, B.J. Modulation of feline immunodeficiency virus infection by stromal cell-derived factor. *J. Virol.* **1998**, *72*, 2097–2104. [PubMed]

60. Willett, B.J.; Adema, K.; Heveker, N.; Brelot, A.; Picard, L.; Alizon, M.; Turner, J.D.; Hoxie, J.A.; Peiper, S.; Neil, J.C.; et al. The second extracellular loop of cxcr4 determines its function as a receptor for feline immunodeficiency virus. *J. Virol.* **1998**, *72*, 6475–6481. [PubMed]

61. Willett, B.J.; Picard, L.; Hosie, M.J.; Turner, J.D.; Adema, K.; Clapham, P.R. Shared usage of the chemokine receptor cxcr4 by the feline and human immunodeficiency viruses. *J. Virol.* **1997**, *71*, 6407–6415. [PubMed]

62. Richardson, J.; Pancino, G.; Merat, R.; Leste-Lasserre, T.; Moraillon, A.; Schneider-Mergener, J.; Alizon, M.; Sonigo, P.; Heveker, N. Shared usage of the chemokine receptor cxcr4 by primary and laboratory-adapted strains of feline immunodeficiency virus. *J. Virol.* **1999**, *73*, 3661–3671. [PubMed]

63. Beebe, A.M.; Dua, N.; Faith, T.G.; Moore, P.F.; Pedersen, N.C.; Dandekar, S. Primary stage of feline immunodeficiency virus infection: Viral dissemination and cellular targets. *J. Virol.* **1994**, *68*, 3080–3091. [PubMed]

64. Brunner, D.; Pedersen, N.C. Infection of peritoneal macrophages in vitro and in vivo with feline immunodeficiency virus. *J. Virol.* **1989**, *63*, 5483–5488. [PubMed]

65. Dow, S.W.; Dreitz, M.J.; Hoover, E.A. Feline immunodeficiency virus neurotropism: Evidence that astrocytes and microglia are the primary target cells. *Vet. Immunol. Immunopathol.* **1992**, *35*, 23–35. [CrossRef]

66. Bucci, J.G.; English, R.V.; Jordan, H.L.; Childers, T.A.; Tompkins, M.B.; Tompkins, W.A. Mucosally transmitted feline immunodeficiency virus induces a CD8+ antiviral response that correlates with reduction of cell-associated virus. *J. Infect. Dis.* **1998**, *177*, 18–25. [CrossRef] [PubMed]

67. Gebhard, D.H.; Dow, J.L.; Childers, T.A.; Alvelo, J.I.; Tompkins, M.B.; Tompkins, W.A. Progressive expansion of an L-selectin-negative CD8 cell with anti-feline immunodeficiency virus (FIV) suppressor function in the circulation of FIV-infected cats. *J. Infect. Dis.* **1999**, *180*, 1503–1513. [CrossRef] [PubMed]

68. Hohdatsu, T.; Miyagawa, N.; Ohkubo, M.; Kida, K.; Koyama, H. Studies on feline cd8+ t cell non-cytolytic anti-feline immunodeficiency virus (FIV) activity. *Arch. Virol.* **2000**, *145*, 2525–2538. [CrossRef] [PubMed]

69. Hohdatsu, T.; Sasagawa, T.; Yamazaki, A.; Motokawa, K.; Kusuhara, H.; Kaneshima, T.; Koyama, H. Cd8+ t cells from feline immunodeficiency virus (FIV) infected cats suppress exogenous fiv replication of their peripheral blood mononuclear cells in vitro. *Arch. Virol.* **2002**, *147*, 1517–1529. [CrossRef] [PubMed]

70. Dow, S.W.; Poss, M.L.; Hoover, E.A. Feline immunodeficiency virus: A neurotropic lentivirus. *J. Acquir. Immune Defic. Syndr.* **1990**, *3*, 658–668. [PubMed]

71. Power, C.; Moench, T.; Peeling, J.; Kong, P.A.; Langelier, T. Feline immunodeficiency virus causes increased glutamate levels and neuronal loss in brain. *Neuroscience* **1997**, *77*, 1175–1185. [CrossRef]

72. Macchi, S.; Maggi, F.; Di Iorio, C.; Poli, A.; Bendinelli, M.; Pistello, M. Detection of feline immunodeficiency proviral sequences in lymphoid tissues and the central nervous system by in situ gene amplification. *J. Virol. Methods* **1998**, *73*, 109–119. [CrossRef]

73. Johnston, J.; Power, C. Productive infection of human peripheral blood mononuclear cells by feline immunodeficiency virus: Implications for vector development. *J. Virol.* **1999**, *73*, 2491–2498. [PubMed]

74. Billaud, J.N.; Selway, D.; Yu, N.; Phillips, T.R. Replication rate of feline immunodeficiency virus in astrocytes is envelope dependent: Implications for glutamate uptake. *Virology* **2000**, *266*, 180–188. [CrossRef] [PubMed]

75. Kawaguchi, Y.; Maeda, K.; Tohya, Y.; Furuya, T.; Miyazawa, T.; Horimoto, T.; Norimine, J.; Kai, C.; Mikami, T. Replicative difference in early-passage feline brain cells among feline immunodeficiency virus isolates. *Arch. Virol.* **1992**, *125*, 347–354. [CrossRef] [PubMed]

76. Yu, N.; Billaud, J.N.; Phillips, T.R. Effects of feline immunodeficiency virus on astrocyte glutamate uptake: Implications for lentivirus-induced central nervous system diseases. *Proc. Natl. Acad. Sci. USA* **1998**, *95*, 2624–2629. [CrossRef] [PubMed]

77. Bragg, D.; Childers, T.; Tompkins, M.; Tompkins, W.; Meeker, R. Infection of the choroid plexus by feline immunodeficiency virus. *J. NeuroVirol.* **2002**, *8*, 211–224. [CrossRef] [PubMed]

78. Steffan, A.M.; Lafon, M.E.; Gendrault, J.L.; Koehren, K.; DeMonte, M.; Royer, C.; Kirn, A.; Gut, J.P. Feline immunodeficiency virus can productively infect cultured endothelial cells from cat brain microvessels. *J. Gen. Virol.* **1994**, *75*, 3647–3653. [CrossRef] [PubMed]

79. Hein, A.; Schuh, H.; Thiel, S.; Martin, J.P.; Dorries, R. Ramified feline microglia selects for distinct variants of feline immunodeficiency virus during early central nervous system infection. *J. NeuroVirol.* **2003**, *9*, 465–476. [CrossRef] [PubMed]

80. Liu, P.; Hudson, L.C.; Tompkins, M.B.; Vahlenkamp, T.W.; Meeker, R.B. Compartmentalization and evolution of feline immunodeficiency virus between the central nervous system and periphery following intracerebroventricular or systemic inoculation. *J. NeuroVirol.* **2006**, *12*, 307–321. [CrossRef] [PubMed]

81. Power, C.; Buist, R.; Johnston, J.B.; Del Bigio, M.R.; Ni, W.; Dawood, M.R.; Peeling, J. Neurovirulence in feline immunodeficiency virus-infected neonatal cats is viral strain specific and dependent on systemic immune suppression. *J. Virol.* **1998**, *72*, 9109–9115. [PubMed]

82. Fletcher, N.F.; Meeker, R.B.; Hudson, L.C.; Callanan, J.J. The neuropathogenesis of feline immunodeficiency virus infection: Barriers to overcome. *Vet. J.* **2011**, *188*, 260–269. [CrossRef] [PubMed]

83. Hudson, L.C.; Bragg, D.C.; Tompkins, M.B.; Meeker, R.B. Astrocytes and microglia differentially regulate trafficking of lymphocyte subsets across brain endothelial cells. *Brain Res.* **2005**, *1058*, 148–160. [CrossRef] [PubMed]

84. Fletcher, N.F.; Bexiga, M.G.; Brayden, D.J.; Brankin, B.; Willett, B.J.; Hosie, M.J.; Jacque, J.M.; Callanan, J.J. Lymphocyte migration through the blood-brain barrier (BBB) in feline immunodeficiency virus infection is significantly influenced by the pre-existence of virus and tumour necrosis factor (TNF)-alpha within the central nervous system (CNS): Studies using an in vitro feline bbb model. *Neuropathol. Appl. Neurobiol.* **2009**, *35*, 592–602. [PubMed]

85. Persidsky, Y.; Stins, M.; Way, D.; Witte, M.H.; Weinand, M.; Kim, K.S.; Bock, P.; Gendelman, H.E.; Fiala, M. A model for monocyte migration through the blood-brain barrier during HIV-1 encephalitis. *J. Immunol.* **1997**, *158*, 3499–3510. [PubMed]

86. Ryan, G.; Grimes, T.; Brankin, B.; Mabruk, M.J.; Hosie, M.J.; Jarrett, O.; Callanan, J.J. Neuropathology associated with feline immunodeficiency virus infection highlights prominent lymphocyte trafficking through both the blood-brain and blood-choroid plexus barriers. *J. Neurovirol.* **2005**, *11*, 337–345. [CrossRef] [PubMed]

87. Poli, A.; Pistello, M.; Carli, M.A.; Abramo, F.; Mancuso, G.; Nicoletti, E.; Bendinelli, M. Tumor necrosis factor-alpha and virus expression in the central nervous system of cats infected with feline immunodeficiency virus. *J. Neurovirol.* **1999**, *5*, 465–473. [CrossRef] [PubMed]

88. Ryan, G.; Klein, D.; Knapp, E.; Hosie, M.J.; Grimes, T.; Mabruk, M.J.; Jarrett, O.; Callanan, J.J. Dynamics of viral and proviral loads of feline immunodeficiency virus within the feline central nervous system during the acute phase following intravenous infection. *J. Virol.* **2003**, *77*, 7477–7485. [CrossRef] [PubMed]

89. Pistello, M.; Menzo, S.; Giorgi, M.; Da Prato, L.; Cammarota, G.; Clementi, M.; Bendinelli, M. Competitive polymerase chain reaction for quantitating feline immunodeficiency virus load in infected cat tissues. *Mol. Cell. Probes* **1994**, *8*, 229–234. [CrossRef] [PubMed]

90. Meeker, R.B.; Bragg, D.C.; Poulton, W.; Hudson, L. Transmigration of macrophages across the choroid plexus epithelium in response to the feline immunodeficiency virus. *Cell Tissue Res.* **2012**, *347*, 443–455. [CrossRef] [PubMed]

91. Steffen, B.J.; Breier, G.; Butcher, E.C.; Schulz, M.; Engelhardt, B. Icam-1, vcam-1, and madcam-1 are expressed on choroid plexus epithelium but not endothelium and mediate binding of lymphocytes in vitro. *Am. J. Pathol.* **1996**, *148*, 1819–1838. [PubMed]

92. Falangola, M.F.; Hanly, A.; Galvao-Castro, B.; Petito, C.K. Hiv infection of human choroid plexus: A possible mechanism of viral entry into the cns. *J. Neuropathol. Exp. Neurol.* **1995**, *54*, 497–503. [CrossRef] [PubMed]

93. Hanly, A.; Petito, C.K. Hla-dr-positive dendritic cells of the normal human choroid plexus: A potential reservoir of HIV in the central nervous system. *Hum. Pathol.* **1998**, *29*, 88–93. [CrossRef]

94. Petito, C.K.; Chen, H.; Mastri, A.R.; Torres-Munoz, J.; Roberts, B.; Wood, C. Hiv infection of choroid plexus in aids and asymptomatic HIV-infected patients suggests that the choroid plexus may be a reservoir of productive infection. *J. Neurovirol.* **1999**, *5*, 670–677. [CrossRef] [PubMed]

95. Ritola, K.; Robertson, K.; Fiscus, S.A.; Hall, C.; Swanstrom, R. Increased human immunodeficiency virus type 1 (HIV-1) env compartmentalization in the presence of hiv-1-associated dementia. *J. Virol.* **2005**, *79*, 10830–10834. [CrossRef] [PubMed]

96. Schnell, G.; Spudich, S.; Harrington, P.; Price, R.W.; Swanstrom, R. Compartmentalized human immunodeficiency virus type 1 originates from long-lived cells in some subjects with HIV-1-associated dementia. *PLoS Pathog.* **2009**, *5*. [CrossRef] [PubMed]

97. Sturdevant, C.B.; Joseph, S.B.; Schnell, G.; Price, R.W.; Swanstrom, R.; Spudich, S. Compartmentalized replication of r5 t cell-tropic HIV-1 in the central nervous system early in the course of infection. *PLoS Pathog.* **2015**, *11*. [CrossRef] [PubMed]

98. Burkala, E.J.; He, J.; West, J.T.; Wood, C.; Petito, C.K. Compartmentalization of HIV-1 in the central nervous system: Role of the choroid plexus. *AIDS* **2005**, *19*, 675–684. [CrossRef] [PubMed]

99. Strain, M.C.; Letendre, S.; Pillai, S.K.; Russell, T.; Ignacio, C.C.; Gunthard, H.F.; Good, B.; Smith, D.M.; Wolinsky, S.M.; Furtado, M.; et al. Genetic composition of human immunodeficiency virus type 1 in cerebrospinal fluid and blood without treatment and during failing antiretroviral therapy. *J. Virol.* **2005**, *79*, 1772–1788. [CrossRef] [PubMed]

100. Chen, H.; Wood, C.; Petito, C.K. Comparisons of HIV-1 viral sequences in brain, choroid plexus and spleen: Potential role of choroid plexus in the pathogenesis of hiv encephalitis. *J. Neurovirol.* **2000**, *6*, 498–506. [CrossRef] [PubMed]

101. Ellis, R.J.; Gamst, A.C.; Capparelli, E.; Spector, S.A.; Hsia, K.; Wolfson, T.; Abramson, I.; Grant, I.; McCutchan, J.A. Cerebrospinal fluid hiv rna originates from both local cns and systemic sources. *Neurology* **2000**, *54*, 927–936. [CrossRef] [PubMed]

102. Shechter, R.; Miller, O.; Yovel, G.; Rosenzweig, N.; London, A.; Ruckh, J.; Kim, K.W.; Klein, E.; Kalchenko, V.; Bendel, P.; et al. Recruitment of beneficial m2 macrophages to injured spinal cord is orchestrated by remote brain choroid plexus. *Immunity* **2013**, *38*, 555–569. [CrossRef] [PubMed]

103. Phillips, T.; Prospero-Garcia, O.; Puaoi, D.; Lerner, D.; Fox, H.; Olmsted, R.; Bloom, F.; Heriksen, S.; Elder, J. Neurological abnormalities associated with feline immunodeficiency virus infection. *J. Gen. Virol.* **1994**, *75*, 979–987. [CrossRef] [PubMed]

104. Phillips, T.R.; Prospero-Garcia, O.; Wheeler, D.W.; Wagaman, P.C.; Lerner, D.L.; Fox, H.S.; Whalen, L.R.; Bloom, F.E.; Elder, J.H.; Henriksen, S.J. Neurologic dysfunctions caused by a molecular clone of feline immunodeficiency virus, FIV-ppr. *J. Neurovirol.* **1996**, *2*, 388–396. [CrossRef] [PubMed]

105. Podell, M.; Hayes, K.; Oglesbee, M.; Mathes, L. Progressive encephalopathy associated with cd4/cd8 inversion in adult FIV-infected cats. *J. Acquir. Immune Defic. Syndr. Hum. Retrovirol.* **1997**, *15*, 332–340. [CrossRef] [PubMed]

106. Podell, M.; Maruyama, K.; Smith, M.; Hayes, K.A.; Buck, W.R.; Ruehlmann, D.S.; Mathes, L.E. Frontal lobe neuronal injury correlates to altered function in FIV-infected cats. *J. Acquir. Immune Defic. Syndr.* **1999**, *22*, 10–18. [CrossRef] [PubMed]

107. Podell, M.; Oglesbee, M.; Mathes, L.; Krakowka, S.; Olmstead, R.; Lafrado, L. Aids-associated encephalopathy with experimental feline immunodeficiency virus infection. *J. Acquir. Immune Defic. Syndr.* **1993**, *6*, 758–771. [PubMed]

108. Henriksen, S.J.; Prospero-Garcia, O.; Phillips, T.R.; Fox, H.S.; Bloom, F.E.; Elder, J.H. Feline immunodeficiency virus as a model for study of lentivirus infection of the central nervous system. *Curr. Top. Microbiol. Immunol.* **1995**, *202*, 167–186. [PubMed]

109. Buck, W.R.; Podell, M. Neuronal loss in fiv-md infected cats. *J. NeuroAIDS.* **1998**, *2*, 69–77. [CrossRef] [PubMed]

110. Phipps, A.J.; Hayes, K.A.; Buck, W.R.; Podell, M.; Mathes, L.E. Neurophysiologic and immunologic abnormalities associated with feline immunodeficiency virus molecular clone FIV-ppr DNA inoculation. *J. Acquir. Immune Defic. Syndr.* **2000**, *23*, 8–16. [CrossRef] [PubMed]

111. Bragg, D.C.; Hudson, L.C.; Liang, Y.H.; Tompkins, M.B.; Fernandes, A.; Meeker, R.B. Choroid plexus macrophages proliferate and release toxic factors in response to feline immunodeficiency virus. *J. NeuroVirol.* **2002**, *8*, 225–239. [CrossRef] [PubMed]

112. Abramo, F.; Bo, S.; Canese, M.G.; Poli, A. Regional distribution of lesions in the central nervous system of cats infected with feline immunodeficiency virus. *AIDS Res. Hum. Retrovir.* **1995**, *11*, 1247–1253. [CrossRef] [PubMed]

113. Boche, D.; Hurtrel, M.; Gray, F.; Claessens-Maire, M.A.; Ganiere, J.P.; Montagnier, L.; Hurtrel, B. Virus load and neuropathology in the FIV model. *J. NeuroVirol.* **1996**, *2*, 377–387. [CrossRef] [PubMed]

114. Hurtrel, M.; Ganiere, J.; Guelifi, J.; Chakrabarti, L.; Maire, M.; Gray, F.; Montagnier, L.; Hurtrel, B. Comparison of early and late feline immunodeficiency virus encephalopathies. *AIDS* **1992**, *6*, 399–406. [CrossRef] [PubMed]

115. Poli, A.; Abramo, F.; Di Iorio, C.; Cantile, C.; Carli, M.A.; Pollera, C.; Vago, L.; Tosoni, A.; Costanzi, G. Neuropathology in cats experimentally infected with feline immunodeficiency virus: A morphological, immunocytochemical and morphometric study. *J. Neurovirol.* **1997**, *3*, 361–368. [CrossRef] [PubMed]

116. Silvotti, L.; Corradi, A.; Brandi, G.; Cabassi, A.; Bendinelli, M.; Magnan, M.; Piedimonte, G. FIV induced encephalopathy: Early brain lesions in the absence of viral replication in monocyte/macrophages. A pathogenetic model. *Vet. Immunol. Immunopathol.* **1997**, *55*, 263–271. [CrossRef]

117. Jacobson, S.; Henriksen, S.J.; Prospero-Garcia, O.; Phillips, T.R.; Elder, J.H.; Young, W.G.; Bloom, F.E.; Fox, H.S. Cortical neuronal cytoskeletal changes associated with FIV infection. *J. Neurovirol.* **1997**, *3*, 283–289. [CrossRef] [PubMed]

118. Koirala, T.R.; Nakagaki, K.; Ishida, T.; Nonaka, S.; Morikawa, S.; Tabira, T. Decreased expression of map-2 and gad in the brain of cats infected with feline immunodeficiency virus. *Tohoku J. Exp. Med.* **2001**, *195*, 141–151. [CrossRef] [PubMed]

119. Meeker, R.B.; Thiede, B.A.; Hall, C.; English, R.; Tompkins, M. Cortical cell loss in asymptomatic cats experimentally infected with feline immunodeficiency virus. *AIDS Res. Hum. Retrovir.* **1997**, *13*, 1131–1140. [CrossRef] [PubMed]

120. Mitchell, T.W.; Buckmaster, P.S.; Hoover, E.A.; Whalen, L.R.; Dudek, F.E. Neuron loss and axon reorganization in the dentate gyrus of cats infected with the feline immunodeficiency virus. *J. Comp. Neurol.* **1999**, *411*, 563–577. [CrossRef]

121. Head, E.; Moffat, K.; Das, P.; Sarsoza, F.; Poon, W.W.; Landsberg, G.; Cotman, C.W.; Murphy, M.P. Beta-amyloid deposition and tau phosphorylation in clinically characterized aged cats. *Neurobiol. Aging* **2005**, *26*, 749–763. [CrossRef] [PubMed]

122. Gunn-Moore, D.A.; McVee, J.; Bradshaw, J.M.; Pearson, G.R.; Head, E.; Gunn-Moore, F.J. Ageing changes in cat brains demonstrated by beta-amyloid and at8-immunoreactive phosphorylated tau deposits. *J. Feline Med. Surg.* **2006**, *8*, 234–242. [CrossRef] [PubMed]

123. Chambers, J.K.; Tokuda, T.; Uchida, K.; Ishii, R.; Tatebe, H.; Takahashi, E.; Tomiyama, T.; Une, Y.; Nakayama, H. The domestic cat as a natural animal model of alzheimer's disease. *Acta Neuropathol. Commun.* **2015**, *3*, 78. [CrossRef] [PubMed]

124. Asproni, P.; Abramo, F.; Millanta, F.; Lorenzi, D.; Poli, A. Amyloidosis in association with spontaneous feline immunodeficiency virus infection. *J. Feline Med. Surg.* **2013**, *15*, 300–306. [CrossRef] [PubMed]

125. Landsberg, G.M.; Denenberg, S.; Araujo, J.A. Cognitive dysfunction in cats: A syndrome we used to dismiss as "old age". *J. Feline Med. Surg.* **2010**, *12*, 837–848. [CrossRef] [PubMed]

126. Gunn-Moore, D.A. Cognitive dysfunction in cats: Clinical assessment and management. *Top. Companion Anim. Med.* **2011**, *26*, 17–24. [CrossRef] [PubMed]

127. Bragg, D.C.; Boles, J.C.; Meeker, R.B. Destabilization of neuronal calcium homeostasis by factors secreted from choroid plexus macrophage cultures in response to feline immunodeficiency virus. *Neurobiol. Dis.* **2002**, *9*, 173–186. [CrossRef] [PubMed]

128. Bragg, D.C.; Meeker, R.B.; Duff, B.A.; English, R.V.; Tompkins, M.B. Neurotoxicity of FIV and fiv envelope protein in feline cortical cultures. *Brain Res.* **1999**, *816*, 431–437. [CrossRef]

129. Meeker, R.; English, R.; Tompkins, M. Enhanced excitotoxicity in primary feline neural cultures exposed to feline immunodeficiency virus (FIV). *J. Neuro-AIDS* **1997**, *1*, 1–27. [CrossRef]

130. Meeker, R.B.; Poulton, W.; Feng, W.H.; Hudson, L.; Longo, F.M. Suppression of immunodeficiency virus-associated neural damage by the p75 neurotrophin receptor ligand, lm11a-31, in an in vitro feline model. *J. Neuroimmune Pharmacol.* **2012**, *7*, 388–400. [CrossRef] [PubMed]

131. Meeker, R.B.; Azuma, Y.; Bragg, D.C.; English, R.V.; Tompkins, M. Microglial proliferation in cortical neural cultures exposed to feline immunodeficiency virus. *J. Neuroimmunol.* **1999**, *101*, 15–26. [CrossRef]

132. Al Ghoul, W.M.; Meeker, R.B.; Greenwood, R.S. Kindling induces a long-lasting increase in brain nitric oxide synthase activity. *NeuroRep.* **1995**, *6*, 457–460. [CrossRef]

133. Hudson, L.C.; Tompkins, M.B.; Meeker, R.B. Endothelial cell suppression of peripheral blood mononuclear cell trafficking in vitro during acute exposure to feline immunodeficiency virus. *Cell Tissue Res.* **2008**, *334*, 55–65. [CrossRef] [PubMed]

134. Jones, G.; Power, C. Regulation of neural cell survival by HIV-1 infection. *Neurobiol. Dis.* **2006**, *21*, 1–17. [CrossRef] [PubMed]

135. Avdoshina, V.; Bachis, A.; Mocchetti, I. Synaptic dysfunction in human immunodeficiency virus type-1-positive subjects: Inflammation or impaired neuronal plasticity? *J. Intern. Med.* **2013**, *273*, 454–465. [CrossRef] [PubMed]

136. Gannon, P.; Khan, M.Z.; Kolson, D.L. Current understanding of hiv-associated neurocognitive disorders pathogenesis. *Curr. Opin. Neurol.* **2011**, *24*, 275–283. [CrossRef] [PubMed]

137. Kolson, D.L. Neuropathogenesis of central nervous system HIV-1 infection. *Clin. Lab. Med.* **2002**, *22*, 703–717. [CrossRef]

138. Perry, S.W.; Norman, J.P.; Gelbard, H.A. Adjunctive therapies for HIV-1 associated neurologic disease. *Neurotox. Res.* **2005**, *8*, 161–166. [CrossRef] [PubMed]

139. Turchan, J.; Sacktor, N.; Wojna, V.; Conant, K.; Nath, A. Neuroprotective therapy for hiv dementia. *Curr. HIV Res.* **2003**, *1*, 373–383. [CrossRef] [PubMed]

140. Meeker, R.B.; Boles, J.C.; Robertson, K.R.; Hall, C.D. Cerebrospinal fluid from human immunodeficiency virus—Infected individuals facilitates neurotoxicity by suppressing intracellular calcium recovery. *J. NeuroVirol.* **2005**, *11*, 144–156. [CrossRef] [PubMed]

141. Epstein, L.G.; Gelbard, H.A. HIV-1-induced neuronal injury in the developing brain. *J. Leukoc. Biol.* **1999**, *65*, 453–457. [PubMed]

142. Gemignani, A.; Paudice, P.; Pittaluga, A.; Raiteri, M. The HIV-1 coat protein gp120 and some of its fragments potently activate native cerebral nmda receptors mediating neuropeptide release. *Eur. J. Neurosci.* **2000**, *12*, 2839–2846. [CrossRef] [PubMed]

143. Haughey, N.J.; Nath, A.; Mattson, M.P.; Slevin, J.T.; Geiger, J.D. HIV-1 tat through phosphorylation of nmda receptors potentiates glutamate excitotoxicity. *J. Neurochem.* **2001**, *78*, 457–467. [CrossRef] [PubMed]

144. Lipton, S.; Sucher, N.; Kaiser, P.; Dreyer, E. Synergistic effects of hiv coat protein and nmda receptor-mediated neurotoxicity. *Neuron* **1991**, *7*, 111–118. [CrossRef]

145. Lipton, S. Models of neuronal injury in aids: Another role for the nmda receptor? *TINS* **1992**, *15*, 75–80. [CrossRef]

146. Self, R.L.; Mulholland, P.J.; Nath, A.; Harris, B.R.; Prendergast, M.A. The human immunodeficiency virus type-1 transcription factor tat produces elevations in intracellular Ca2+ that require function of an n-methyl-d-aspartate receptor polyamine-sensitive site. *Brain Res.* **2004**, *995*, 39–45. [CrossRef] [PubMed]

147. Fine, S.M.; Angel, R.A.; Perry, S.W.; Epstein, L.G.; Rothstein, J.D.; Dewhurst, S.; Gelbard, H.A. Tumor necrosis factor alpha inhibits glutamate uptake by primary human astrocytes. Implications for pathogenesis of HIV-1 dementia. *J. Biol. Chem.* **1996**, *271*, 15303–15306. [PubMed]

5

Prevalence and Multilocus Genotyping Analysis of *Cryptosporidium* and *Giardia* Isolates from Dogs in Chiang Mai, Thailand

Sahatchai Tangtrongsup [1,2,*], A. Valeria Scorza [3], John S. Reif [4], Lora R. Ballweber [5], Michael R. Lappin [3] and Mo D. Salman [2]

[1] Department of Companion Animal and Wildlife Clinic, Faculty of Veterinary Medicine, Chiang Mai University, Chiang Mai 50100, Thailand

[2] Animal Population Health Institute, Department of Clinical Sciences, College of Veterinary Medicine and Biomedical Sciences, Colorado State University, Fort Collins, CO 80523, USA; mo.salman@colostate.edu

[3] Center for Companion Animal Studies, Department of Clinical Sciences College of Veterinary Medicine and Biomedical Sciences, Colorado State University, Fort Collins, CO 80523, USA; andrea.scorza@colostate.edu (A.V.S.); michael.lappin@colostate.edu (M.R.L.)

[4] Department of Environmental and Radiological Health Sciences, College of Veterinary Medicine and Biomedical Sciences, Colorado State University, Fort Collins, CO 80523, USA; john.reif@colostate.edu

[5] Department of Microbiology, Immunology and Pathology, College of Veterinary Medicine and Biomedical Sciences, Colorado State University, Fort Collins, CO 80523, USA; lora.ballweber@colostate.edu

* Correspondence: sahatchai.t@cmu.ac.th

Academic Editor: Katharina D. C. Stärk

Abstract: The occurrence and zoonotic potential of *Cryptosporidium* spp. and *Giardia duodenalis* isolated from dogs in Chiang Mai, Thailand were determined. Fecal samples were collected from 109 dogs between July and August 2008. *Cryptosporidium* spp. infection was determined by immunofluorescent assay (IFA), PCR assays that amplify *Cryptosporidium* heat-shock protein 70 kDa (hsp70), and two PCR assays that amplify a small subunit-ribosomal RNA (SSU-rRNA). *Giardia duodenalis* infection was identified using zinc sulfate centrifugal flotation, IFA, and four PCR assays that amplify the *Giardia* glutamate dehydrogenase (gdh), beta-giardin (bg), and generic and dog-specific assays of triosephosphate isomerase (tpi) genes. Overall prevalence of *Cryptosporidium* spp. and *G. duodenalis* was 31.2% and 45.9%, respectively. Sequence analysis of 22 *Cryptosporidium*-positive samples and 21 *Giardia*-positive samples revealed the presence of *C. canis* in 15, and *C. parvum* in 7, *G. duodenalis* Assemblage C in 8, D in 11, and mixed of C and D in 2 dogs. Dogs in Chiang Mai were commonly exposed to *Cryptosporidium* spp. and *G. duodenalis*. *Cryptosporidium parvum* can be isolated from the feces of dogs, and all *G. duodenalis* assemblages were dog-specific. Dogs could be a reservoir for a zoonotic *Cryptosporidium* infection in humans, but further studies will be required to determine the clinical and zoonotic importance.

Keywords: *Cryptosporidium*; *Giardia*; dogs; Chiang Mai; Thailand

1. Introduction

Cryptosporidium spp. and *Giardia duodenalis* are common intestinal protists that can infect humans and animals worldwide [1]. The clinical signs of cryptosporidiosis and giardiasis in dogs vary from sub-clinical to severe diarrhea [2,3].

At least 27 species of *Cryptosporidium* spp. and eight assemblages (A–H) of *G. duodenalis* have been described [4,5]. Although dogs are commonly infected with species-specific *C. canis* and *G. duodenalis* (Assemblages C and D), the occurrence of zoonotic *C. parvum* and *G. duodenalis* (Assemblages A and B) in dogs have raised concern that these animals may serve as a potential reservoir for human transmission [6].

In Thailand, studies regarding cryptosporidiosis and giardiasis in dogs and their zoonotic potential are limited. In one study, *C. canis* was identified in 2 of 95 temple dogs in central Thailand using PCR that amplify an 830-bp fragment of small subunit-ribosomal RNA (SSU-rRNA) gene [7]. The prevalence of *G. duodenalis* infection in temple dogs in the Bangkok area varied from 7.9–56.8% depending on the test used [8,9]. The majority of *G. duodenalis* isolates recovered in these samples were Assemblages A and D. It has been noted that similar genotypes (Assemblage A) were recovered from dogs and humans in the same monastery. In another study in a shelter in Nakornnayok province, the prevalence of *Giardia* infection in shelter dogs using a formalin-ether concentrating technique was 2.8% [10]. To our knowledge, there has been no previous research concerning *Cryptosporidium* spp. and *G. duodenalis* infections and their zoonotic potential in dogs in this area. Since these protist infections are a potential public health concern, determining the prevalence and genotypes of these organisms in dogs living in close proximity to humans and other animals is a priority. Therefore, the aims of this study were to estimate the prevalence of *Cryptosporidium* spp. and *G. duodenalis* infections in dogs in Chiang Mai, Thailand, and to characterize the organism isolates using molecular techniques in order to determine the potential for zoonotic transmission.

2. Materials and Methods

2.1. Study Location

Chiang Mai is the second largest province of Thailand. It is located in the northern part of the country at geographic coordinates 18°47′ N and 98°59′ E. The city of Chiang Mai maintains its deep roots of traditional community culture in a hybrid landscape of rural and urban city development, and includes agricultural, industrial, and tourism areas. Chiang Mai also represents a tropical environment, which exists in many parts of the world.

2.2. Sample Collection

Between July and August 2008, 109 canine fecal samples were obtained from animals visiting the Small Animal Hospital of the Faculty of Veterinary Medicine, Chiang Mai University ($n = 36$), private clinics ($n = 9$), a shelter ($n = 15$), or breeders ($n = 49$) in Chiang Mai province, Thailand. The samples were collected on a volunteer basis regardless of the health status of the animals. Demographic information (age, sex, and housing types) was recorded. Fecal consistency was determined using the Nestle Purina Fecal Scoring System for Dogs and Cats (Nestle-Purina Pet Food Co, St. Louis, MO, USA). Fecal scores of 1–3 were considered as normal, with 4–7 classified as diarrheic.

2.3. Determination of Cryptosporidium and Giardia Infections

Cryptosporidium spp. infection was determined using immunofluorescent assay (IFA) and PCR techniques. *Giardia duodenalis* infection was determined using zinc sulfate centrifugal flotation, immunofluorescent assay, and PCR techniques.

2.3.1. Zinc Sulfate Centrifugal Flotation and Microscopy

Fecal consistency was determined upon the receipt of the sample, and all fecal samples were stored in closed plastic containers at 4 °C. Microscopic examination of feces after the performance of a conventional zinc sulfate centrifugal flotation was used to determine intestinal parasitic infection within 5 days of collection, and the remaining fecal samples were stored at −20 °C until being shipped to Colorado State University for IFA and molecular analysis. All fecal samples were shipped to the USA on dry ice and stored at −20 °C until processed.

2.3.2. Fecal Concentration and Immunofluorescent Assay

Prior to IFA and DNA extraction, all fecal samples were concentrated using sucrose gradient centrifugation technique as previously described [11,12]. The IFA slides were processed according to the manufacturer's instructions (Merifluor® *Cryptosporidium*/*Giardia* IFA kit, Meridian Diagnostic Corporation, Cincinnati, OH, USA). The remaining concentrated fecal material was stored at $-20\,°C$ until DNA extraction was performed.

2.3.3. Molecular Detection of *Cryptosporidium* spp. and *Giardia duodenalis* Infection

Three hundred microliters of each fecal concentrate were subjected to DNA extraction following an established protocol [13]. Three PCR assays for *Cryptosporidium* identification were performed. PCR assays amplify a 325-bp fragment of the heat-shock protein (hsp70), a ~290-bp fragment (one-step PCR), and an ~830-bp fragment (nested PCR) of the small subunit-ribosomal RNA (SSU-rRNA) genes were utilized to detect the presence of *Cryptosporidium* spp. [14–16]. For *Giardia* molecular identification, four nested PCR assays targeting a 432-bp fragment of glutamate dehydrogenase (gdh), a 510-bp fragment of beta-giardin (bg), and a 511-bp fragment of triose phosphate isomerase genes using generic primers (tpigen) and dog-specific primers (tpiD) were performed as previously described [17–20]. All PCR assays had several modifications from original publication. PCR mix consisted of $1\times$ HotStarTaq Master Mix (Qiagen, Valencia, CA, USA), 10 pmol of each primer, and 1 µL of template DNA in a final volume of 25 µL for each targeting gene. PCR positive and negative controls were included in every PCR reaction. The *Giardia* positive control was obtained from a dog sample that tested positive for *G. duodenalis* by all four *Giardia* PCR assays, and was subsequently sequenced. The *Cryptosporidium* positive control was obtained from a *C. parvum*-positive cow. The negative control contained the PCR reagents but no DNA. In addition, in nested PCR assays, the negative controls from primary PCRs were included in the secondary PCR assays to evaluate the possibility of contamination.

2.4. DNA Sequencing and Genotyping Analysis

The PCR products were evaluated by nucleotide sequencing using a commercially available service (Proteomics and Metabolomics Facility, Colorado State University). The obtained sequences were compared with nucleotide sequences from the nucleotide database from the GenBank by BLAST analysis (http://blast.ncbi.nlm.nih.gov/Blast.cgi).

2.5. Data Analysis

A sample was considered positive for *Cryptosporidium* if the sample was positive by either IFA or any of the *Cryptosporidium* PCR assays, and considered positive for *Giardia* if the sample was positive by either zinc sulfate fecal flotation, IFA, or any of the *Giardia* PCRs. Overall prevalence and 95% confidence intervals (CI) were calculated [21]. Associations between *G. duodenalis* or *Cryptosporidium* spp. infections and age (less than one year or one year or more), sex, diarrhea status (yes or no), and housing type (household or breeding kennel/shelter) were assessed using Fisher's exact test [21]. Odds ratios and 95% CI were estimated using univariate logistic regression analysis to measure the strength of association of each independent variable including age, sex, diarrhea status, housing type, and the presence of co-infection (having both *Cryptosporidium* and *Giardia*). A multivariate logistic regression model against either *Cryptosporidium* spp. or *G. duodenalis* infection in dogs was constructed using a backward stepwise elimination procedure [22]. Variables found to be associated with *Cryptosporidium* spp. or *G. duodenalis* infection in the univariate logistic regression ($p < 0.25$) were included in the multivariable logistic regression analysis. Variables were retained in the model based on the likelihood ratio χ^2 statistic, at $p \leq 0.05$. All statistical analyses were performed using the Stata statistical software release 10.1 (Stata Corp., College Station, TX, USA).

3. Results

3.1. Detection of Cryptosporidium spp. and Giardia duodenalis Isolates

A single fecal sample was collected from 109 dogs. The characteristics of the samples are shown in Table 1. Fourteen samples (12.8%) were positive for *Cryptosporidium* by IFA; 21 samples (19.3%) were positive by any of the *Cryptosporidium* PCR assays. Thirty-three samples (30.3%) were positive for *Giardia* by fecal centrifugal flotation test; 14 samples (12.8%) were positive by IFA; 21 samples (19.3%) were positive by any of the *Giardia* PCR assays. The overall prevalence of *Cryptosporidium* spp. and *G. duodenalis* infections were 31.2% (95% CI: 22.4–40.0) and 45.9% (95% CI: 36.4–55.4), respectively (Table 2). In addition, in dogs, single infections with *Cryptosporidium* spp. or *G. duodenalis* were 14.7% (16/109) and 29.4% (32/109), respectively. Co-infection of *G. duodenalis* and *Cryptosporidium* spp. was shown in 16.5% (18/109) of the samples.

Table 1. Characteristics of samples included in the current study (*n* = 109).

Variable	No. of Samples in This Study (%)
Age	
<1 year	23 (21.1)
≥1 year	83 (76.1)
Unknown	3 (2.8)
Sex	
Male	34 (31.2)
Female	66 (60.6)
Unknown	9 (8.3)
Diarrhea status	
Yes	17 (15.6)
No	89 (81.7)
Unknown	3 (2.8)
Housing type	
Breeder and Shelter	64 (58.7)
Household	45 (41.3)

Table 2. Prevalence of *Giardia* and *Cryptosporidium* infections by age, sex, diarrhea status, and housing type. Number in parentheses represents the number of samples in each category.

Variable	*Cryptosporidium* spp. % (95% CI *)	*p* Value	*G. duodenalis* % (95% CI *)	*p* Value
Dog (109)	31.2 (22.4–40.0)		45.9 (36.4–55.4)	
Age		0.003		0.003
<1 year (23)	56.5 (34.6–78.4)		73.9 (54.5–93.3)	
≥1 year (83)	24.1 (14.7–33.5)		38.5 (29.9–49.2)	
Sex		0.140		0.666
Male (34)	20.6 (6.3–34.9)		50.0 (32.3–67.7)	
Female (66)	34.8 (23.0–46.0)		45.5 (33.1–57.8)	
Diarrhea status		0.575		0.065
Yes (17)	23.5 (1.0–46.0)		64.7 (39.4–90.0)	
No (89)	32.6 (22.7–42.5)		40.4 (30.1–50.8)	
Housing type		0.392		0.070
Breeder and Shelter (64)	34.4 (22.4–46.3)		53.1 (40.6–65.7)	
Household (45)	26.7 (13.2–40.1)		35.6 (21.0–50.1)	

* 95% CI = 95% confidence interval.

3.2. Genotyping of Cryptosporidium spp. and Giardia duodenalis Isolates

Eleven sequences from *Cryptosporidium* hsp70, eleven sequences from *Cryptosporidium* one step SSU-rRNA, and eight sequences from *Cryptosporidium* nested SSU-rRNA PCR positive samples were available for genotyping analysis. Using BLAST analyses, 15 dog isolates were typed as *C. canis* and seven were typed as *C. parvum* (Table 3).

Table 3. *Cryptosporidium* genotypes determined by nucleotide sequence analyses of heat shock protein 70 (hsp70), one-step small subunit-rRNA (SSU-rRNA), and nested SSU-rRNA PCR products from dog samples in Chiang Mai, Thailand.

Sample	hsp70	One-Step SSU-rRNA	Nested SSU-rRNA
TH08Dog5	n/a	*C. canis*	n/a
TH08Dog7	n/a	*C. canis*	*C. canis*
TH08Dog22	n/a	*C. parvum*	n/a
TH08Dog28	n/a	*C. canis*	*C. canis*
TH08Dog 42	n/a	*C. canis*	*C. canis*
TH08Dog43	*C. parvum*	n/a	n/a
TH08Dog46	*C. canis*	*C. canis*	*C. canis*
TH08Dog54	*C. parvum*	n/a	n/a
TH08Dog55	*C. canis*	*C. canis*	*C. canis*
TH08Dog58	*C. canis*	n/a	n/a
TH08Dog61	n/a	n/a	*C. canis*
TH08Dog68	n/a	n/a	*C. canis*
TH08Dog69	n/a	*C. canis*	n/a
TH08Dog71	n/a	*C. canis*	n/a
TH08Dog76	*C. parvum.*	n/a	n/a
TH08Dog86	*C. parvum.*	n/a	n/a
TH08Dog87	*C. parvum.*	n/a	n/a
TH08Dog92	*C. canis*	n/a	n/a
TH08Dog96	*C. canis*	n/a	n/a
TH08Dog101	*C. parvum.*	n/a	n/a
TH08Dog102	n/a	*C. canis*	n/a
TH08Dog107	n/a	*C. canis*	*C. canis*

n/a = not available.

Twenty-one sequences from gdh, 18 sequences from bg, 8 from generic tpi, and 15 dog-specific tpi PCR positive samples were available for analysis. Eight dog isolates were typed as *G. duodenalis* Assemblage C, 12 were typed as D, and one C or D depending on target genes (Table 4).

Table 4. *Giardia* genotypes determined by nucleotide sequence analyses of glutamate dehydrogenase (gdh), β-giardin (bg), and triose phosphate isomerase (tpi) PCR products from dog samples in Chiang Mai, Thailand.

ID	gdh	bg	tpigen [a]	tpid [b]
TH08Dog5	D	D	n/a	D
TH08Dog15	D	D	n/a	n/a
TH08Dog17	D	D	C	D
TH08Dog19	C	C	C	C
TH08Dog22	C	C	C	C
TH08Dog23	D	D	n/a	D
TH08Dog24	D[ash]	D	n/a	D
TH08Dog30	C	C	C	C
TH08Dog33	D	D	n/a	D
TH08Dog36	D[ash]	D	n/a	D
TH08Dog40	D	n/a	n/a	n/a
TH08Dog43	D	D	n/a	D
TH08Dog45	D[ash]	D	n/a	D
TH08Dog73	C	C	C	C
TH08Dog93	D	n/a	n/a	n/a
TH08Dog96	D	n/a	n/a	n/a
TH08Dog100	C	C	n/a	n/a
TH08Dog101	C	C	C	C
TH08Dog103	C	C	n/a	n/a
TH08Dog107	D[ash]	C[ash]	C[ash]	D
TH08Dog108	C[ash]	C	C	C[ash]

[a] tpi with generic primers; [b] tpi with dog specific primers; n/a = not available; ash = allelic sequence heterogeneity.

3.3. Statistical Analysis

Using χ^2 or Fisher's exact tests, age was significantly associated with the prevalence of both *Cryptosporidium* spp. and *G. duodenalis* (Table 2). Other variables were not associated with infection.

Univariate and Multivariate Logistic Regression Analyses for Risk Associated with *Cryptosporidium* spp. and *Giardia duodenalis* Infection

Univariate logistic regression analyses for categorical variables showed dogs aged less than one year were more likely to be infected with *Cryptosporidium* spp. (OR = 4.10, 95% CI: 1.56–10.76) or *G. duodenalis* (OR = 4.52, 95% CI: 1.61–12.65) than dogs age one year or older (Table 5).

Table 5. Univariate logistic regression analysis of variables associated with *Cryptosporidium* and *Giardia* infections in dogs in Chiang Mai, Thailand.

Variable	Odds Ratio (OR)	95% CI *	*p* Value
Cryptosporidium spp.			
Age < 1 year (*n* = 106)	4.10	1.56–10.76	0.004
Sex (male) (*n* = 100)	0.48	0.18–1.28	0.145
Diarrhea (*n* = 106)	0.64	0.19–2.12	0.463
Breeder and Shelter (*n* = 109)	1.44	0.62–3.33	0.393
Presence of *Giardia* infection	1.51	0.67–3.41	0.320
Giardia duodenalis			
Age < 1 year (*n* = 106)	4.52	1.61–12.65	0.004
Sex (male) (*n* = 100)	1.20	0.52–2.75	0.666
Diarrhea (*n* = 106)	2.70	0.92–7.96	0.072
Breeder and Shelter (*n* = 109)	2.05	0.94–4.50	0.072
Presence of *Cryptosporidium* infection	1.51	0.67–3.41	0.320

* 95% CI = 95% confidence interval.

The variables remaining in the model following multivariate logistic regression for *G. duodenalis* infection were age less than one year (OR = 4.11, 95% CI: 1.33–12.70), having diarrhea (OR = 4.59, 95% CI: 1.14–18.49), and residing in breeding kennels or a shelter (OR = 3.723, 95% CI: 1.35–10.26) (Table 6).

Table 6. Multivariate logistic regression analysis of variables associated with *Giardia duodenalis* infection in dogs in Chiang Mai, Thailand (*n* = 97).

Variable	Odds Ratios	95% CI *	*p* Value
Age < 1 year	4.11	1.33–12.70	0.004
Diarrhea	4.59	1.14–18.49	0.032
Breeder/Shelter	3.72	1.35–10.26	0.011

* 95% CI = 95% confidence interval.

4. Discussion

The current study represents the first report of the *Cryptosporidium* spp. and *G. duodenalis* prevalence rates and genotypes/species in dogs in Chiang Mai, Thailand. The global prevalence of *Cryptosporidium* spp. and *G. duodenalis* infection in dogs varies depending on the test used, geographic location, and population tested [4,23]. In the present study, overall *Cryptosporidium* spp. and *G. duodenalis* prevalence was 31.2% and 45.9%, respectively. These high prevalences were derived by considering detection in parallel from four tests for *Cryptosporidium* spp. and six tests for *G. duodenalis*.

The prevalence of *Cryptosporidium* spp. is comparable to a previous report of sled dogs from Poland [24], and the prevalence of *Giardia* found in this study is comparable to a previous report of 56.8% in Bangkok [9] and similarly high rates in other countries such as Japan [25], Mexico [26], Brazil [27], Italy [28], and Belgium [29], where most of the studies were from breeding kennels, shelters or abandoned dogs. Nevertheless, the prevalence of these two organisms in this study may have been overestimated due to selection bias. The samples available for this study were not randomly selected, but depended on voluntary participation of the owner visiting the small animal hospital and caregivers of breeders and a shelter. Therefore, the sample may have been biased towards infected and diarrheic animals, resulting in an overestimation of the apparent prevalence.

Zoonotic species or genotypes of *Cryptosporidium* spp. and *G. duodenalis* cannot be distinguished from host-adapted organisms using morphological differentiation. Therefore, molecular characterization using PCR assay and sequence analysis is suggested due to its rapidity and specificity to differentiate the species or genotypes of these organisms. However, not all PCR assays have the same sensitivity for detecting *Cryptosporidium* or *Giardia* nucleotides in fecal samples. In the current study, hsp70 and SSU-rRNA are not in agreement. Of 22 *Cryptosporidium* PCR positive samples, nine were identified from hsp70 only, five from one-step SSU-rRNA only, and two from nested SSU-rRNA only, four from both one-step and nested SSU-rRNA, and two from all three PCRs. It is unclear whether hsp70 or SSU-rRNA have an advantage over each other due to the limitation on the PCR of biological or fecal samples. Of three targeting genes for *Giardia* detection, *Giardia* gdh PCR had the highest amplification rate compared to bg and tpi genes (Table 4). This observation was similar to the study by Scorza and colleagues [12], which showed that the gdh PCR had higher amplification rate than bg or tpi. However, this observation contrasted with the studies by Covacin et al. [30] and Sprong et al. [31], which showed that gdh PCR had the least amplification rate compared to bg, tpi, and SSU-rRNA. In addition, the discrepancies of genotype determination among these three genes have also been reported. Based on this study and our experiences, PCR for the gdh gene may be suggested if the multilocus PCR assay is not affordable.

The majority of genotypes of *G. duodenalis* that infect dogs are host-adapted (Assemblages C or D); however, the pattern can differ geographically [4,12,32]. For example, in the Western United states, zoonotic genotypes of *Giardia* Assemblages A and B were highly prevalent [30], whereas in temple dogs in Bangkok, Thailand, the majority of *Giardia* isolates were identified as Assemblage A [9]. In the current study, all of the *G. duodenalis* isolates were dog-adapted assemblages (C or D). Therefore, the potential of zoonotic *Giardia* transmission from pet dogs in this location is possibly low.

In the current study, from 22 *Cryptosporidium* PCR-positive dogs, 15 specimens were identified as *C. canis* (68%) and 7 specimens (32%) were identified as *C. parvum*. The rate of *C. canis* detection in this study was relevant to previous studies of *Cryptosporidium* isolates from dogs worldwide; 41 *Cryptosporidium* isolates that had been previously reported in dogs, 76% of the isolates were identified as *C. canis*, 22% as *C. parvum*, and 2% as *C. meleagridis* [33,34]. Due to the nature of the cross-sectional study, we are not certain whether the isolated *C. parvum* was a pathogen circulating in the dog population, or transmitted from other animals or humans. The presence of *C. parvum* in the dog samples suggests that dogs could be a potential reservoir for the zoonotic transmission of *Cryptosporidium* spp. While *C. parvum* and *C. hominis* are significant causes of human cryptosporidiosis, the detection of *C. canis* in HIV patients in Thailand [35–37] and elsewhere [38,39], as well as the detection of *C. canis* in children [40] have raised concerns regarding the transmission of protozoal diseases from pets to humans even when they harbor the host-adapted pathogens. Further investigation of these parasites among humans and animals living in the same household or in close proximity are needed to confirm this relationship. However, good sanitary practices are highly recommended for all pet owners to avoid zoonotic transmission to humans.

Cryptosporidium and *Giardia* genotypes/species isolates from dogs in this study may not reflect the majority of genotypes/species for the dog population as a whole in Chiang Mai, Thailand, since we made our interpretation in the light of the available nucleotide sequences. The information regarding the genotype/species for 35% of *Cryptosporidium*-infected samples and 46% of *Giardia*-infected samples was unknown. Failure of PCR assays to amplify the organisms' target genes may be from the presence of a PCR inhibitor [41], or degradation of DNA material in the samples which may result from international shipment or long-term storage before PCR processing. Therefore, the failure to amplify

Cryptosporidium or *Giardia* genes in the fecal samples using PCR did not rule out *Cryptosporidium* or *Giardia* infection. Thus, a PCR should not be used as the primary test for *Cryptosporidium* or *Giardia* clinical diagnosis for practical and cost effective reasons, but it certainly has an important role for confirmation and in research.

Young age, presence of diarrhea, feeding a home-cooked diet, presence of other enteric parasites, being an abandoned or stray dog, and having been kept in a kennel are risk factors that have been reported to be associated with *Cryptosporidium* and *Giardia* in previous studies [42–45]. Similarly, in this study, *G. duodenalis* infection was shown to be associated with young age, the presence of diarrhea, and coming from a breeder or a shelter. However, to help in prevention and control of these pathogens in dogs in Chiang Mai area, the important risk factors mentioned above including history of the pet's acquisition, season, and source of drinking water could be applied to this population.

5. Conclusions

The current information suggests that the *Cryptosporidium* and *Giardia* infections in young dogs in Chiang Mai are common. Dogs may be a reservoir for zoonotic transmission of *Cryptosporidium*; however, dogs may not be a primary reservoir for zoonotic transmission of *G. duodenalis*. Further investigation using molecular analysis of *Cryptosporidium* and *Giardia* species/genotypes isolated from animals and humans (pets and owners or shelter animals with the caregivers) may clarify the transmission cycle of these organisms between humans and animals in the same environmental setting.

Acknowledgments: This study was supported by the CSU Program of Economically Important Infectious Animal Diseases through a special grant from USDA-NIFA, the PVM Student Grant Program in the Center for Companion Animal Studies, and the Research Council of the College of Veterinary Medicine and Biomedical Sciences, Colorado State University.

Author Contributions: Sahatchai Tangtrongsup, Mo D. Salman, Michael R. Lappin, John S. Reif and Lora R. Ballweber conceived and designed the experiments; Sahatchai Tangtrongsup performed the experiments; Sahatchai Tangtrongsup and Mo D. Salman analyzed the data; Sahatchai Tangtrongsup and A. Valeria Scorza performed the molecular analyses; Michael R. Lappin contributed reagents. Sahatchai Tangtrongsup wrote the paper.

References

1. Thompson, R.C.; Smith, A. Zoonotic enteric protozoa. *Vet. Parasitol.* **2011**, *182*, 70–78. [CrossRef] [PubMed]
2. Scorza, V.; Tangtrongsup, S. Update on the diagnosis and management of *Cryptosporidium* spp. infections in dogs and cats. *Top. Companion Anim. Med.* **2010**, *25*, 163–169. [CrossRef] [PubMed]
3. Tangtrongsup, S.; Scorza, V. Update on the diagnosis and management of *Giardia* spp. infections in dogs and cats. *Top. Companion Anim. Med.* **2010**, *25*, 155–162. [CrossRef] [PubMed]
4. Feng, Y.; Xiao, L. Zoonotic potential and molecular epidemiology of *Giardia* species and giardiasis. *Clin. Microbiol. Rev.* **2011**, *24*, 110–140. [CrossRef] [PubMed]
5. Slapeta, J. Cryptosporidiosis and *Cryptosporidium* species in animals and humans: A thirty colour rainbow? *Int. J. Parasitol.* **2013**, *43*, 957–970. [CrossRef] [PubMed]
6. Xiao, L.; Fayer, R. Molecular characterisation of species and genotypes of *Cryptosporidium* and *Giardia* and assessment of zoonotic transmission. *Int. J. Parasitol.* **2008**, *38*, 1239–1255. [CrossRef] [PubMed]
7. Koompapong, K.; Mori, H.; Thammasonthijarern, N.; Prasertbun, R.; Pintong, A.R.; Popruk, S.; Rojekittikhun, W.; Chaisiri, K.; Sukthana, Y.; Mahittikorn, A. Molecular identification of *Cryptosporidium* spp. in seagulls, pigeons, dogs, and cats in Thailand. *Parasite* **2014**, *21*, 52. [CrossRef] [PubMed]
8. Inpankaew, T.; Traub, R.; Thompson, R.C.; Sukthana, Y. Canine parasitic zoonoses in Bangkok Temples. *Southeast Asian J. Trop. Med. Public Health* **2007**, *38*, 247–255. [PubMed]

9.   Traub, R.J.; Inpankaew, T.; Reid, S.A.; Sutthikornchai, C.; Sukthana, Y.; Robertson, I.D.; Thompson, R.C. Transmission cycles of *Giardia duodenalis* in dogs and humans in temple communities in Bangkok—A critical evaluation of its prevalence using three diagnostic tests in the field in the absence of a gold standard. *Acta Trop.* **2009**, *111*, 125–132. [CrossRef] [PubMed]

10.   Rojekittikhun, W.; Chaisiri, K.; Mahittikorn, A.; Pubampen, S.; Sa-Nguankiat, S.; Kusolsuk, T.; Maipanich, W.; Udonsom, R.; Mori, H. Gastrointestinal parasites of dogs and cats in a refuge in Nakhon Nayok, Thailand. *Southeast Asian J. Trop. Med. Public Health* **2014**, *45*, 31–39. [PubMed]

11.   O'Handley, R.M.; Olson, M.E.; Fraser, D.; Adams, P.; Thompson, R.C. Prevalence and genotypic characterisation of *Giardia* in dairy calves from Western Australia and Western Canada. *Vet. Parasitol.* **2000**, *90*, 193–200. [CrossRef]

12.   Scorza, A.V.; Ballweber, L.R.; Tangtrongsup, S.; Panuska, C.; Lappin, M.R. Comparisons of mammalian *Giardia duodenalis* assemblages based on the beta-giardin, glutamate dehydrogenase and triose phosphate isomerase genes. *Vet. Parasitol.* **2012**, *189*, 182–188. [CrossRef] [PubMed]

13.   da Silva, A.J.; Caccio, S.; Williams, C.; Won, K.Y.; Nace, E.K.; Whittier, C.; Pieniazek, N.J.; Eberhard, M.L. Molecular and morphologic characterization of a *Cryptosporidium* genotype identified in lemurs. *Vet. Parasitol.* **2003**, *111*, 297–307. [CrossRef]

14.   Morgan, U.M.; Monis, P.T.; Xiao, L.; Limor, J.; Sulaiman, I.; Raidal, S.; O'Donoghue, P.; Gasser, R.; Murray, A.; Fayer, R.; et al. Molecular and phylogenetic characterisation of *Cryptosporidium* from birds. *Int. J. Parasitol.* **2001**, *31*, 289–296. [CrossRef]

15.   Morgan, U.M.; Constantine, C.C.; Forbes, D.A.; Thompson, R.C. Differentiation between human and animal isolates of *Cryptosporidium parvum* using rdna sequencing and direct PCR analysis. *J. Parasitol.* **1997**, *83*, 825–830. [CrossRef] [PubMed]

16.   Xiao, L.; Morgan, U.M.; Limor, J.; Escalante, A.; Arrowood, M.; Shulaw, W.; Thompson, R.C.; Fayer, R.; Lal, A.A. Genetic diversity within *Cryptosporidium parvum* and related *Cryptosporidium* species. *Appl. Environ. Microbiol.* **1999**, *65*, 3386–3391. [PubMed]

17.   Caccio, S.M.; De Giacomo, M.; Pozio, E. Sequence analysis of the beta-giardin gene and development of a polymerase chain reaction-restriction fragment length polymorphism assay to genotype *Giardia duodenalis* cysts from human faecal samples. *Int. J. Parasitol.* **2002**, *32*, 1023–1030. [CrossRef]

18.   Sulaiman, I.M.; Jiang, J.; Singh, A.; Xiao, L. Distribution of *Giardia duodenalis* genotypes and subgenotypes in raw urban wastewater in Milwaukee, Wisconsin. *Appl. Environ. Microbiol.* **2004**, *70*, 3776–3780. [CrossRef] [PubMed]

19.   Read, C.M.; Monis, P.T.; Thompson, R.C. Discrimination of all genotypes of *Giardia duodenalis* at the glutamate dehydrogenase locus using PCR-RFLP. *Infect. Genet. Evol.* **2004**, *4*, 125–130. [CrossRef] [PubMed]

20.   Lebbad, M.; Mattsson, J.G.; Christensson, B.; Ljungstrom, B.; Backhans, A.; Andersson, J.O.; Svard, S.G. From mouse to moose: Multilocus genotyping of *Giardia* isolates from various animal species. *Vet. Parasitol.* **2010**, *168*, 231–239. [CrossRef] [PubMed]

21.   Fleiss, J.L. *Statistical Methods for Rates and Proportions*; Wiley-Interscience: Hoboken, NJ, USA, 2003.

22.   Dohoo, I.; Martin, W.; Stryhn, H. *Veterinary Epidemiologic Research*, 2nd ed.; AVC, Inc.: Charlotte, NC, Canada, 2007.

23.   Lucio-Forster, A.; Griffiths, J.K.; Cama, V.A.; Xiao, L.; Bowman, D.D. Minimal zoonotic risk of cryptosporidiosis from pet dogs and cats. *Trends Parasitol.* **2010**, *26*, 174–179. [CrossRef] [PubMed]

24.   Bajer, A.; Bednarska, M.; Rodo, A. Risk factors and control of intestinal parasite infections in sled dogs in Poland. *Vet. Parasitol.* **2011**, *175*, 343–350. [CrossRef] [PubMed]

25.   Itoh, N.; Muraoka, N.; Saeki, H.; Aoki, M.; Itagaki, T. Prevalence of *Giardia intestinalis* infection in dogs of breeding kennels in Japan. *J. Vet. Med. Sci.* **2005**, *67*, 717–718. [CrossRef] [PubMed]

26.   Ponce-Macotela, M.; Peralta-Abarca, G.E.; Martinez-Gordillo, M.N. *Giardia intestinalis* and other zoonotic parasites: Prevalence in adult dogs from the southern part of Mexico City. *Vet. Parasitol.* **2005**, *131*, 1–4. [CrossRef] [PubMed]

27.   Mundim, M.J.; Rosa, L.A.; Hortencio, S.M.; Faria, E.S.; Rodrigues, R.M.; Cury, M.C. Prevalence of *Giardia duodenalis* and *Cryptosporidium* spp. in dogs from different living conditions in Uberlandia, Brazil. *Vet. Parasitol.* **2007**, *144*, 356–359. [CrossRef] [PubMed]

28.   Papini, R.; Gorini, G.; Spaziani, A.; Cardini, G. Survey on giardiosis in shelter dog populations. *Vet. Parasitol.* **2005**, *128*, 333–339. [CrossRef] [PubMed]

29. Claerebout, E.; Casaert, S.; Dalemans, A.C.; De Wilde, N.; Levecke, B.; Vercruysse, J.; Geurden, T. *Giardia* and other intestinal parasites in different dog populations in Northern Belgium. *Vet. Parasitol.* **2009**, *161*, 41–46. [CrossRef] [PubMed]

30. Covacin, C.; Aucoin, D.P.; Elliot, A.; Thompson, R.C. Genotypic characterisation of *Giardia* from domestic dogs in the USA. *Vet. Parasitol.* **2011**, *177*, 28–32. [CrossRef] [PubMed]

31. Sprong, H.; Caccio, S.M.; van der Giessen, J.W. Identification of zoonotic genotypes of *Giardia duodenalis*. *PLoS Negl. Trop. Dis.* **2009**, *3*, e558. [CrossRef] [PubMed]

32. Ballweber, L.R.; Xiao, L.; Bowman, D.D.; Kahn, G.; Cama, V.A. Giardiasis in dogs and cats: Update on epidemiology and public health significance. *Trends Parasitol.* **2010**, *26*, 180–189. [CrossRef] [PubMed]

33. Palmer, C.S.; Traub, R.J.; Robertson, I.D.; Devlin, G.; Rees, R.; Thompson, R.C. Determining the zoonotic significance of *Giardia* and *Cryptosporidium* in Australian dogs and cats. *Vet. Parasitol.* **2008**, *154*, 142–147. [CrossRef] [PubMed]

34. Santin, M.; Trout, J.M. Companion animals. In *Cryptosporidium and Cryptosporidiosis*; Fayer, R., Xiao, L., Eds.; CRC Press: Boca Raton, FL, USA, 2008; pp. 437–449.

35. Gatei, W.; Suputtamongkol, Y.; Waywa, D.; Ashford, R.W.; Bailey, J.W.; Greensill, J.; Beeching, N.J.; Hart, C.A. Zoonotic species of *Cryptosporidium* are as prevalent as the anthroponotic in HIV-infected patients in Thailand. *Ann. Trop. Med. Parasitol.* **2002**, *96*, 797–802. [CrossRef] [PubMed]

36. Srisuphanunt, M.; Saksirisampant, W.; Karanis, P. Prevalence and genotyping of *Cryptosporidium* isolated from HIV/AIDS patients in urban areas of Thailand. *Ann. Trop. Med. Parasitol.* **2011**, *105*, 463–468. [CrossRef] [PubMed]

37. Tiangtip, R.; Jongwutiwes, S. Molecular analysis of *Cryptosporidium* species isolated from HIV-infected patients in Thailand. *Trop. Med. Int. Health* **2002**, *7*, 357–364. [CrossRef] [PubMed]

38. Cama, V.A.; Bern, C.; Sulaiman, I.M.; Gilman, R.H.; Ticona, E.; Vivar, A.; Kawai, V.; Vargas, D.; Zhou, L.; Xiao, L. *Cryptosporidium* species and genotypes in HIV-positive patients in Lima, Peru. *J. Eukaryot. Microbiol.* **2003**, *50*, 531–533. [CrossRef] [PubMed]

39. Alves, M.; Matos, O.; Pereira Da Fonseca, I.; Delgado, E.; Lourenco, A.M.; Antunes, F. Multilocus genotyping of *Cryptosporidium* isolates from human HIV-infected and animal hosts. *J. Eukaryot. Microbiol.* **2001**, 17S–18S. [CrossRef]

40. Xiao, L.; Bern, C.; Limor, J.; Sulaiman, I.; Roberts, J.; Checkley, W.; Cabrera, L.; Gilman, R.H.; Lal, A.A. Identification of 5 types of *Cryptosporidium* parasites in children in Lima, Peru. *J. Infect. Dis.* **2001**, *183*, 492–497. [CrossRef] [PubMed]

41. da Silva, A.J.; Bornay-Llinares, F.J.; Moura, I.N.; Slemenda, S.B.; Tuttle, J.L.; Pieniazek, N.J. Fast and reliable extraction of protozoan parasite DNA from fecal specimens. *Mol. Diagn.* **1999**, *4*, 57–64. [CrossRef]

42. Mircean, V.; Gyorke, A.; Cozma, V. Prevalence and risk factors of *Giardia duodenalis* in dogs from Romania. *Vet. Parasitol.* **2012**, *184*, 325–329. [CrossRef] [PubMed]

43. Katagiri, S.; Oliveira-Sequeira, T.C. Prevalence of dog intestinal parasites and risk perception of zoonotic infection by dog owners in Sao Paulo State, Brazil. *Zoonoses Public Health* **2008**, *55*, 406–413. [CrossRef] [PubMed]

44. Upjohn, M.; Cobb, C.; Monger, J.; Geurden, T.; Claerebout, E.; Fox, M. Prevalence, molecular typing and risk factor analysis for *Giardia duodenalis* infections in dogs in a central London rescue shelter. *Vet. Parasitol.* **2010**, *172*, 341–346. [CrossRef] [PubMed]

45. Scaramozzino, P.; Di Cave, D.; Berrilli, F.; D'Orazi, C.; Spaziani, A.; Mazzanti, S.; Scholl, F.; De Liberato, C. A study of the prevalence and genotypes of *Giardia duodenalis* infecting kennelled dogs. *Vet. J.* **2009**, *182*, 231–234. [CrossRef] [PubMed]

6

Detection and Characterization of Histamine-Producing Strains of *Photobacterium damselae* subsp. *damselae* Isolated from Mullets

Marcello Trevisani [1,*]**, Rocco Mancusi** [1]**, Matilde Cecchini** [1]**, Claudia Costanza** [1]
and Marino Prearo [2]

[1]   Dipartimento di Scienze Mediche Veterinarie, Università degli Studi di Bologna, Alma Mater Studiorum, via Tolara di Sopra 50, Ozzano Emilia 40064, Italy; mancusirocco@virgilio.it (R.M.); matilde.cecchini@unibo.it (M.C.); claudia.costanza.vet@gmail.com (C.C.)

[2]   S.S. Laboratorio Specialistico Ittiopatologia, Istituto Zooprofilattico Sperimentale del Piemonte, Liguria e Valle d'Aosta, Torino 10154, Italy; Marino.Prearo@izsto.it

*   Correspondence: marcello.trevisani@unibo.it

Academic Editors: Chrissanthy Papadopoulou, Vangelis Economou and Hercules Sakkas

Abstract: *Photobacterium damselae* subsp. *damselae* (*Pdd*) is considered to be an emerging pathogen of marine fish and has also been implicated in cases of histamine food poisoning. In this study, eight strains isolated from mullets of the genera *Mugil* and *Liza* captured in the Ligurian Sea were characterized, and a method to detect histamine-producing *Pdd* from fish samples was developed. The histamine-producing potential of the strains was evaluated in culture media (TSB+) using a histamine biosensor. Subsequently, two strains were used to contaminate mackerel fillets (4 or 40 CFU/g), simulating a cross-contamination on the selling fish stalls. Sample homogenates were enriched in TSB+. The cultures were then inoculated on thiosulfate-citrate-bile salts-sucrose agar (TCBS) and the dark green colonies were cultured on Niven agar. The violet isolates were characterized using specific biochemical and PCR based tests. All *Pdd* strains were histamine producers, yielding concentration varying from 167 and 8977 μg/mL in TSB+ cultures incubated at 30 °C for 24 h. *Pdd* colonies were detected from the inoculated mackerel samples and their histidine decarboxylase gene was amplified using species-specific primer pairs designed for this study. The results indicate that mullets can be source of *Pdd* and the fish retailers needs to evaluate the risk posed by cross-contamination on the selling fish stalls.

Keywords: *Photobacterium damselae* subsp. *damselae*; histidine decarboxylase; cross contamination; mullets; histamine biosensor

---

1. Introduction

Histamine fish poisoning is among the most common food borne diseases related to fish consumption. Fifty-six of the 71 food borne disease outbreaks (78.9%) that have been notified in Europe in 2011 were due to histamine fish poisoning [1]. The risk is correlated with the number and the histidine decarboxylase activity of the contaminating bacteria that grow in the flesh of fishes that are rich of free histidine, such as tuna, mackerel, and bonito.

Bacteria of the genus *Photobacterium*, i.e., *P. damselae* subsp. *damselae* (*Pdd*) and *P. phosphoreum*, are strong histamine producers [2–4].

Photobacterium damselae subsp. *damselae* is considered to be an emerging pathogen of marine fish of importance in aquaculture, with a notable increase in its geographical distribution during the last several years [5].

Kanki et al. [2] demonstrated that *Pdd* inoculated on tuna can produce toxic levels of histamine even at 4 °C. These authors observed that *Pdd* displayed the highest performance in accumulating histamine in fish samples stored at refrigeration temperature in comparison with other psychrotolerant marine bacteria, namely *P. phosphoreum* and *Raoultella planticola*. They demonstrated that *Pdd* (strain JCM 8968) can produce more than 500 mg/kg histamine at 4 °C in 24 h and maintain 60% and 50% of the initial activity in tuna and dried saury for up to 12 weeks at −20 °C, respectively. The presence of *Pdd* in the fish that are stored in melting ice or at chilling temperature and even in the de-frozen and processed seafood can thus pose a significant hazard if the contamination is carried on fish species which are rich in free histidine.

The histidine decarboxylase activity of bacteria that are present in fish samples can be assessed in enrichment broth supplemented with histidine using different analytical methods, including immuno-enzymatic (ELISA) tests, chromatographic methods, or bio-sensing devices [3,6–8]. The detection of histamine-producing bacteria (HPB) is possible by plating the fish homogenates on differential grow media, such as the Niven agar plates [9] and the screening of the suspect colonies with PCR assays for the histidine decarboxylase encoding genes [10], but these analytical methods did not allow the isolation of HPB in a number of samples that developed high level of histamine in the enrichment broth supplemented with histidine [7]. Many studies have demonstrated that among HPB there are some species that are not able to grow on the Niven medium and consequently false negative results occur [11]. In order to isolate the halophilic *Photobacterium* spp., the use of specific culture medium is needed.

There are few studies concerning the histidine-decarboxylase encoding genes of *P. damselae* and *P. phosphoreum* [11], and the variability of phenotype expression (histidine-decarboxylase activity) [3,4]. Biosensor technology allows fast, cost effective, and specific detection of histamine in seafood spoilage [12] and histamine biosensors can be useful in assessing the microbiological quality of fish. The enzyme diaminoxidase is known to catalyse the conversion of histamine to imidazole acetaldehyde by means of a bi-enzyme system, used by various researchers [13–15]. The co-substrate, molecular oxygen, is reduced to hydrogen peroxide (Equation (1)). The reduction of hydrogen peroxide to water is catalysed by the enzyme peroxidase using potassium hexacyanoferrate(II) (or other redox systems) as the mediator (Equation (2)). The introduction of a mediator in the bi-enzymatic system (DAO/HRP) leads to an acceleration of the electron transfer, a decrease in the applied working potential (the reduction of the mediator is detected at the electrode), and an increase in sensitivity [15–17].

$$RCH_2NH_2 + O_2 + H_2O \rightarrow (DAO) \rightarrow RCHO + NH_3 + H_2O_2 \quad (1)$$

$$H_2O_2 + Fe(CN)_6{}^{-4} \rightarrow HRP \rightarrow H_2O + Fe(CN)_6{}^{-3} + e^- \quad (2)$$

The working electrode of a potentiostat acts as an oxidant and the oxidation current increases. The aims of this study were to develop a simple and rapid method to detect histamine-producing *P. damselae* subsp. *damselae* from fish samples and characterize their histidine decarboxylase activity.

2. Materials and Methods

2.1. Characterization of Pdd Strains

Eight strains of *Pdd* that have been isolated from different samples of fish of the species *Mugil cephalus*, *Liza aurata*, *L. ramada,* and *L. saliens*, which were captured at the estuary of the river Magra in the Eastern Ligurian Sea (Bocche di Magra and Fiumaretta, Amelia municipality, La Spezia province, Italy) [18], were used in this study. The isolates were characterized with biochemical tests for their oxidase, catalase, urease activities, and the ability of fermenting glucose and galactose. In addition, the presence of specific target genes *ure*C and *16S* rRNA was assessed by PCR using the primers designed by Osorio et al. [19] (Table 1).

Table 1. Primers and PCR protocols used for the identification of *P. damselae* subsp. *damselae* and its histidine decarboxylase gene.

Gene/Primers	Nucleotide Sequences	Thermal Cycling Conditions	Reference
ureC Ure-5' Ure-3'	5'-TCCGGAATAGGTAAAGCGGG-3' 5'-CTTGAATATCCATCTCATCTGC-3'	95 °C 4 min; 30× (95 °C 60 s; 60 °C 60 s; 72 °C 40 s); 72 °C 5 min	Osorio et al., 2000
16S rRNA Car1 Car2	5'-GCTTGAAGAGATTCGAGT-3' 5'-CACCTCGCGGTCTTGCTG-3'		
hdc dp [a] HIS2-F HIS2-R	5'-AAYTSNTTYGAYTTYGARAARGARGT-3' 5'-TANGGNSANCCDATCATYTTRTGNCC-3'	95 °C 3 min; 35× (95 °C 15 s; 53 °C * 30 s; 72 °C 40 s); 72 °C 5 min	De Las Rivas et al., 2005
*hdc*Pdd [b] hdcPdd-F hdcPdd-R	5'-GGATTAGCGGCCATGGATTGGT-3' 5'-AACGCCTAAGAAAACCCCACA-3'	95 °C 3 min; 30× (95 °C 10 s; 60 °C 45 s)	(Genebank accession number JCM 8968)

Notes: [a] dp, degenerate primers targeting multiple sequences of the Gram-histidine decarboxylase (*hdc*) genes; [b] primers targeting specific sequence of *Photobacterium damselae* subsp. *damselae hdc* gene. * gradient in the range from 49 to 53 °C.

In order to detect the histidine decarboxylase gene of *P. damselae* subsp. *damselae* two primer pairs were used. The primers *HIS*2-F and *HIS*2-R designed by De Las Rivas et al. [10] allow the amplification of a specific 531-bp DNA fragment from gram-negative histamine-producing bacteria including *P. damselae*, strain CECT 626T (ATCC 33539) [20].

In this study, target-specific primers for *Pdd* were designed to be specific for Genbank accession AB259289.1 (HDC, Histidine decarboxylase gene of *Photobacterium damselae* (strain JCM 8968)) [2]. The designed PCR primers (*hdc*Pdd, Table 1) were checked for specificity with Primer-Blast software (NCBI, Cambridge, UK).

2.2. DNA Extraction and PCR Procedures

Strains were grown on Tryptone Soy Agar (TSA, Thermofisher, Milano, Italy) supplemented with NaCl (2%) at 25 °C for 48 h. Two colonies were randomly picked for each strain using a sterile toothpick and the DNA was extracted by boiling suspensions of cells in a 5% suspension of Chelex 100 (Bio-Rad Laboratories, Hercules, CA, USA) following the producer protocol.

Real-Time PCR was performed on a MiniOpticon Real-Time PCR System (Bio-Rad Laboratories) using SsoFast EvaGreen Supermix (Bio-Rad). Total reaction volume of 20 μL included: 300 nM of each forward and reverse primers, 1 μL of template DNA and the SsoFast EvaGreen Supermix (according to the manufacturer's instructions). Each run included a non-template control (NTC). Two laboratory reference strains characterized as *Morganella morganii* and *Photobacterium damselae* subsp. *damselae* in accordance with their colony characteristics, biochemical tests (API20E and API20NE systems) and genetic characterization were used as positive controls [19,21]. Real-time amplification for each gene, including controls and samples, was performed in duplicate under identical PCR conditions. Thermal cycle was set as reported in Table 1. At the end of the PCR cycles, a melting curve was conducted between 65 °C and 95 °C with a 0.5 °C/5 s increment read and continuous fluorescence measurement. The effect of annealing temperature was analyzed using gradient PCR amplification in the range from 49 to 53 °C.

2.3. Assay for Histamine Production: A Biosensor Fabrication

To confirm histamine production by each HPB isolate, single colonies were suspended in Tryptone Soy Broth (Thermofisher, Milano, Italy) supplemented with NaCl (2%) and L-Histidine hydrochloride (1%) (Sigma-Aldrich, Milano, Italy) (TSB+) and incubated at 30 °C for 24 h. After the incubation, the cultures were sterilized at 121 °C for 15 min and the supernatant was used for histamine quantitative detection.

To comparatively assess histamine production ability of each strain, the microbial suspensions were diluted with TSB+ to have 40% optical density at 540 nm, corresponding to approximately 10^8 CFU/mL. The concentration of bacteria was subsequently assessed by plating the appropriate dilutions on Tryptone Soy Agar (TSA, Thermofisher, Milano, Italy) with 2% NaCl.

Quantitative detection of histamine in the enriched broth cultures and standardized microbial suspensions was made using an amperometric enzymatic biosensor. The histamine biosensor is based on the co-immobilization diamine-oxidase (DAO, from Porcine Kidney, 0.11 U/mg) and peroxidase (HRP, from horseradish, 25 KU/mg) (Sigma-Aldrich, Milano, Italy) on the surface of a glassy carbon electrode (diameter 3 mm, BAS, West Lafayette, IN, USA). The enzymes were immobilized by chemical cross-linking with glutaraldehyde (GA, 25%) and bovine serum albumin (BSA, fraction V, purity 96–99%). All reagents were purchased from Sigma-Aldrich (Milano, Italy). Briefly, 10 mg of DAO, 6 mg of HRP and 4 mg of BSA were dissolved in 100 μL of Phosphate Buffer (PB, 0.1 M Ph = 7.4). Five μL of GA diluted in water (2.5%) were mixed with 15 μL of the DAO-HRP-BSA solution. Ten μL of the final solution was put on the cleaned surface of the working electrode and allowed to dry for 30 min at 25 °C. After the BSA enzyme solution were cross-linked with GA and a consistent gel has developed on the electrode surface, the enzymatic sensor was washed in PB and stored in the same medium at refrigeration temperature.

The response of the biosensor to the histamine concentration in the bacterial cultures was calculated as the difference between the amperometric signal in inoculated and non-inoculated medium. The values were recorded in millivolts by a potentiostat (Metrhom Autolab PGSTAT10, EcoChemie, Utrecht, The Netherlands) connected to a personal computer using the Autolab GPES 4.9 software. The calibration data was obtained with a series of standard histamine solutions (1, 2, 4, 6, 8, 10, and 20 ppm) were fitted using the software Excel (Microsoft, Redmond, WA, USA). The concentration of histamine in the enriched cultures was calculated by interpolation of the amperometric responses for the samples into the calibration plot constructed with histamine standards.

2.4. Detection of Pdd from Fish Samples

A procedure to detect *Pdd* in fish was developed and tested. With this aim mackerel samples were inoculated in duplicate with two *Pdd* strains that produced more than 1000 µg/mL of histamine in TSB+ culture incubated at 30 °C for 24 h (high HPB). The test were carried out independently with each of the two strains. Fresh mackerels were purchased from the market and samples (25 g) were inoculated with either 100 µL of *Pdd* suspensions standardized to approximately 10^3 and 10^4 CFU/mL (4 and 40 CFU/g) and control samples (taken from the same mackerels) were analyzed in parallel (controls).

The samples were homogenized (1:10 w/v) in TSB+ and the contaminating bacteria were enriched at 25 °C for 48 h and subsequently plated on thiosulfate-citrate-bile salts-sucrose agar (TCBS, Thermofisher, Milano, Italy). Dark green colonies with smooth edges were picked and inoculated on plates of modified Niven Agar [9]. Isolated purple colonies developed within 48 h (suspect HPB) were picked and seeded on TSA with 2% NaCl.

Isolates were analyzed for the oxidase activity (oxidase detection strips Oxoid, Thermofisher, Milano, Italy) and by Gram stain, then the Gram-oxidase positive strains were characterized for the ability to ferment glucose and galactose and the urease activity with the API 20E kit (bioMérieux Italia, Bagno di Ripoli, FI, Italy). DNA of the strains that gave positive reactions was extracted by boiling suspensions of cells in a 5% suspension of Chelex 100 (Bio-Rad Laboratories) following the producer protocol. DNA extracts were analyzed to detect the presence or absence of specific nucleotide sequence of the genes *ure*C e *16S* rRNA of *Pdd* by using the PCR protocols described (Table 1).

3. Results

All the strains isolated from the fish of the genera *Mugil* and *Liza* captured in the Ligurian Sea grew on TCBS producing dark green colonies with smooth edges, tested positive at the glucose, galactose, and urease tests, and produced typical amplicons after PCR, with melting temperatures (*Tm*) of 84 °C and 86 °C for the genes *ure*C and *16S* rRNA, respectively. The primers *his*1 and *his*2 produced positive PCR tests only with three of the eight strains analyzed and the level of amplification (cycle threshold, Ct values was higher than 33). The *Tm* of the amplicons of *Pdd* was 80 °C and was different from the amplicon produced by *M. morganii* (Tm 84.5 °C) (Figure 1). The level of amplification improved when the annealing temperature of PCR was reduced from 53 to 49 °C and amplicon melting temperature remained at 80 °C for *Pdd* strains.

All the strains produced good amplification levels by using the primers couple HDC*Pdd* designed for this study and the PCR amplicons produced had a melting temperature of 80.5 °C (Figure 2).

Molecular sequence analysis with BLAST software were used to compare the HDC*Pdd* primers sequences with the genomes of Gram-bacteria. The primers showed 100% similarity with a known nucleotide sequence of *Pdd* histidine decarboxylase gene and no similarity with other known sequences of Gram-bacteria.

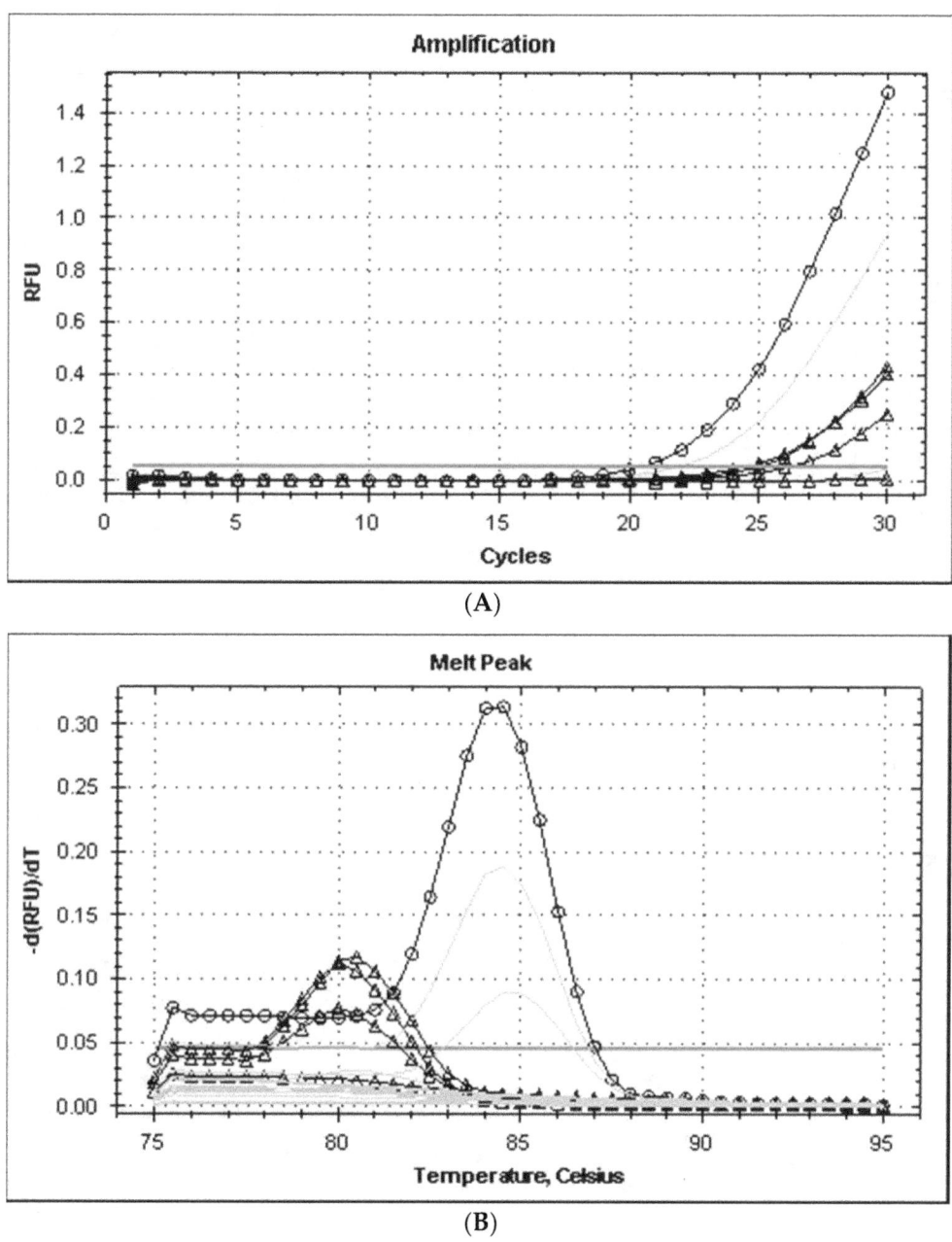

Figure 1. Amplification plot (**A**) and melt curves (**B**) from rt-PCR of histidine decarboxylase genes of Gram-negative bacteria (primers hdc-dp). Legend: annealing temperature for gradient PCR amplification ranged from 49 (dark lines) to 53 °C (grey lines); lines with symbols Δ and ○ correspond to *Pdd* (3 strains)and *M. morgani*, respectively.

All these strains gave positive results with the assay for histamine production in TSB+ at 30 °C. The concentration of histamine produced in 24 h was between 167 and 8977 µg/mL (median = 1053).

Histamine producing *Pdd* strains were isolated from all the inoculated samples and typical colonies can be easily detected and characterized using the procedure described even at the lower concentration (4 CFU/g) used in this study. Other Gram-bacteria, subsequently identified as *Proteus* spp., grew on the TCBS and also on the Niven plates, but they did not show swarming behavior. The colonies on the TCBS plates were green, but not dark as those of *Pdd*. The PCR and biochemical assays can easily discriminate the *Pdd* strains.

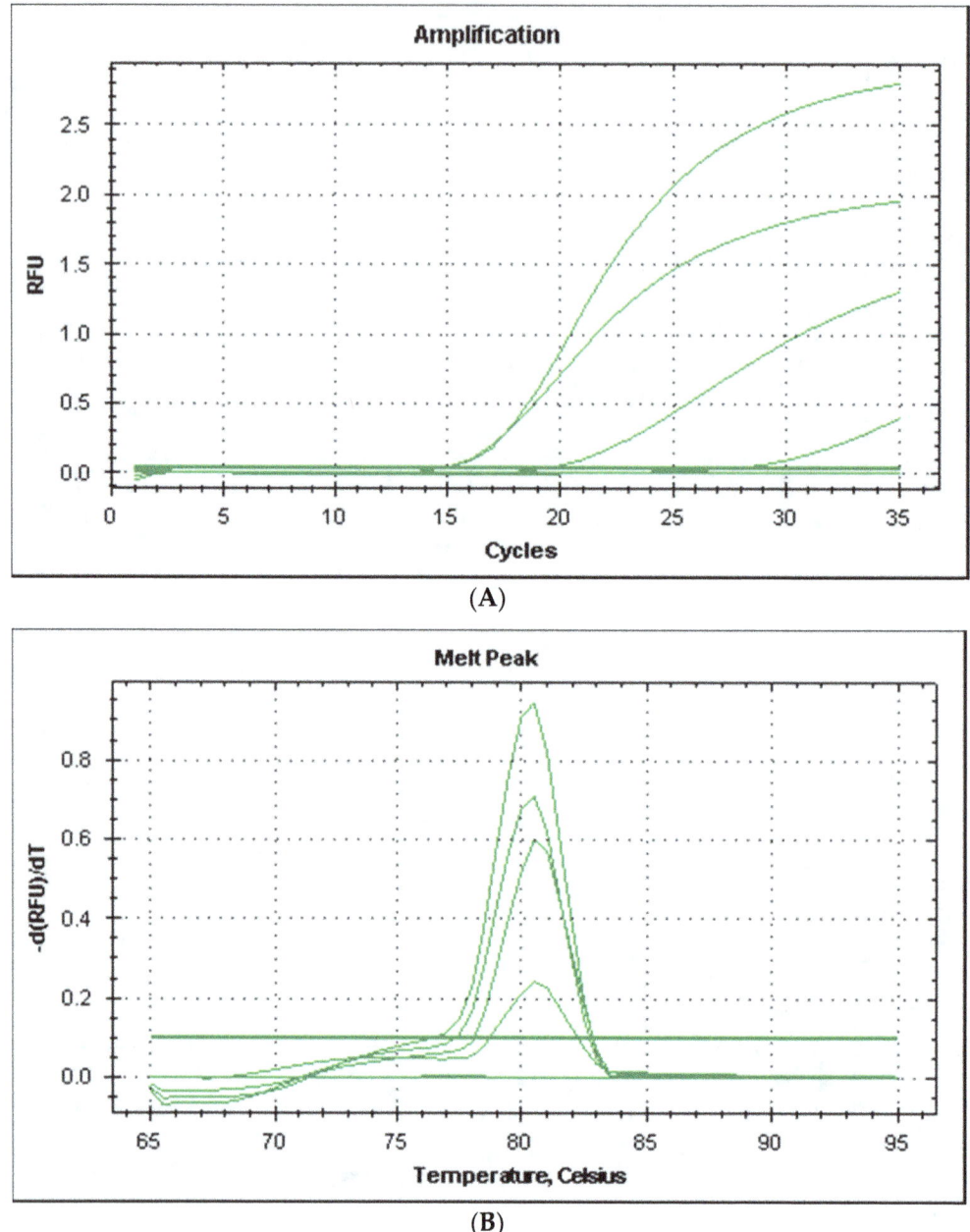

Figure 2. Amplification plot (**A**) and melt curves (**B**) from rt-PCR of histidine decarboxylase gene of *Photobacterium damselae* subsp. *damselae*.

4. Discussion

Contamination of fish meat with histamine-producing bacteria that can grow at refrigeration temperature pose a risk for the marine species that have high concentration of free histidine.

The presence of psychrototrophic bacteria that are strong producers of histamine of the genus *Morganella*, *Photobacterium* e *Raoultella* was observed in fish during surveys or in the many outbreaks of intoxication [22–24]. Their presence has been frequently detected also in surveys carried out in the Italian fish market [7,25].

Photobacterium damselae subsp. *damselae* do not grow at the temperature of melting ice, but their role in accumulation of histamine in tuna and dried saury was clearly documented and was correlated to the high stability of its histidine decarboxylase also in defrozen and dried fish [2] and can persist even if its viability is reduced [21]. Recent studies have reported a notable increase in the *Pdd* geographical distribution during the last several years, especially in marine aquaculture [5,26].

Contamination can occur after the harvest, due to manipulations, and during processing. Development of histamine is favored by the spread of bacteria and HDC resulting from the loss of integrity and the post mortem decay of natural barriers (skin, gut, and gills). The risk of histamine (scombroid) intoxication is correlated with the number of HPB and their enzymatic activity of the microbial species, other than to the temperature and time [27,28].

The screening of fish samples to detect HPB and characterize their HDC activity is of utmost importance for the food business operators (FBO) and the food safety authorities that verify the effectiveness of the FBO's controls [29,30].

Differential culture method [9], conductance method [31], and also culture independent Real-Time PCR Method [32] have been used to detect and quantify HPB. Immunological and chromatographic methods, and also biosensors, can be used to measure the histamine produced in the culture media and distinguish the phenotype of HPB strains (i.e., strong or weak histamine producers). Biosensors offer a cheaper alternative to the immunoenzymatic methods [2] or HPLC [3]. The specific detection of HPB strains is needed to characterize the risk, but many studies have reported that the detection of HPB from enriched samples that have tested positive by the assays for histamine can be hampered by the use of the Niven differential culture media, which do not allow the growth of strict halophilic species or other species which are sensitive to its low pH, producing a number of false negative results [4,7,33]. In addition, Niven medium is not selective, producing false positive isolates that must be subsequently discriminated by PCR assays or labelled DNA probes for the *hdc* gene [4,10,34].

Multiple primers sets have been reported for amplification of the histidine decarboxylase gene from Gram-negative bacteria [10,33], but this study has revealed that the degenerate primers designed by De Las Rivas et al. [10] to amplify several similar genetic sequences of the Gram-*hdc* gene do not give a good performance with the *Pdd* strains analyzed in this study. A PCR amplification was obtained only by lowering annealing temperature, thus allowing primers with many mismatches with templates to provide amplification [35].

In order to detect *Pdd* from fish samples that have tested strongly positive by the assays for histamine, the use of a selective and differential medium like TCBS in combination with the Niven medium for the selective detection of HPB allowed improvement of the performance of the detection method and the presence of *Pdd* can be confirmed by a PCR assay targeted toward the species-specific sequence of *hdc* gene.

An excellent correlation between the histamine amount values obtained with biosensors and the histamine amount values obtained by ELISA (enzyme-linked immunosorbent assay) and HPLC has been established [14,36,37]. Therefore, its use for screening purpose is suitable to analyze the sample enrichments and detect those contaminated with strong HPB active at low or ambient temperatures. Nevertheless, comparative analysis of HPB are usually carried out at 30 °C for 24 h and the *Pdd* isolates can be categorized as high histamine (>1000 ppm) producers (three strains), intermediate (501 to 999 ppm) histamine producers (four strains), and low histamine (126 to 500 ppm) producer (one strain) [3].

The widespread distribution of *P. damselae* subsp. *damselae* was reported in farmed fish in Spain (*Pagrus auriga*) [38] and South-eastern Black Sea (*Dicentrarchus labrax*) [5] where it has been associated with high mortalities. Sea bream and sea bass or mullet are not fish species implicated in histamine poisoning cases, but these farmed fishes are commonly exposed on the selling fish stalls close to tuna and mackerel fillets and manipulated, and even the ice used in the stalls has been reported to be contaminated with HPB [39].

5. Conclusions

Fish retailers and other operators should review the risk management practices employed throughout the fish processing chain in relation to controlling histamine formation in at-risk fish species and consider that other fish species, such as mullets of the genera Mugil and Liza, can be considered potential carriers of Pdd. Therefore, they must ensure good hygienic practices to prevent cross contamination.

Acknowledgments: We wish to thank the Ictiopathology Laboratory of the Istituto Zooprofilattico Sperimentale del Piemonte, Liguria e Valle d'Aosta for supplying *Photobacterium damselae* strains.

Author Contributions: Marcello Trevisani conceived, designed the experiments, wrote the paper, contributed reagents/materials/analysis tools and analyzed the data; Rocco Mancusi performed the microbiological experiments and designed the set of primers for PCR detection of P. damselae; Matilde Cecchini performed the analysis for quantification of histamine; Claudia Costanza helped in the microbiological experiments; Marino Prearo provided the Pdd strains and helped reviewing the paper.

References

1. European Food Safety Authority (EFSA); European Centre for Disease Prevention and Control (ECDC). The European Union Summary Report on Trends and Sources of Zoonoses, Zoonotic Agents and Food-Borne Outbreaks in 2011. *EFSA J.* **2013**, *11*, 3129.

2. Kanki, M.; Yoda, T.; Tsukamoto, T.; Baba, E. Histidine Decarboxylases and Their Role in Accumulation of Histamine in Tuna and Dried Saury. *Appl. Environ. Microbiol.* **2007**, *73*, 1467–1473. [CrossRef] [PubMed]

3. Bjornsdottir, K.; Bolton, G.E.; McClellan-Green, P.D.; Jaykus, L.-A.; Green, D.P. Detection of Gram-Negative Histamine-Producing Bacteria in Fish: A Comparative Study. *J. Food Prot.* **2009**, *72*, 1987–1991. [CrossRef] [PubMed]

4. Björnsdóttir-Butler, K.; Bolton, G.E.; Jaykus, L.A.; McClellan-Green, P.D.; Green, D.P. Development of Molecular-Based Methods for Determination of High Histamine Producing Bacteria in Fish. *Int. J. Food Microbiol.* **2010**, *139*, 161–167. [CrossRef] [PubMed]

5. Terceti, M.S.; Ogut, H.; Osorio, R. In the Black Sea: Evidence of a Multiclonal Origin. *Appl. Environ. Microbiol.* **2016**, *82*, 3736–3745. [CrossRef] [PubMed]

6. Chen, H.C.; Kung, H.F.; Chen, W.C.; Lin, W.F.; Hwang, D.F.; Lee, Y.C.; Tsai, Y.H. Determination of Histamine and Histamine-Forming Bacteria in Tuna Dumpling Implicated in a Food-Borne Poisoning. *Food Chem.* **2008**, *106*, 612–618. [CrossRef]

7. Costanza, C.; Cecchini, M.; Mancusi, R.; Mosso, A.; Giani, G.; Rosmini, R.; Trevisani, M. Evaluation and Identification of Histamine-Forming Bacteria on Fish Products of Middle Adriatic Sea. *Ital. J. Food Saf.* **2013**, *1*, 17–20. [CrossRef]

8. Marcobal, A.; De Las Rivas, B.; Muñoz, R. Methods for the Detection of Bacteria Producing Biogenic Amines on Foods: A Survey. *J. Verbraucherschutz Lebensmittelsicherheit* **2006**, *1*, 187–196. [CrossRef]

9. Mavromatis, P.; Quantick, P.C. Modication of Niven's Medium for the Enumeration of Histamine-Forming Bacteria and Discussion of the Parameters Associated with Its Use. *J. Food Prot.* **2002**, *65*, 546–551. [CrossRef] [PubMed]

10. De Las Rivas, B.; Marcobal, Á.; Muñoz, R. Improved Multiplex-PCR Method for the Simultaneous Detection of Food Bacteria Producing Biogenic Amines. *FEMS Microbiol. Lett.* **2005**, *244*, 367–372. [CrossRef] [PubMed]

11. Landete, J.M.; De las Rivas, B.; Marcobal, A.; Muñoz, R. Updated Molecular Knowledge about Histamine Biosynthesis by Bacteria. *Crit. Rev. Food Sci. Nutr.* **2008**, *48*, 697–714. [CrossRef] [PubMed]

12. Male, K.B.; Bouvrette, P.; Luong, J.H.T.; Gibbs, B.F. Amperometric Biosensor for Total Histamine, Putrescine and Cadaverine Using Diamine Oxidase. *J. Food Sci.* **1996**, *61*, 1012–1016. [CrossRef]

13. Niraj, M.M.G.; Pandey, S. Histamine Biosensor: A Review. *Int. J. Pharm. Sci. Res.* **2012**, *3*, 4158–4168.

14. Pérez, S.; Bartrolí, J.; Fàbregas, E. Amperometric Biosensor for the Determination of Histamine in Fish Samples. *Food Chem.* **2013**, *141*, 4066–4072. [CrossRef] [PubMed]

15. Tombelli, S.; Mascini, M. Electrochemical Biosensors for Biogenic Amines—A Comparison between Different Approaches. *Anal. Chim. Acta* **1998**, *358*, 277–285. [CrossRef]

16. Grieshaber, D.; Mackenzie, R.; Vörös, J.; Reimhult, E. Electrochemical Biosensors—Sensor Principles and Architectures. *Sensors* **2008**, *8*, 1400–1458. [CrossRef] [PubMed]

17. Rondeau, A.; Larsson, N.; Boujtita, M.; Gorton, L.; El Murr, N. The Synergetic Effect of Redox Mediators and Peroxidase in a Bienzymatic Biosensor for Glucose Assays in FIA. *Analusis* **1999**, *27*, 649–656. [CrossRef]

18. Serracca, L.; Ercolini, C.; Rossini, I.; Battistini, R.; Giorgi, I.; Prearo, M. E Photobacterium Damselae Subsp. Piscicida in Cefali Del Fiume Magra (Italia) Detection of Photobacterium Damselae Subsp. Damselae and Photobacterium Damselae Subsp. Piscicida in Mullets Caught in the Magra River (Italy). *Ittiopatologia* **2009**, *6*, 221–228.

19. Osorio, C.R.; Toranzo, A.E.; Romalde, J.L.; Barja, J.L. Multiplex PCR Assay for ureC and 16S rRNA Genes Clearly Discriminates between Both Subspecies of Photobacterium Damselae. *Dis. Aquat. Org.* **2000**, *40*, 177–183. [CrossRef] [PubMed]

20. Landete, J.M.; de las Rivas, B.; Marcobal, A.; Muñoz, R. Molecular Methods for the Detection of Biogenic Amine-Producing Bacteria on Foods. *Int. J. Food Microbiol.* **2007**, *117*, 258–269. [CrossRef] [PubMed]

21. Podeur, G.; Dalgaard, P.; Leroi, F.; Prévost, H.; Emborg, J.; Martinussen, J.; Hansen, L.H.; Pilet, M.F. Development of a Real-Time PCR Method Coupled with a Selective Pre-Enrichment Step for Quantification of Morganella Morganii and Morganella Psychrotolerans in Fish Products. *Int. J. Food Microbiol.* **2015**, *203*. [CrossRef] [PubMed]

22. Lin, C.S.; Kung, H.F.; Lin, C.M.; Tsai, H.C.; Tsai, Y.H. Histamine Production by Raoultella Ornithinolytica in Mahi-Mahi Meat at Various Storage Temperatures. *J. Food Drug Anal.* **2016**, *24*, 305–310. [CrossRef]

23. Emborg, J.; Dalgaard, P. Formation of Histamine and Biogenic Amines in Cold-Smoked Tuna: An Investigation of Psychrotolerant Bacteria from Samples Implicated in Cases of Histamine Fish Poisoning. *J. Food Prot.* **2006**, *69*, 897–906. [CrossRef] [PubMed]

24. Kanki, M.; Yoda, T.; Ishibashi, M.; Tsukamoto, T. Photobacterium Phosphoreum Caused a Histamine Fish Poisoning Incident. *Int. J. Food Microbiol.* **2004**, *92*, 79–87. [CrossRef] [PubMed]

25. Mancusi, R.; Bini, R.M.; Cecchini, M.; Delle Donne, G.; Rosmini, R.; Trevisani, M. Presenza D'istamina Nei Prodotti Ittici in Commercio. *Ital. J. Food Saf.* **2012**, *1*, 35–39. [CrossRef]

26. Rivas, A.J.; Lemos, M.L.; Osorio, C.R. Photobacterium Damselae Subsp. Damselae, a Bacterium Pathogenic for Marine Animals and Humans. *Front. Microbiol.* **2013**, *4*, 1–6. [CrossRef] [PubMed]

27. Agence Nationale de Sécurité Sanitaire de L'Alimentation, de L'Environnement et du Travail. Caractéristiques et Sources de L'histamine. In *Fiches de Dangers Biologiques Transmissibles par les Aliments "Histamine"*; ANSES: Maisons-Alfort Cedex, France, 2012; Available online: https://www.anses.fr/fr/system/files/MIC2010sa0261.pdf (accessed on 8 June 2017).

28. Canadian Food Inspection Agency. *Lookup Results of CFIA Fish List*; Canadian Food Inspection Agency: Ottawa, ON, Canada, 2016; Available online: http://www.inspection.gc.ca/active/scripts/fssa/fispoi/fplist/fpresults.asp?lang=e&q=&cmbIn=e&cbShowAll=on (accessed on 8 June 2017).

29. Hwang, C.C.; Kung, H.F.; Lin, C.S.; Hwang, D.F.; Tsai, Y.H. Bacteriological Quality and Histamine-Forming Bacteria Associated with Fish Meats and Environments in HACCP and Non-HACCP Fish Processing Factories. *Food Control* **2011**, *22*, 1657–1662. [CrossRef]

30. Hungerford, J.M. Scombroid Poisoning: A Review. *Toxicon* **2010**, *56*, 231–243. [CrossRef] [PubMed]

31. Dalgaard, P.; Mejlhom, O.; Huss, H.H. Conductance Method for Quantitative Determination of Photobacterium Phosphoreum in Fish Products. *J. Appl. Microbiol.* **1996**, *81*, 57–64.

32. Macé, S.; Mamlouk, K.; Chipchakova, S.; Prévost, H.; Joffraud, J.J.; Dalgaard, P.; Pilet, M.F.; Dousset, X. Development of a Rapid Real-Time PCR Method as a Tool to Quantify Viable Photobacterium Phosphoreum Bacteria in Salmon (Salmo Salar) Steaks. *Appl. Environ. Microbiol.* **2013**, *79*, 2612–2619. [CrossRef] [PubMed]

33. Takahashi, H.; Kimura, B.; Yoshikawa, M.; Fujii, T. Cloning and Sequencing of the Histidine Decarboxylase Genes of Gram-Negative, Histamine-Producing Bacteria and Their Application in Detection and Identification of These Organisms in Fish. *Appl. Environ. Microbiol.* **2003**, *69*, 2568–2579. [CrossRef] [PubMed]

34. Wongsariya, K.; Bunyapraphatsara, N.; Yasawong, M. Development of Molecular Approach Based on PCR Assay for Detection of Histamine Producing Bacteria. *J. Food Sci. Technol.* **2016**, *53*, 640–648. [CrossRef] [PubMed]

35. Green, S.J.; Venkatramanan, R.; Naqib, A. Deconstructing the Polymerase Chain Reaction: Understanding and Correcting Bias Associated with Primer Degeneracies and Primer-Template Mismatches. *PLoS ONE* **2015**, *10*, e0128122. [CrossRef] [PubMed]

36. Apetrei, I.M.; Apetrei, C. Amperometric Biosensor Based on Diamine Oxidase/platinum Nanoparticles/graphene/chitosan Modified Screen-Printed Carbon Electrode for Histamine Detection. *Sensors* **2016**, *16*, 422. [CrossRef] [PubMed]

37. Keow, C.M.; Bakar, F.A.; Salleh, A.B.; Heng, L.Y.; Wagiran, R.; Siddiquee, S. Screen-Printed Histamine Biosensors Fabricated from the Entrapment of Diamine Oxidase in a Photocured poly(HEMA) Film. *Int. J. Electrochem. Sci.* **2012**, *7*, 4702–4715.

38. Labella, A.; Berbel, C.; Manchado, M.; Castro, D.; Borrego, J.J. Photobacterium Damselae Subsp. Damselae, an Emerging Pathogen Affecting New Cultured Marine Fish Species in Southern Spain. *Recent Adv. Fish Farms* **2011**, 136–152.

39. Economou, V.; Gousia, P.; Kemenetzi, D.; Sakkas, H.; Papadopoulou, C. Microbial Quality and Histamine Producing Microflora Analysis of the Ice Used for Fish Preservation. *J. Food Saf.* **2016**, *37*, e12285. [CrossRef]

7

Myocardial Adiponectin Isoform Shift in Dogs with Congestive Heart Failure-A Comparison to Hibernating Brown Bears (*Ursus arctos horribilis*)

O. Lynne Nelson [1,*], Rachael M. Wood [1], Jens Häggström [2], Clarence Kvart [3] and Charles T. Robbins [4]

[1] Department of Veterinary Clinical Sciences, Washington State University, Pullman, WA 99164, USA; rwood@vetmed.wsu.edu
[2] Department of Clinical Sciences and Anatomy, Physiology and Biochemistry, Swedish University of Agricultural Sciences, Uppsala 750 07, Sweden; jens.haggstrom@slu.se
[3] Faculty of Veterinary Medicine and Animal Science, Swedish University of Agricultural Sciences, Uppsala 750 07, Sweden; clarence.kvart@slu.se
[4] School of the Environment and School of Biological Sciences, Washington State University, Pullman, WA 99164, USA; ctrobbins@wsu.edu
* Correspondence: olnelson@vetmed.wsu.edu

Academic Editors: Sonja Fonfara and Lynne O'Sullivan

Abstract: Adiponectin is the most abundant plasma adipokine, and is well known for its role in energy homeostasis and cardiac protection. In humans with dilated cardiomyopathy, myocardial adiponectin protein expression is reduced compared to normal hearts and has been implicated in the pathology of cardiomyopathy. Serum adiponectin levels are often conflicting, with higher levels associated with poor survival in humans with congestive heart failure (CHF). We evaluated adiponectin serum concentrations and myocardial protein expression in dogs with naturally occurring myxomatous mitral valve disease and CHF. We compared the findings to active and hibernating brown bears as bears are adapted to endure an extreme period of low cardiac output during their annual hibernation. Bears exhibited largely the active high-molecular weight (HMW) versus the low-molecular weight isoforms of myocardial adiponectin (HMW:LMW = 6.3) during both the active period and hibernation, while healthy dogs exhibited a more balanced mix of isoforms. Dogs with CHF expressed predominately HMW isoforms of adiponectin (HMW:LMW = 12.5), appearing more similar to bears. In contrast to humans, serum adiponectin was significantly lower in dogs with CHF and lowest levels in the severest CHF class. In both dogs and bears, myocardial adiponectin was expressed independent of circulating adiponectin concentrations, suggesting a local regulatory mechanism within the heart.

Keywords: low molecular weight adiponectin; high molecular weight adiponectin; chronic valvular heart disease; endocardiosis; hibernation

1. Introduction

Adiponectin is a primarily adipose tissue-derived cytokine that plays a key role in both metabolic and cardiac health. Adiponectin is the most abundant plasma adipokine, and is well known for its role in energy homeostasis and insulin sensitivity [1–3]. It is an essential protein for animals living in highly seasonal environments which must rely on annually switching from lipogenic to lipolytic states [4–7]. In contrast to other adipokines, serum adiponectin is inversely related to visceral obesity in humans [1,8]. Clinically, serum adiponectin concentrations are also inversely related to the risk of developing type II diabetes and cardiovascular disease, but directly related to decompensated congestive heart failure (CHF) [1,8–13]. Thus, these seemingly conflicting results are generating much interest into the systemic modulatory effects of this adipokine.

Adiponectin regulates metabolism in part by promoting the phosphorylation and activation of AMP-activated protein kinase (AMPK) via the AdipoR1 receptor in skeletal muscle, adipose, and endothelial cells where it regulates glucose and lipid metabolism. The AdipoR2 receptor is expressed primarily in the liver, and its activation leads to increased insulin sensitivity [10,14–16]. The third adiponectin receptor—T-cadherin—is expressed predominantly in the heart and vasculature, and produces diverse myocardial and vascular protective effects, such as suppression of myocardial remodeling, and reduction of reactive oxygen species and pro-inflammatory cytokines [17,18]. There are multiple oligomeric forms of adiponectin that affect its activity. The isoforms are grouped into low-molecular weight (LMW, predominately in serum) and high-molecular weight (HMW, predominantly intracellular) [19,20]. Levels of the HMW isoform have better correlations with insulin sensitivity than total adiponectin, suggesting that the HMW isoform is the active form [21–25]. T-cadherin exclusively binds with HMW adiponectin. Studies in rodents deficient in T-cadherin have demonstrated pathologic cardiac hypertrophy, and worsening of inflammation and myocardial reperfusion injury [17]. Additional studies in animal models have demonstrated that increased expression of adiponectin can improve systolic function, inhibit protein synthesis, and retard cardiac remodeling [25–28]. In humans with dilated cardiomyopathy (DCM), myocardial adiponectin protein expression is reduced compared to normal hearts, and has been implicated in the pathology of cardiomyopathy [29]. Adiponectin is produced by the myocardium, and is released in proportion to the extent of left ventricular dysfunction which may in part explain the increased serum levels seen in humans with CHF [30].

Heart failure is no longer considered to be a single organ disease, but is now seen as a complex multisystem syndrome involving hemodynamic, neurohormonal, and metabolic alterations. Adiponectin has recently emerged as an important metabolic component [2,31]; however, interpretation of serum adiponectin concentration in human heart disease has been conflicting. On one hand, higher levels of serum adiponectin in the general population are considered healthy and are associated with reduced risk of diabetes mellitus, insulin resistance, systemic hypertension, and cardiovascular events [1,13,32–34]. On the other hand, low adiponectin levels are observed in heart disease without CHF, while the highest concentrations are seen in patients with CHF from any cause and are associated with poor survival. Along with the knowledge of adiponectin's reputed beneficial effects on the heart, this U-shaped relationship of serum adiponectin in cardiac disease has been designated as "the adiponectin paradox" [34,35]. It is unclear if adiponectin has a negative impact on cardiac pathophysiology or if levels may rise to mitigate robust neurohormonal and metabolic impairment in CHF.

We were curious as to the roles of adiponectin in non-human species that manifest cardiac disease and CHF compared to species that might be considered to endure a natural hemodynamic "stress" of extremely low cardiac output. We compared naturally occurring canine CHF due to myxomatous mitral valve disease (MMVD) to hibernating brown bears (*Ursus arctos horribilis*). The reduction in cardiac output of these two conditions has been previously well documented. We felt it could be valuable to contrast native compensatory processes of disease manifestation to a natural physiologic process, as oftentimes the naturally adaptive response may shed light on the potential mechanisms underpinning the maladaptive response. Additionally, bears and dogs are close relatives in the Carnivora clade of mammals, and in general adiponectin appears to be well-conserved across species. We chose to compare canine MMVD (also known as endocardiosis or chronic valvular heart disease), as it is the most common acquired heart disease in dogs that presents for management of CHF. The prevalence of MMVD is high in older smaller breed dogs, with up to 85% showing some evidence of the disease at necropsy by 13 years of age [36,37]. The cause of MMVD is unknown, but the age of onset appears to have an inherited component in some dog breeds [38,39]. Bears are well known for their annual hibernation, where heart rate and cardiac output are reduced to 25% of the active season and maintained at this level for 4–6 months without feeding [40–43]. Hibernation is a natural physiological condition, and thus cardiovascular compensatory adaptations must occur for the myocardium to remain healthy and efficient during a long period of extremely low cardiac output. We hypothesized that active HMW myocardial adiponectin would increase in bears during hibernation if its presence is cardioprotective and associated with an altered myocardial workload. We hypothesized that myocardial HMW adiponectin would decrease and serum adiponectin would increase in dogs with CHF, reflecting decompensated CHF status similar to humans. Comparing a natural bradycardic state in bears that would create cardiac failure in other animals to a pathologic cardiac state in dogs may highlight adaptive processes.

2. Materials and Methods

2.1. Dogs

Healthy dogs ($n = 18$) and dogs with CHF ($n = 18$) were used to assess serum adiponectin. Dogs were included for sampling in the healthy group if the dog had no reported signs of systemic or cardiopulmonary illness and had a normal cardiovascular examination. The breeds of dogs included were: Beagle, Chihuahua (2), Maltese, Miniature Australian shepherd (2), Miniature Dachshund (2), Norfolk terrier, Pug, and eight mix-breeds. These dogs ranged in age from 4–12 years (mean weight: 8.7 kg). Dogs in the CHF group presented with clinical signs consistent with pulmonary edema and were ultimately diagnosed with decompensated MMVD by radiography and echocardiography. Dogs included for sampling in this study were classified into stage C or D (nine in each stage) according to the guidelines for the diagnosis and treatment of MMVD [36]. The breeds of CHF dogs included were: American Cocker Spaniel (2), Beagle, Brittany, Brussels Griffon (2), French Bulldog, Maltese (2), Miniature Schnauzer (2), Pembroke Welsh Corgi, Silky Terrier, Toy Poodle, and four mix-breeds. These dogs ranged in age from 9–14 years (mean weight: 9.4 kg). Blood samples were collected, spun, and stored at −80 °C.

Canine left ventricular (LV) myocardium was collected from six normal dogs euthanized for reasons unrelated to this study and six dogs that died or were euthanized due to CHF caused by MMVD. The normal dogs ranged in age from 4–9 years and were all mixed-breed (mean weight: 14.3 kg).

The normal dogs did not have an echocardiogram performed prior to death, but no gross cardiac abnormalities were noted on necropsy. The CHF dogs breeds were: Cavalier King Charles Spaniel (3), Miniature Dachshund, Toy Poodle, and terrier-mix. The CHF dogs ranged in age from 9–14 years (mean weight: 9.3 kg). All samples were snap frozen in liquid nitrogen within 30 min of death, and then stored at −80 °C until use. Dogs were client-owned, and owner consent was required for all sampling.

2.2. Bears

Sixteen brown bears (*Ursus arctos horribilis*) were used to assess serum adiponectin (4 males, 12 females). The age range was 2–22 years. All animals were housed at the Washington State University Bear Research, Education and Conservation Center. The animals were maintained according to the Bear Care and Colony Health Standard Operating Procedures approved by the Washington State Institutional Animal Care and Use Committee (Animal Subject Approval Form #3054) based on the U.S. National Institutes of Health guidelines. Hibernation began in early November, and feeding resumed the second week of March. Bears hibernated in pairs in unheated pens with continuous access through a small door to an outdoor area. The dens were monitored with surveillance cameras (Silent Witness, Surrey, BC, Canada) which confirmed that bears were recumbent for the hibernation period. Bears were anesthetized with tiletamine HCl/zolazepam HCl (5 mg/kg during the active phase and 2 mg/kg during hibernation) given intramuscularly. Due to the unique seasonal physiology of this species, blood samples were collected in serum tubes monthly throughout the year, spun and stored at −80 °C within 1 h. Body weights were recorded monthly from April to November in ten bears to correlate weight gain with circulating adiponectin levels in this species. Percent monthly weight gain was recorded to correct for the wide individual variation in size of bears.

Left ventricular (LV) myocardium was collected from 12 grizzly bears (6 male, 6 female) euthanized for reasons unrelated to this project, generally the completion of ecology-related projects. The bears were considered healthy at the time of euthanasia. The age range was 3–22 years. Tissue collection was during active and hibernation periods (n = 6 for each group). The active period tissue collection was during the months of June, July, and August. The hibernation collection period was during the months of December and January. All samples were snap frozen in liquid nitrogen within 30 min of death, and then stored at −80 °C until use. All animal protocols were approved by Washington State University's Institutional Animal Care and Use Committee (Animal Subject Approval Form #3054).

2.3. Serum Adiponectin

Circulating adiponectin concentrations were quantified using a Mouse/Rat Adiponectin ELISA kit (B-Bridge International Inc., Mountain View, CA, USA) that has been previously validated in dogs and bears [44]. We chose to use one kit/method for both species versus using a canine ELISA kit which have been validated for dogs but not for bears. Additionally, we avoided using two different test kits, which could introduce assay variability.

2.4. Western Blot Protocol

Left ventricular free wall myocardium samples were used to evaluate protein levels of adiponectin by Western Blot. Approximately 150 mg of tissue was frozen in liquid nitrogen and ground to a fine powder using a mortar and pestle. The tissue was transferred to a 7 mL tissue homogenizer and allowed to temper in a −20 °C freezer for 30 min, then homogenized in 1 mL Pierce IP lysis buffer with 10 µL Halt Protease Inhibitor cocktail (Thermo Fisher Scientific, Rockford, IL, USA). The tissue lysate was transferred to a 1.5 mL Eppendorf tube and centrifuged at 13,000 × g at 4 °C for 10 min. The supernatant was collected, and protein concentration determined by the bicinchoninic acid assay (BCA) method and stored at −80 °C until use.

Velocity sedimentation was used to separate the adiponectin isomers as previously described [45]. Five-hundred micrograms of protein was diluted in 10 mM HEPES, pH 8, 125 mM NaCl, and layered on a 5–20% sucrose gradient in 10 mM HEPES, pH 8, 125 mM NaCl. The gradient was spun on an ultracentrifuge at 55,000 rpm for 4 h at 4 °C. Fractions were removed in 150 µL aliquots (labeled fractions 1–14), taken from the top of the gradient, and stored at −80 °C until use.

Ten microliters of each fraction was added to 6× Laemmli buffer and heated to 95 °C for 5 min to denature the protein. Protein samples were loaded onto a precast gel (12% Tris-HCL ReadyGel, Bio-Rad Laboratories, Inc., Hercules, CA, USA) along with a protein standard (Precision Plus Protein Standards, Bio-Rad Laboratories, Inc., Hercules, CA, USA) and run at 150 V for one hour in 1× Tris/Glycine/SDS (TGS, Bio-Rad Laboratories, Inc., Hercules, CA, USA). The protein was then transferred to 0.2 µm pore nitrocellulose membrane in 20% methanol in 1× TGS transfer buffer for 3 h at 200 mA. The membrane was blocked in 5% nonfat dry milk in Tris Buffered Saline with 0.05% Tween 20 (TBS-T) at room temperature for one hour. The membrane was washed three times for 3 min with TBS-T and primary antibody 1:1000 rabbit anti-adiponectin (Sigma-Aldrich, St Louis, MO, USA) and 1:1000 anti-adipoR1 (Thermo Fisher Scientific, Rockford, IL, USA) diluted in 1% bovine serum albumin (BSA) in TBS-T was placed on the membrane and allowed to incubate overnight at 4 °C on a rocker. The membrane was washed five times in TBS-T for 5 min and then allowed to incubate in secondary antibody (1:20,000 Immun-Star Goat anti-rabbit HRP conjugate and 1:10,000 Precision Protein StrepTactin-HRP conjugate, Bio-Rad Laboratories, Inc., Hercules, CA, USA) diluted in TBS-T at room temperature for one hour on a shaker. A commercial kit (Immun-Star WesternC Chemiluminescent kit, Bio-Rad Laboratories, Inc., Hercules, CA, USA) was used according to manufacturer's instructions for the detection of secondary antibody. Images were captured using a gel imaging system (ChemiDoc XRS Imager,

Bio-Rad Laboratories, Inc., Hercules, CA, USA). Band density targeting adiponectin was determined for fractions obtained from sucrose gradients and plotted for each sample. Fractions 3–6 contained the LMW isoforms of adiponectin, and fractions 9–12 contained the HMW isoforms (Figure 1).

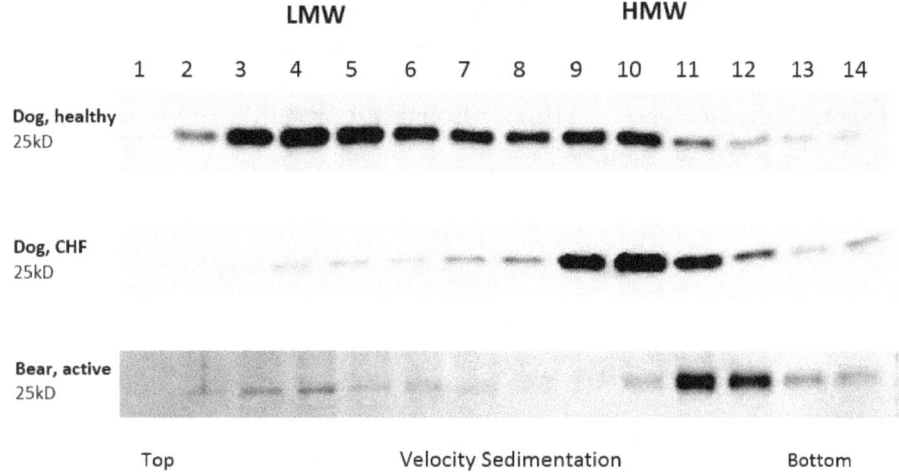

Figure 1. Identification of myocardial adiponectin fractions from velocity sucrose gradient sedimentation in a healthy dog, dog with congestive heart failure (CHF), and an active bear. Fractions 3–6 contain the low-molecular weight form (LMW) and 9–12 contain the high-molecular weight form (HMW).

2.5. Statistical Analysis

Analysis was performed using commercial statistical software (JMP SAS, Cary, NC, USA). For serum samples and Western blot samples, statistical analysis was performed using a decision tree. For paired data (measured on the same animal), the normality of the protein differences was assessed using the Shapiro–Wilk test. If significant at a level of 0.05, the nonparametric Wilcoxon signed rank test was used. If not significant, the paired t-test was used. Both tests were conducted to evaluate differences in protein between hibernating and active bears, and healthy dogs and dogs with CHF. Paired-samples t-tests have been shown to be appropriate with extremely small sample size, specifically when the within-pair Pearson coefficient is high [46]. For unpaired data, equal variances were assessed using Levene's test, and normality of residuals were assessed using the Shapiro-Wilk test. If normality was achieved, then a two-sample t-test with either equal variances (Levene's test not significant) or unequal variances (Levene's test significant) was used. If normality was not achieved, the nonparametric Wilcoxon rank-sum test was used. A p-value of <0.05 was considered significant. All data are presented as mean $\pm$ standard deviation.

3. Results

Mean serum adiponectin concentration was significantly higher in healthy dogs (12.1 $\pm$ 2.9 µg/mL, n = 18) than in dogs with all classes of CHF (8.4 $\pm$ 2.6 µg/mL, n = 18, p = 0.001; Figure 2).

The serum concentration of adiponectin in bears varied seasonally, and was significantly lower during hibernation (November–February, 2.6 $\pm$ 0.8 µg/mL) than during the summer active period (April–August, 6.5 $\pm$ 0.5 µg/mL) (Figure 3). Its concentration increased dramatically in September (12.1 $\pm$ 1.5 µg/mL) after rapid weight gain occurred in August (fall hyperphagia). Adiponectin declined rapidly in October and November.

Healthy dogs expressed similar myocardial concentrations of HMW (10.8 $\pm$ 3.4 µg/mL) and LMW (9.2 $\pm$ 2.9 µg/mL, p = 0.46) adiponectin isoforms, whereas CHF dogs expressed significantly greater concentrations of HMW isoforms (18.8 $\pm$ 2.6 µg/mL, p < 0.001) and significantly lower concentrations of LMW isoforms (1.5 ± 0.2 μg/mL, $p = 0.005$) adiponectin (Figures 4 and 5). The ratio of HMW:LMW adiponectin expression in the healthy dog myocardium was 1.2, whereas the ratio of HMW:LMW adiponectin expression in dogs with CHF was 12.5. The increase in myocardial HMW adiponectin in CHF dogs was contrary to the decreasing circulating serum concentration in this group. Bears expressed a higher concentration of HMW isoforms in both the active: (19.5 ± 3.8 μg/mL) and hibernation states (18.9 ± 2.6 μg/mL) relative to LMW isoforms (active: 3.1 ± 1.8 μg/mL, hibernation: 3.0 ± 1.6 μg/mL, $p \leq 0.0001$; Figures 4 and 5), and the ratio of HMW:LMW isoforms did not change seasonally ($p = 0.93$). Cardiac adiponectin protein expression was independent of circulating adiponectin seasonal changes.

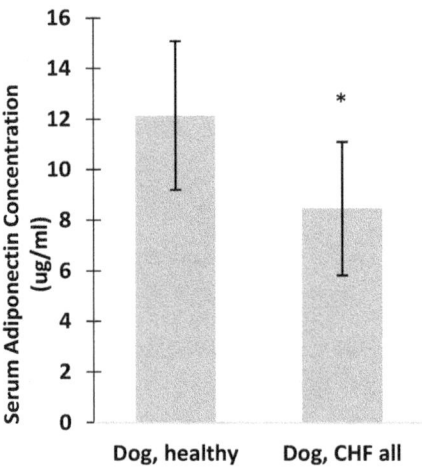

Figure 2. Mean serum adiponectin concentration was significantly higher in healthy dogs ($n = 18$) than in dogs with all classes of CHF ($n = 18$), * $p = 0.001$.

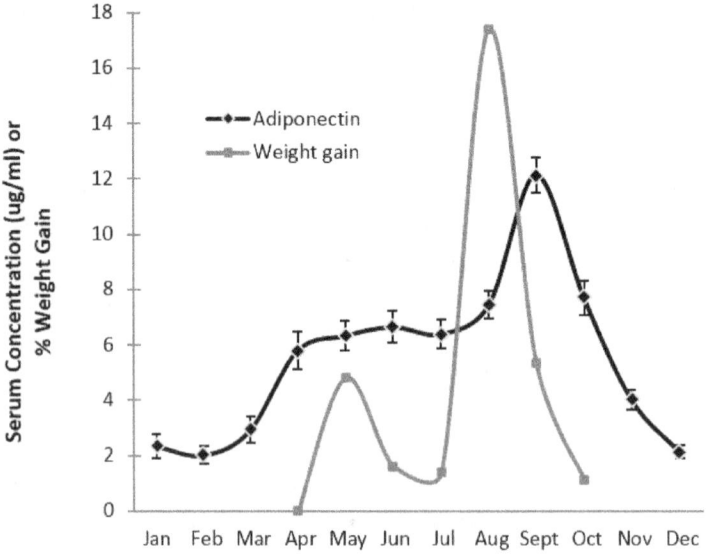

Figure 3. Monthly measurement of serum adiponectin compared to percent weight gain in 16 brown bears. Adiponectin data presented as means ± SD. The concentration of adiponectin mirrored weight gain through the active season (April–October) and peaked as rapid weight gain occurred in August and September. Serum adiponectin was significantly lower during hibernation (November–February) relative to the summer active period.

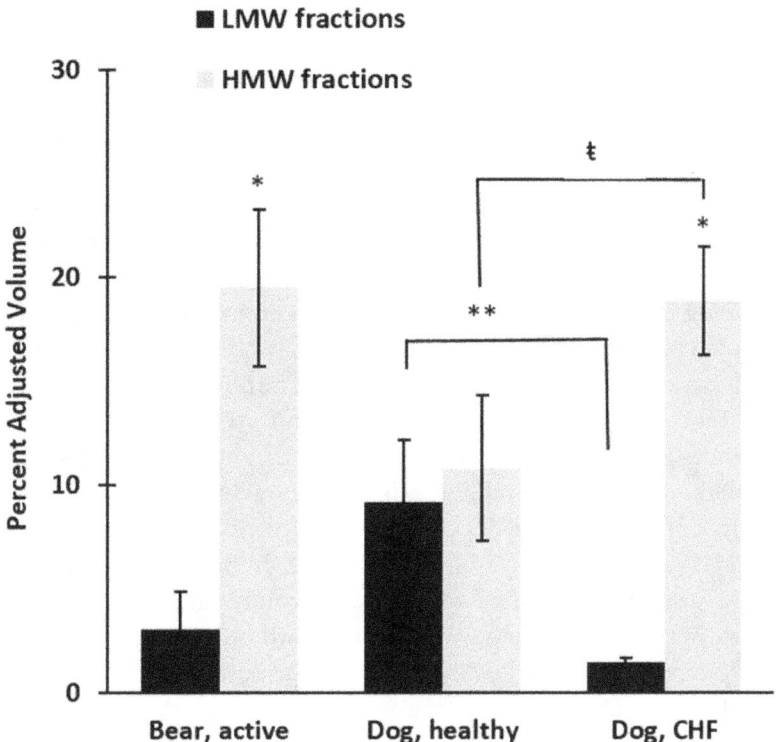

Figure 4. Pooled LMW and HMW fractions of myocardial adiponectin protein in six active bears, six healthy dogs, and six dogs with congestive heart failure (CHF). Fractions 3–6 contain the LMW isoforms of adiponectin and fractions 9–12 contain the HMW isoforms. Bears expressed 6.3 times greater concentration of HMW isoforms relative to LMW isoforms in both active period and hibernation. Healthy dogs expressed similar amounts of adiponectin isoforms, but dogs with CHF expressed 12 times greater concentrations of the HMW isoforms. * $p < 0.0001$; ** $p = 0.005$; ŧ $p < 0.001$.

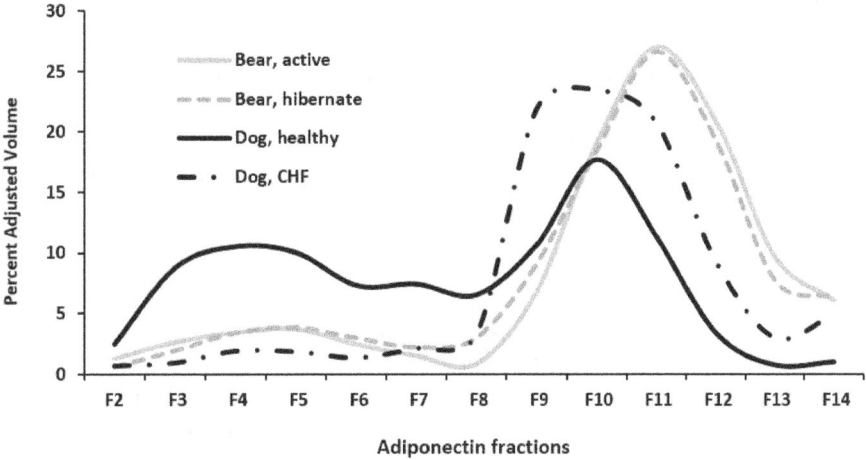

Figure 5. Band density targeting myocardial adiponectin was determined for fractions obtained from sucrose gradients and plotted for each group. Fractions 3–6 contain the LMW isoforms of adiponectin and fractions 9–12 contain the HMW isoforms. All bears expressed a higher concentration of HMW isoforms relative to LMW isoforms of adiponectin, and no significant difference was found between the active ($n = 6$) and hibernating bears ($n = 6$). Healthy dogs ($n = 6$) expressed similar myocardial concentrations of LMW and HMW adiponectin isoforms, whereas CHF dogs ($n = 6$) expressed significantly greater concentrations of HMW relative to LMW adiponectin.

4. Discussion

The healthy dog myocardium expressed similar concentrations of HMW versus LMW adiponectin proteins, while CHF dogs expressed predominately the HMW isoforms (more than 12 times the LMW isoforms). The CHF dogs mirrored the bears' myocardial adiponectin expression, as bears exhibited a predominance of HMW adiponectin in both the active and hibernating seasons (Figures 4 and 5). High molecular weight adiponectin is the more active form, and could serve as a compensatory response for myocardial pathology in the dog. Animal model studies have demonstrated that increased expression of myocardial adiponectin can improve systolic function, inhibit protein synthesis, and retard cardiac remodeling [25–28]. As such, HMW adiponectin may be compensatory or protective in dogs with MMVD. In humans with DCM, myocardial adiponectin expression is reduced compared to normal individuals, independent of serum concentrations, implicating adiponectin in the pathology of the disease [29]. Since cardiomyocytes synthesize and secrete adiponectin, and blockage of protein secretion induces upregulation of adiponectin receptors, this suggests the existence of an auto/paracrine regulation within the heart [29,30]. It is unclear why myocardial adiponectin expression is increased dogs with CHF due to MMVD compared to the decrease seen in humans. The reason may be linked to a species-specific physiologic response or due to the different type of cardiac condition evaluated. Myxomatous mitral valve disease is a condition that causes volume overload and compensatory eccentric hypertrophy of otherwise normal cardiomyocytes, whereas DCM is a primary dysfunction of the cardiomyocyte [29,36]. A dysfunctional response may be more likely to result from primary muscle defect such as DCM.

In addition, adiponectin expression in humans with cardiac disease may be confounded by high body mass index or type II diabetes, as there are more clear effects on adiponectin in humans with these conditions than in dogs [1,15,47,48]. High molecular weight adiponectin is also predominately expressed in the bear. Brown bears may need to maintain HMW adiponectin, as they have dramatically reduced cardiac output during hibernation, have evolved to accumulate large fat deposits in the fall, and subsequently switch from a lipogenic to lipolytic state as they enter hibernation [5]. In both the bear and dog, myocardial adiponectin is expressed independent of circulating adiponectin levels suggesting a local regulatory mechanism within the heart.

In contrast to humans, dogs with CHF had significantly reduced serum adiponectin concentrations (Figure 2). It is unknown if the discordance in serum level represents a species-related difference, a difference in cardiac disease evaluated, increased adiponectin utilization, or perhaps a decompensatory process. Discrepant studies suggest body condition score and neuter status of dogs may be important in interpreting serum adiponectin levels. These factors were not accounted for in this study. Total adiponectin is measured in serum, which consists of mainly the LMW isoform [1,19,20]. Total adiponectin could theoretically decline due to utilization of the HMW isoform and clearance from the serum, although this has not been evaluated in dogs or humans.

Serum adiponectin in bears mirrored the change in weight gain over the summer months, then serum levels rapidly declined once hibernation began (Figure 3). The annual requirements for massive fat accumulation and maintenance of glucose metabolism to survive hibernation imply that adiponectin is directly related to weight gain and differs from the negative relationship that is found in humans. The association of adiponectin to percent body fat in active bears has been described [5]. Adiponectin is then uncoupled with adiposity in bears during hibernation, and marks the switch to insulin resistance, facilitating a lipolytic state [5]. In winter, bears show some similarity to humans, as very low levels of serum adiponectin are also used as a marker of insulin resistance in humans [1]. Due to the multiple metabolic functions of adiponectin (in heart, fat, vascular, liver, and muscle tissue), serum levels are not likely to be an adequate marker of tissue stores in the heart. We suspect myocardial adiponectin to be more directly related to cardiac physiology requirements and less affected by peripheral factors. For example, cardiac expression of adiponectin is maintained during extremely low cardiac output in hibernation (despite low circulating levels), implying that adiponectin is necessary for cardiac metabolism during this time. Thus, the upregulation of cardiac HMW adiponectin in the dog could suggest that adiponectin is also desirable in CHF due to MMVD. These data underscore the value of comparative physiology research by highlighting the value of contrasting native compensatory responses to disease manifestation. This approach could detect potential mechanisms of pathology or adaptation.

Study Limitations

The authors acknowledge that this is a small study with few numbers of animals, particularly of myocardial tissues. The diseases and states compared are somewhat different between species and patho/physiology observed. The proportion of measured serum adiponectin isoforms (LMH vs. HMW) is unknown, as only total serum adiponectin is measured.

Acknowledgments: We are indebted to the talented and dedicated graduate, undergraduate, and veterinary students at the Washington State University Bear Research Education and Conservation Center who have participated in this work.

Author Contributions: O. Lynne Nelson and Rachael M. Wood conceived and designed the experiments; O. Lynne Nelson and Rachael M. Wood performed the experiments; O. Lynne Nelson and Charles T. Robbins analyzed the data; Jens Häggström and Clarence Kvart contributed samples to the project; O. Lynne Nelson wrote the paper.

References

1. Balsan, G.A.; Vieira, J.L.; Oliveira, A.M.; Portal, V.L. Relationship between adiponectin, obesity and insulin resistance. *Rev. Assoc. Med. Bras.* **2015**, *61*, 72–80. [CrossRef] [PubMed]

2. Parker-Duffen, J.L.; Walsh, K. Cardiometabolic effects of adiponectin. *Best Pract. Res. Clin. Endocrinol. Metab.* **2014**, *28*, 81–91. [CrossRef] [PubMed]

3. Oh, D.K.; Ciaraldi, T.; Henry, R.R. Adiponectin in health and disease. *Diabetes Obes. Metab.* **2007**, *9*, 282–289. [CrossRef] [PubMed]

4. Florant, G.L.; Porst, H.; Peiffer, A.; Hudachek, S.F.; Pittman, C.; Summers, S.A.; Rajala, M.W.; Scherer, P.E. Fat-cell mass, serum leptin and adiponectin changes during weight gain and loss in yellow-bellied marmots (Marmota flaviventris). *J. Comp. Physiol. B* **2004**, *174*, 633–639. [CrossRef] [PubMed]

5. Rigano, K.S.; Gehring, J.L.; Evans Hutzenbiler, B.D.; Chen, A.V.; Nelson, O.L.; Vella, C.A.; Robbins, C.T.; Jansen, H.J. Life in the fat lane: Seasonal regulation of insulin sensitivity, food intake, and adipose biology in brown bears. *J. Comp. Physiol. B* **2017**, *187*, 649–676. [CrossRef] [PubMed]

6. Wong, G.W.; Wang, J.; Hug, C.; Tsao, T.S.; Lodish, H.F. A family of Acrp30/adiponectin structural and functional paralogs. *Proc. Natl. Acad. Sci. USA* **2004**, *101*, 10302–10307. [CrossRef] [PubMed]

7. Weitten, M.; Robin, J.P.; Oudart, H.; Pévet, P.; Habold, C. Hormonal changes and energy substrate availability during the hibernation cycle of Syrian hamsters. *Horm. Behav.* **2013**, *64*, 611–617. [CrossRef] [PubMed]

8. Steffes, M.W.; Gross, M.D.; Schreiner, P.J.; Yu, X.; Hilner, J.E.; Gingerich, R.; Jacobs, D.R., Jr. Serum adiponectin in young adults—Interactions with central adiposity, circulating levels of glucose, and insulin resistance: The CARDIA study. *Ann. Epidemiol.* **2004**, *14*, 492–498. [CrossRef] [PubMed]

9. Hopkins, T.A.; Ouchi, N.; Shibata, R.; Walsh, K. Adiponectin actions in the cardiovascular system. *Cardiovasc. Res.* **2007**, *74*, 11–18. [CrossRef] [PubMed]

10. Berg, A.H.; Combs, T.P.; Du, X.; Brownlee, M.; Scherer, P.E. The adipocyte-secreted protein Acrp30 enhances hepatic insulin action. *Nat. Med.* **2001**, *7*, 947–953. [CrossRef] [PubMed]

11. Weyer, C.; Funahashi, T.; Tanaka, S.; Hotta, K.; Matsuzawa, Y.; Pratley, R.E.; Tataranni, P.A. Hypoadiponectinemia in obesity and type 2 diabetes: Close association with insulin resistance and hyperinsulinemia. *J. Clin. Endocrinol. Metab.* **2001**, *86*, 1930–1935. [CrossRef] [PubMed]

12. Lee, Y.; Kim, B.K.; Lim, Y.H.; Kim, M.K.; Choi, B.Y.; Shin, J. The relationship between adiponectin and left ventricular mass index varies with the risk of left ventricular hypertrophy. *PLoS ONE* **2013**, *8*, e70246. [CrossRef] [PubMed]

13. George, J.; Patal, S.; Wexler, D.; Sharabi, Y.; Peleg, E.; Kamari, Y.; Grossman, E.; Sheps, D.; Keren, G.; Roth, A. Circulating adiponectin concentrations in patients with congestive heart failure. *Heart* **2006**, *92*, 1420–1424. [CrossRef] [PubMed]

14. Kadowaki, T.; Yamauchi, T. Adiponectin and adiponectin receptors. *Endocr. Rev.* **2005**, *26*, 439–451. [CrossRef] [PubMed]

15. Kadowaki, T.; Yamauchi, T.; Kubota, N.; Hara, K.; Ueki, K. Adiponectin and adiponectin receptors in obesity-linked insulin resistance. *Novartis Found. Symp.* **2007**, *286*, 164–176, discussion 76–82, 200–203. [PubMed]

16. Yamauchi, T.; Nio, Y.; Maki, T.; Kobayashi, M.; Takazawa, T.; Iwabu, M.; Okada-Iwabu, M.; Kawamoto, S.; Kubota, N.; Kubota, T.; et al. Targeted disruption of AdipoR1 and AdipoR2 causes abrogation of adiponectin binding and metabolic actions. *Nat. Med.* **2007**, *13*, 332–339. [CrossRef] [PubMed]

17. Denzel, M.S.; Scimia, M.C.; Zumstein, P.M.; Walsh, K.; Ruiz-Lozano, P.; Ranscht, B. T-cadherin is critical for adiponectin-mediated cardioprotection in mice. *J. Clin. Invest.* **2010**, *120*, 4342–4352. [CrossRef] [PubMed]

18. Hug, C.; Wang, J.; Ahmad, N.S.; Bogan, J.S.; Tsao, T.S.; Lodish, H.F. T-cadherin is a receptor for hexameric and high-molecular-weight forms of Acrp30/adiponectin. *Proc. Natl. Acad. Sci. USA* **2004**, *101*, 10308–10313. [CrossRef] [PubMed]

19. Tsao, T.S.; Tomas, E.; Murrey, H.E.; Hug, C.; Lee, D.H.; Ruderman, N.B.; Heuser, J.E.; Lodish, H.F. Role of disulfide bonds in Acrp30/adiponectin structure and signaling specificity. Different oligomers activate different signal transduction pathways. *J. Biol. Chem.* **2003**, *278*, 50810–50817. [CrossRef] [PubMed]

20. Waki, H.; Yamauchi, T.; Kamon, J.; Kita, S.; Ito, Y.; Hada, Y.; Uchida, S.; Tsuchida, A.; Takekawa, S.; Kadowaki, T. Generation of globular fragment of adiponectin by leukocyte elastase secreted by monocytic cell line THP-1. *Endocrinology* **2005**, *146*, 790–796. [CrossRef] [PubMed]

21. Han, S.H.; Quon, M.J.; Kim, J.A.; Koh, K.K. Adiponectin and cardiovascular disease: Response to therapeutic interventions. *J. Am. Coll. Cardiol.* **2007**, *49*, 531–538. [CrossRef] [PubMed]

22. Pajvani, U.B.; Hawkins, M.; Combs, T.P.; Rajala, M.W.; Doebber, T.; Berger, J.P.; Wagner, J.A.; Wu, M.; Knopps, A.; Xiang, A.H.; Utzschneider, K.M.; Kahn, S.E.; Olefsky, J.M.; Buchanan, T.A.; Scherer, P.E. Complex distribution, not absolute amount of adiponectin, correlates with thiazolidinedione-mediated improvement in insulin sensitivity. *J. Biol. Chem.* **2004**, *279*, 12152–12162. [CrossRef] [PubMed]

23. Kissebah, A.H.; Sonnenberg, G.E.; Myklebust, J.; Goldstein, M.; Broman, K.; James, R.G.; Marks, J.A.; Krakower, G.R.; Jacob, H.J.; Weber, J.; Martin, L.; Blangero, J.; Comuzzie, A.G. Quantitative trait loci on chromosomes 3 and 17 influence phenotypes of the metabolic syndrome. *Proc. Natl. Acad. Sci. USA* **2000**, *97*, 14478–14483. [CrossRef] [PubMed]

24. Heidemann, C.; Sun, Q.; van Dam, R.M.; Meigs, J.B.; Zhang, C.; Tworoger, S.S.; Mantzoros, C.S.; Hu, F.B. Total and high-molecular-weight adiponectin and resistin in relation to the risk for type 2 diabetes in women. *Ann. Intern. Med.* **2008**, *149*, 307–316. [CrossRef] [PubMed]

25. Nanayakkara, G.; Kariharan, T.; Wang, L.; Zhong, J.; Amin, R. The cardio-protective signaling and mechanisms of adiponectin. *Am. J. Cardiovasc. Dis.* **2012**, *2*, 253–266. [PubMed]

26. Ouchi, N.; Shibata, R.; Walsh, K. Cardioprotection by adiponectin. *Trends Cardiovasc. Med.* **2006**, *16*, 141–146. [CrossRef] [PubMed]

27. Liao, Y.; Takashima, S.; Maeda, N.; Ouchi, N.; Komamura, K.; Shimomura, I.; Hori, M.; Matsuzawa, Y.; Funahashi, T.; Kitakaze, M. Exacerbation of heart failure in adiponectin-deficient mice due to impaired regulation of AMPK and glucose metabolism. *Cardiovasc. Res.* **2005**, *67*, 705–713. [CrossRef] [PubMed]

28. Shibata, R.; Ouchi, N.; Ito, M.; Kihara, S.; Shiojima, I.; Pimentel, D.R.; Kumada, M.; Sato, K.; Schiekofer, S.; Ohashi, K.; et al. Adiponectin-mediated modulation of hypertrophic signals in the heart. *Nat. Med.* **2004**, *10*, 1384–1389. [CrossRef] [PubMed]

29. Skurk, C.; Wittchen, F.; Suckau, L.; Witt, H.; Noutsias, M.; Fechner, H.; Schultheiss, H.P.; Poller, W. Description of a local cardiac adiponectin system and its deregulation in dilated cardiomyopathy. *Eur. Heart J.* **2008**, *29*, 1168–1180. [CrossRef] [PubMed]

30. Takano, H.; Obata, J.E.; Kodama, Y.; Kitta, Y.; Nakamura, T.; Mende, A.; Kawabata, K.; Saito, Y.; Fujioka, D.; Kobayashi, T.; et al. Adiponectin is released from the heart in patients with heart failure. *Int. J. Cardiol.* **2009**, *132*, 221–226. [CrossRef] [PubMed]

31. Park, M.; Sweeney, G. Direct effects of adipokines on the heart: Focus on adiponectin. *Heart Fail. Rev.* **2013**, *18*, 631–644. [CrossRef] [PubMed]

32. Shinmura, K. Is adiponectin a bystander or a mediator in heart failure? The tangled thread of a good-natured adipokine in aging and cardiovascular disease. *Heart Fail. Rev.* **2010**, *15*, 457–466. [CrossRef] [PubMed]

33. Hao, G.; Li, W.; Guo, R.; Yang, J.G.; Wang, Y.; Tian, Y.; Liu, M.Y.; Peng, Y.G.; Wang, Z.W. Serum total adiponectin level and the risk of cardiovascular disease in general population: A meta-analysis of 17 prospective studies. *Atherosclerosis* **2013**, *228*, 29–35. [CrossRef] [PubMed]

34. Sente, T.; Gevaert, A.; Van Berendoncks, A.; Vrints, C.J.; Hoymans, V.Y. The evolving role of adiponectin as an additive biomarker in HFrEF. *Heart Fail. Rev.* **2016**, *21*, 753–769. [CrossRef] [PubMed]

35. Ohara, T.; Hashimura, K.; Asakura, M.; Ogai, A.; Amaki, M.; Hasegawa, T.; Kanzaki, H.; Sonoda, M.; Nishizawa, H.; Funahashi, T.; Kitakaze, M. Dynamic changes in plasma total and high molecular weight adiponectin levels in acute heart failure. *J. Cardiol.* **2011**, *58*, 181–190. [CrossRef] [PubMed]

36. Atkins, C.; Bonagura, J.; Ettinger, S.; Fox, P.; Gordon, S.; Haggstrom, J.; Hamlin, R.; Keene, B.; Luis-Fuentes, V.; Stepien, R. Guidelines for the diagnosis and treatment of canine chronic valvular heart disease. *J. Vet. Intern. Med.* **2009**, *23*, 1142–1150. [CrossRef] [PubMed]

37. Borgarelli, M.; Savarino, P.; Crosara, S.; Santilli, R.A.; Chiavegato, D.; Poggi, M.; Bellino, C.; La Rosa, G.; Zanatta, R.; Haggstrom, J.; Tarducci, A. Survival characteristics and prognostic variables of dogs with mitral regurgitation attributable to myxomatous valve disease. *J. Vet. Intern. Med.* **2008**, *22*, 120–128. [CrossRef] [PubMed]

38. Olsen, L.H.; Fredholm, M.; Pedersen, H.D. Epidemiology and inheritance of mitral valve prolapse in Dachshunds. *J. Vet. Intern. Med.* **1999**, *13*, 448–456. [CrossRef] [PubMed]

39. Swenson, L.; Häggström, J.; Kvart, C.; Juneja, R.K. Relationship between parental cardiac status in Cavalier King Charles spaniels and prevalence and severity of chronic valvular disease in offspring. *J. Am. Vet. Med. Assoc.* **1996**, *208*, 2009–2012. [PubMed]

40. Laske, T.G.; Garshelis, D.L.; Iaizzo, P.A. Monitoring the wild black bear's reaction to human and environmental stressors. *BMC Physiol.* **2011**, *11*, 13. [CrossRef] [PubMed]

41. Nelson, O.L.; Robbins, C.T. Cardiac function adaptations in hibernating grizzly bears (Ursus arctos horribilis). *J. Comp. Physiol. B* **2010**, *180*, 465–473. [CrossRef] [PubMed]

42. Nelson, O.L.; Robbins, C.T. Cardiovascular function in large to small hibernators: Bears to ground squirrels. *J. Comp. Physiol. B* **2015**, *185*, 265–279. [CrossRef] [PubMed]

43. Toien, O.; Blake, J.; Edgar, D.M.; Grahn, D.A.; Heller, H.C.; Barnes, B.M. Hibernation in black bears: Independence of metabolic suppression from body temperature. *Science* **2011**, *331*, 906–909. [CrossRef] [PubMed]

44. Lusby, A.L.; Kania, S.A.; Abd-Eldaim, M.; Bartges, J.W.; Kirk, C.A. Detection of serum adiponectin in the cat, bear, and horse using antibody from a commerical ELISA kit. *J. Anim. Physiol. Anim. Nutr.* **2008**, *92*, 220–221. [CrossRef]

45. Pajvani, U.B.; Du, X.; Combs, T.P.; Berg, A.H.; Rajala, M.W.; Schulthess, T.; Engel, J.; Brownlee, M.; Scherer, P.E. Structure-function studies of the adipocyte-secreted hormone Acrp30/adiponectin. Implications fpr metabolic regulation and bioactivity. *J. Biol. Chem.* **2003**, *278*, 9073–9085. [CrossRef] [PubMed]

46. De Winter, J.C. Using the Student's *t*-test with extremely small sample sizes. *Pract. Assess. Res. Eval.* **2013**, *18*, 1–12.

47. Tvarijonaviciute, A.; Ceron, J.J.; Holden, S.L.; Cuthbertson, D.J.; Biourge, V.; Morris, P.J.; German, A.J. Obesity-related metabolic dysfunction in dogs: A comparison with human metabolic syndrome. *BMC Vet. Res.* **2012**, *8*, 147. [CrossRef] [PubMed]

48. Tvarijonaviciute, A.; Carrillo-Sanchez, J.D.; García-Martinez, J.D.; Tecles, F.; Martinez-Subiela, S.; German, A.J.; Ceron, J.J. Measurement of salivary adiponectin concentrations in dogs. *Vet. Clin. Pathol.* **2014**, *43*, 416–421. [CrossRef] [PubMed]

8

Inquiring into the Gaps of *Campylobacter* Surveillance Methods

Maria Magana [1], Stylianos Chatzipanagiotou [1], Angeliki R. Burriel [2] and Anastasios Ioannidis [1,2,*]

[1] Department of Biopathology and Clinical Microbiology, Aeginition Hospital, Athens Medical School, Athens 15772, Greece; mariamgn91@gmail.com (M.M.); schatzi@med.uoa.gr (S.C.)

[2] Department of Nursing, Faculty of Human Movement and Quality of Life Sciences, University of Peloponnese, Sparta 23100, Greece; aburriel@uop.gr

* Correspondence: tasobi@uop.gr

Academic Editors: Chrissanthy Papadopoulou, Vangelis Economou and Hercules Sakkas

Abstract: *Campylobacter* is one of the most common pathogen-related causes of diarrheal illnesses globally and has been recognized as a significant factor of human disease for more than three decades. Molecular typing techniques and their combinations have allowed for species identification among members of the *Campylobacter* genus with good resolution, but the same tools usually fail to proceed to subtyping of closely related species due to high sequence similarity. This problem is exacerbated by the demanding conditions for isolation and detection from the human, animal or water samples as well as due to the difficulties during laboratory maintenance and long-term storage of the isolates. In an effort to define the ideal typing tool, we underline the strengths and limitations of the typing methodologies currently used to map the broad epidemiologic profile of campylobacteriosis in public health and outbreak investigations. The application of both the old and the new molecular typing tools is discussed and an indirect comparison is presented among the preferred techniques used in current research methodology.

Keywords: Campylobacteriosis; methodology; molecular typing; human infection; zoonosis; surveillance; epidemiology

1. Introduction

Campylobacter is one of the most common pathogen-related causes in diarrheal illnesses globally and has been recognized as a significant factor of human disease for over three decades [1]. Campylobacteriosis is a self-limiting infection with enteritis, abdominal cramps, fever, nausea and vomiting as the main manifestations. Besides the gastrointestinal symptoms of *Campylobacter* infection, the extra-gastrointestinal manifestations include cases of reactive arthritis, septicemia, endocarditis, meningitis, brain abscesses, bone and soft-tissue infections, periodontitis and the Guillain–Barré and Miller Fisher neurological syndromes [2]. Due to the self-limiting character of the disease, most campylobacteriosis cases simply require supportive therapy including hydration and maintenance of electrolytes balance [3]. Antibiotic therapy is indicated only in severe and persisting infections in sensitive populations including children, the elderly, pregnant women and immunocompromised patients, as well as in cases of extra-gastrointestinal manifestations. Ciprofloxacin is used for the empirical treatment of travel-related gastroenteritis but macrolides are the treatment of choice [4].

The majority of campylobacteriosis cases go undiagnosed or under-reported due to the self-limiting character of the disease. However, according to the Foodborne Diseases Active Surveillance Network (FoodNet), 14 cases of campylobacteriosis are diagnosed per 100,000 population in the United States (U.S.) (approximately 1.3 million persons) and 71 cases per 100,000 population in the European Union (EU) (approximately 200,000 persons) annually [5,6]. Campylobacteriosis is rarely a fatal disease, and rare mortality reports are usually confined to extreme age groups and/or immunocompromised patients [7]. It has been estimated that approximately 76 persons in the US with *Campylobacter* infection die annually, while in the EU the reported deaths in 2015 accounted for 59 in a total number of 229,213 human cases [5,6].

For years, *Salmonella* was the number one cause of enteric infections within the EU representing a significant challenge to public health; however, the scenery has changed since the increased trend of *Campylobacter* spp. infections [8,9]. According to recent data from the European Food Safety Authority (EFSA) and the European Centre for Disease Prevention and Control (ECDC), in terms of zoonoses and foodborne outbreaks, human campylobacteriosis is the most commonly detected zoonosis in the EU exceeding salmonellosis cases [9]. Most animals serve as reservoirs of *Campylobacter* species and only a small number is afflicted by campylobacteriosis [10]. In fact, a decreasing rate of campylobacteriosis cases is reported in animals compared to 2014 in the EU, due to an overall lack of surveillance data. In general, spatiotemporal comparisons of campylobacteriosis incidence rates in various animals among the EU countries are difficult; variations in data acquisition stem from inconsistent sampling procedures and testing methodologies [6].

The diverse members of the *Campylobacter* genus, most commonly represented by *Campylobacter jejuni* and *Campylobacter coli* in both humans and animals, constitute a large number of either unknown or newly identified species. Among the *Campylobacter* species, *Campylobacter jejuni* subsp. *jejuni* is most frequently isolated in human gastroenteritis accounting for approximately 90% of campylobacteriosis cases, followed by *C. coli* [11–13]. According to previous reports, the *Campylobacter* genus consists of 16 species and six subspecies, while the total species number has been rearranged to 36 species including both the "emerging" human and animal pathogens (*Campylobacter upsaliensis, Campylobacter hyointestinalis, Campylobacter ureolyticus, Campylobacter concisus, Campylobacter lari, Campylobacter fetus*) and the novel *Campylobacter hepaticus* sp. nov. [2,14,15].

However, it is of great significance that there has been a failure of phenotypic markers to differentiate isolates at family and genus level, which has historically changed the "map" of the order of Campylobacterales. The exclusion of several species from the *Campylobacter* genus and their new taxonomy into different genera, according to the distance among species in phylogenetic analyses, has gone silent in the past two decades [16]. Namely, *Campylobacter pyloris, Campylobacter cinaedi* and *Campylobacter fennelliae* are now transferred to the *Helicobacter* genus (family of Helicobacteraceae), while *Campylobacter butzleri, Campylobacter nitrofigilis,* and *Campylobacter cryaerophila* are now members of the *Arcobacter* genus (family of Campylobacteraceae) [16–19].

Despite the confusing status regarding the true number of *Campylobacter* species, molecular techniques and their combinations have allowed for species identification among members of the *Campylobacter* genus at a rather increased resolution rate, but the same tools usually fail to proceed to subtyping of closely related species due to high sequence similarity [20]. Typing and subtyping failure does not apply for *C. jejuni* and *C. coli* which are the most popular campylobacters in the research milieu; numerous studies involve the two pathogens and this fact could probably stem from the fact that other clinically significant pathogens have been transferred from the *Campylobacter* genus to another genus as previously discussed. Additionally, there is a gap in determining the link between human infection and the source of infection. The pathogenicity and clinical relevance of the emerged campylobacters are still unidentified and the interrelationship of the environmental reservoirs with the human host remains ambiguous [11].

In an effort to shed light on the above-mentioned inquiries, this review aims to (i) discuss the absence of ideal storage conditions of campylobacters that could facilitate a more comprehensive sample analysis; (ii) critically revisit the inadequacies of detection/identification methods used in laboratory routine; and (iii) underline the strengths and limitations of currently used molecular typing methodologies in mapping the broad epidemiologic profile of campylobacteriosis.

2. Gaps in *Campylobacter* spp. Identification

The argument that we still have no proper appreciation of the relative importance of the emerging species hampers further development of subtyping methods. Greater focus should be placed on closer detection of the emerging species and improved microbiological methods for enhanced cell recovery from clinical and environmental samples. Determination of the relative prevalence of these species in clinical specimens will provide answers regarding the necessity for subtyping methods development for epidemiological investigations.

The first observations suggesting that *Campylobacter*-like isolates are potential human pathogens associated with gastrointestinal infections in both healthy and immunocompromised hosts stems back to the 1980s [21]. Since then, a multitude of novel *Campylobacter* species has emerged, linked with campylobacteriosis manifestations, colonizing a diverse number of niches in human. Reports implicate *C. concisus*, *Campylobacter curvus*, *C. fetus* subsp. *fetus*, *Campylobacter gracilis*, *Campylobacter helveticus*, *Campylobacter hominis*, *C. hyointestinalis*, *C. insulaenigrae*, *C. lari*, *Campylobacter lanienae*, *Campylobacter peloridis*, *Campylobacter mucosalis*, *Campylobacter showae*, *Campylobacter sputorum* biovar *paraureolyticus*, *C. upsaliensis* and *C. ureolyticus* in diarrhea and vomiting [22–33], and most of them have been recovered from blood samples of bacteremic patients [24,28,34–37]. There are also case reports of hospitalized humans due to life-threatening complications by *Campylobacter*-related species (namely *C. concisus*, *C. curvus*, *C. fetus* subsp. *fetus*, *C. gracilis*, *C. rectus*, *C. peloridis*, *C. showae*, *C. sputorum* biovar *sputorum*, *C. upsaliensis* and *C. ureolyticus*) isolated from the cerebrospinal and peritoneal fluid, the axillary nerve, hepatic, lung, genitalia and brain abscesses as well as from soft tissue lesions, bone infections and thoracic empyema [28,38–47]. In animals, the species *C. avium* has been isolated from the cecal contents of chickens and turkeys, *C. canadensis* from the cloacal swabs of whooping crane, *Campylobacter cuniculorum* from the cecal contents of rabbits, *C. subantarcticus* from the fecal swabs of albatross chicks and gentoo penguins, *Campylobacter troglodytis* from the stools of chimpanzees, and *Campylobacter volucris* from the cloacal swabs of gulls [48–53]. In humans, there is one case reporting bacteremia associated with *C. volucris* in a cirrhotic patient with polycythemia vera and one case of *C. troglodytis* isolated from infants' diarrheic stool samples in Tanzania, Bangladesh, and Peru [54,55]. All other *Campylobacter* species found in human are also isolated mostly from the feces of domestic and wild animals implying the fecal-oral route of transmission; however, the complete mechanisms of the human host infection are not completely understood.

The similarity in the isolated species found both in humans and in animals indicate that the environment, including food and water products, plays a significant role in the transmission of emerging *Campylobacter* species. However, their isolation and identification are not easy and always successful procedures. Robust assays targeting features conserved in each species and that can be used to differentiate it from other species would improve the procedure of identification of the various campylobacters [56,57]. But why do emerging *Campylobacter* spp. detection and identification fail? Apart from the protocols for the laboratory growth and isolation of the fastidious *Campylobacter* spp. that may not be routinely followed (hydrogen-enriched atmospheric conditions, antibiotic-enriched culture media, incubation for up to 7 days with close monitoring of growth), the contamination from non-fastidious microorganisms, the delayed specimens handling, as well as the isolates loss during extensive freeze-thaw cycles and suboptimal storage of the bacterial samples set inevitable risk factors for detection and identification failure. The isolates loss is a "silent risk" that affects the survival and the identification at species and strain-level, and has raised concerns to the scientific community, creating the need for optimal storage and maintenance conditions. The thermophilic *Campylobacter* is particularly sensitive in temperature changes, thus extensive freeze—thaw procedures lead to reduction of the population of *Campylobacter* spp., entrance in the viable but non-culturable (VBNC) state, and potential loss of novel species and/or strains [14,58].

For years, the *Campylobacter* storage has been a hot issue and several protocols have emerged. Additionally, the existence of the "protective shield" of a multispecies biofilm community could hide a wide array of emerging *Campylobacter* species, while the metabolically inactive persister cells which can effectively "escape" adverse environments and regain the ability to cause infection when found in optimal circumstances may also lead the identification process to erroneous results [11,59]. Finally, the VBNC campylobacters that retain their virulence and physiology—but cannot be cultured in standard culture media—are highly resistant to external stresses such as pasteurization, and their presence in food sets a serious challenge for public health [60–62].

Laboratory diagnosis of campylobacteriosis caused by species other than *C. jejuni* and *C. coli* is complicated due to the demanding growth and identification procedures of the various subsets of species. Both the culture-dependent (biochemical tests) and culture-independent (PCR-polymerase chain reaction, immunological assays) methodologies present inconsistent and suboptimal data regarding sensitivity, providing evidence that there is not a single gold standard method for *Campylobacter* identification, but the preferred path is the combinatorial application of the available molecular methods [2]. Traditional culture-dependent methods based on colony appearance on charcoal cefoperazone deoxycholate agar (CCDA) or other *Campylobacter*-specific media in the presence of antibiotics, microaerobically incubated at 41.5 °C for 48 h, followed by typical biochemical testing (oxidase/catalase tests, hippurate hydrolysis) in pure cultures, often fail to properly identify pathogens at species and strain level [63–65]. Culture-dependent methods serve in the identification of phenotypic traits but fail to overcome the burden of high sequence similarity of the *Campylobacter* species.

Culture-independent methods include molecular identification by using nucleic acid amplification tests (NAATs), offering enhanced sensitivity in the determination of the bacterial genetic traits [2,65]. PCR amplification of the 16S rRNA gene is a popular tool for *Campylobacter* detection; however, PCR is a labor-intensive and time-consuming methodology and the fact that the 16S rRNA gene needs species-specific primers fails to differentiate closely related *Campylobacter* species [66–68]. A costly yet reliable solution to this problem is the construction of a phylogenetic tree by combining the 16S and 23S rRNA genes with the internal transcribed spacer (ITS) region, offering a high-resolution differentiation at a species and strain level [31]. Another culture-independent method is protein composition analysis of the bacterial cell by using the principle of the matrix-assisted laser desorption ionization time of flight mass spectrometry (MALDI-TOF MS). This method offers pure bacteria culture identification at the species-level in a time-efficient manner, requires less effort than the DNA-based methods, is cost-effective and provides reproducible results with high sensitivity [69]. Another key property of this method is its ability to identify multiple members of the *Campylobacter* genus in mixed cultures [70]. MALDI-TOF MS has been applied for species-level identification for a wide array of campylobacters as they are the well-known *C. jejuni, C. coli,* as well as for the emerging *C. lari, C. fetus, C. hyointestinalis, C. upsaliensis, and C. sputorum* [70,71]. Novel taxa differentiation at the subspecies level in the emerging campylobacters group would be difficult by applying conventional phenotypic tests. However, MALDI-TOF MS enables such a discrimination through phenotypic biomarkers [72].

3. Molecular Typing Tools: Getting to Know Each Other

Molecular typing tools (i) are widely applied in the identification of novel bacterial strains, (ii) aid the discrimination of closely related isolates, (iii) aim at the study of the bacterial organization at the genome level, and (iv) track infection patterns and routes of transmission [57,73]. Molecular methodologies for the differentiation of *Campylobacter* at species and strain level have overcome the burdens of traditional phenotype-based techniques and have enhanced the discrimination power in epidemiology surveillance and outbreak detection; nevertheless, the reported cases of *Campylobacter* infections to date reflect only partially the actual magnitude of the disease [56,74]. Accuracy is the number one factor in strain differentiation and identification, therefore, careful processing of data is a necessity for molecular epidemiology regarding both human infections and environmental surveys. In general, high quality typeability is mandatory for all typing methods, yet the choice of the ideal method should be based on the epidemiological and spatiotemporal context to be applied and should incorporate several features in order to meet specific practical requirements [75,76].

In the clinical setting as well as in research laboratories, the implementation of molecular typing methods requires rapid and easy-to-perform analysis. Another significant characteristic of the ideal typing method should be deployability, therefore offering high-throughput techniques by using standard and inexpensive laboratory equipment [56,76]. The validation of the tools applied for molecular typing must meet performance criteria referring to the stability, reproducibility and the portability of the analysis [57]. Molecular typing tools allow accessibility from electronic databases offering surveillance at a larger scale. Improved bioinformatics algorithms for data mining and sharing have made it possible for *Campylobacter* typing networks to universally communicate the results of phylogenetic analyses.

Typing methods should incorporate versatility by providing high discriminatory power to identify the isolates relatedness in order to link the causative agent with the outcome either for foodborne outbreaks detection or longitudinal surveillance [76]. In this section we will focus on the most widely used molecular typing techniques that are at the forefront of current research (Figure 1). Molecular methods based on DNA electrophoresis or single loci analysis, including pulsed-field gel electrophoresis (PFGE) fingerprinting, restriction fragment length polymorphism (RFLP) analysis and *flaA* short variable region (SVR) typing, as well as the multi-locus sequence typing (MLST), the major outer membrane protein (MOMP) schemes and the whole-genome sequencing (WGS) have provided significant insights into the similarities among *Campylobacter* isolates stemming from human disease and environmental reservoirs such as farm animals and water [77,78].

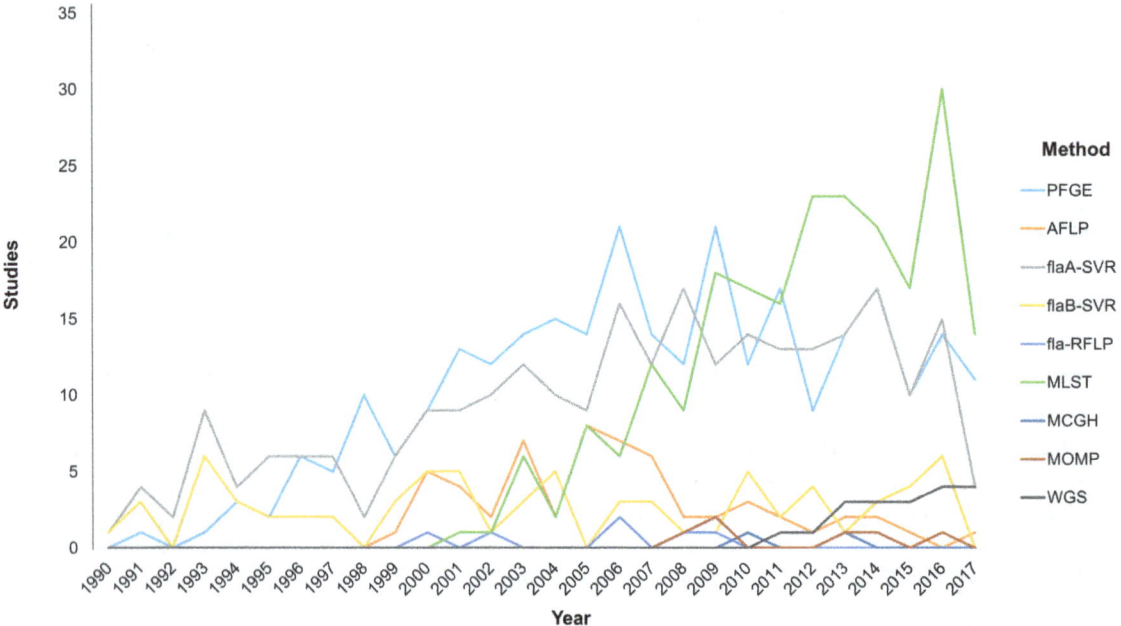

Figure 1. Graphical analysis of the applied molecular typing methodologies over time based on PubMed search. The use of molecular methodologies for the differentiation of *Campylobacter* at species and strain level has been modified during the last decades according to the new trends in technology, the improvements in bioinformatics, and the needs of the scientific community. Pulsed-field gel electrophoresis (PFGE), amplified fragment length polymorphism (AFLP), fla short variable region (fla-SVR), fla restriction fragment length polymorphism (fla-RFLP), multi-locus sequence typing (MLST), microarray comparative genomic hybridization (MCGH), major outer membrane protein (MOMP), whole genome sequencing (WGS).

PFGE is the first DNA-based typing method applied for *Campylobacter* spp. and is generally considered as the "gold standard" technique for the typing of a multitude of important pathogens [79,80]. With a total of 283 hits in a PubMed search using the query ("PFGE" and "*Campylobacter*"), the PFGE method has been the most widely adopted epidemiological tool from 1991 to present. The success of PFGE stems from the high discriminatory power it offers in both outbreak investigation and epidemiological surveillance. PFGE has remained the primary molecular typing method for almost for three decades, and is a cost-effective tool with high reproducibility among different laboratories. Bioinformatics, in accordance with the standardized protocols of PFGE, have offered substantial help in a worldwide fingerprinting of *Campylobacter* and other foodborne isolates as well as for the monitoring of emerging clones; this method actually set the basis for the implementation of PulseNet in the U.S. [81]. Despite the significant advantages of PFGE, the increased difficulty in workload, the lack of rapidity in analysis, the difficulty in intralaboratory communication of the results, as well as the low resolution of the method in distinguishing bands of relatively same size has set several serious limitations [73,75]. The amplified fragment length polymorphism (AFLP) typing method offers high discriminatory power, portability of the analysis results and high reproducibility, but the costly equipment and the difficulties in its use set serious limitations [73,75]. These limitations along with the fact that it is a more recent method than PFGE may partially explain the reduced application frequency.

Studying bacterial isolates relatedness based on a single target gene is the field of the single locus sequence typing (SLST) method. For *Campylobacter*, nucleotide sequencing of a short variable region (SVR) of a gene provides significant information for the *Campylobacter* "fingerprint" [75,76,82]. The widely applied sequencing of the SVR of the flagellin A (*flaA*) and flagellin B (*flaB*) genes is a simple, rapid and low-cost method with high discriminatory power that supersedes the previously performed flagellin-based restriction fragment length polymorphism analysis (*fla*-RFLP) for *Campylobacter* isolates discrimination [76,83–85]. The potential low-reliability of the SLST methods for *Campylobacter* spp. lies in the highly variable genome of the isolates due to the naturally occurring genetic elements uptake, recombination and alleles instability [86,87]. Therefore, questions have been raised whether SLST methods are appropriate for long-term and large-scale investigation of closely related *Campylobacter* strains.

The first *Campylobacter* MLST scheme was developed to discriminate between *C. jejuni* and *C. coli*; this scheme required the sequencing of seven stable housekeeping genes (*asp, glnA, gltA, glyA, pgm, uncA, tkt*) [88,89]. For other *Campylobacter* spp. the MLST with variant (rMLST) scheme presented slightly different substitutions of several genetic loci among the various species [90,91]. Although a rather new technique, MLST has gained attention due to the excellent reproducibility when used in epidemiological studies on a large-scale and in genetic studies of the *Campylobacter* population. An interesting notification that needs to be addressed is the numerical advantage of MLST publications over PFGE, despite the fact that the latter is the first typing method applied for *Campylobacter* spp. and is widely accepted to be a "gold-standard" typing technique. MLST seems to have been more widely and rapidly adopted during the last decade (Figure 1). More specifically, MLST data applied for the genetic structure of the *Campylobacter* population have improved our understanding on the various routes of transmission leading to human disease. These data are electronically portable and sequence type profiles are available online in two central databases (http://pubmlst.org and www.mlst.net), while the eBURST online software is used in the determination of bacterial genetic relatedness and clinical relevance, offering a valuable tool in designing prevention strategies to promote the reduction of human campylobacteriosis and its sequelae [75,92–94]. Additionally, the ability of the widely studied *C. jejuni* to adapt in adverse environments has led to genetic instability and phenotypic diversity, thus enhancing the survival of the species and this characteristic can be studied by the MLST method [95,96]. Albeit its contribution for a deeper insight into the structure, evolution, sequence diversity and genetic instability of the *Campylobacter* population, MLST presents limitations in its implementation in outbreaks due to the high-cost and time-consuming analysis [76].

Further characterization of the isolates based on gene encoding for the bacterial outer membrane protein content is known to improve *Campylobacter* epidemiological identification through genetic discrimination [97]. Specifically, for *C. jejuni* and *C. coli*, the presence of the the *porA* gene encoding for the MOMP porin A has been demonstrated, while for *C. fetus* the genes *cmp1* and *cmp2* encode for two porin-like activity MOMPs other than porin A [97,98]. Regional outbreak investigations regarding foodborne human campylobacteriosis underline the usefulness of MOMP typing to triage environmental *Campylobacter* isolates before conducting more laborious molecular typing analysis [99]. The MOMP typing method is very recent and is mostly used for *C. jejuni* typing. To date, the *cmp*-based typing method is considered a tool with high discriminatory power which is simple in use [98,100].

DNA microarrays using probes that are complementary to specific bacterial nucleotide sequences, represent a rapid method for detecting genes or alleles of particular bacterial species in a single experiment [75,76]. Extensively used in *C. jejuni* research studies, microarray comparative genomic hybridization (MCGH) has yielded successful genomic analysis of the highly variable genome of this pathogen. However, microarrays are ultimately abandoned and cannot be considered as optimal tools for subtyping because they offer limited throughput in real-time outbreak investigation and constitute a costly and a technique that is difficult to standardize. Another method of comparative genomics is the recent typing method of comparative genomic fingerprinting (CGF), which has improved routine campylobacteriosis surveillance [101]. The CGF is the preferred method for the detection of *Campylobacter* genes with high variability among the different species of bacterial clusters that have been previously identified by the MCGH method [102].

Finally, the revolutionary next generation sequencing (NGS) methods promise a broader application of high-resolution bacterial WGS, which, however, remains a laborious tool in the daily routine of research and clinical laboratories. Genome data deriving from WGS will soon comprise useful information for detection and evaluation of the bacterial pathogens that are close phylogenetic neighbors and play an important role in public health [75,103]. In the era of metagenomic sequencing-based tools, public health microbiology is undergoing substantial changes; WGS replaces traditional phenotypic tests and narrowed-spectrum genetic methods that apply to universal or species-specific markers with low discriminatory power for subtyping analyses. The application of high quality WGS provides the research community a wider array of *Campylobacter* reference genomes for exploitation. In fact, WGS enables the analysis of multiple strains within a bacterial sample and offers a comprehensive genome sequence data set, a property previously unavailable given that routine subtyping methods provided restricted discriminatory power in non-clonal populations with high genetic diversity [104]. WGS will allow the detection of epidemiological variations among strains and will progressively replace traditional typing methods, but before this, issues related to genetic diversity have to be addressed in order to define the cut off values and criteria that determine which infections stem from clonal isolates or a common source [56,105].

In general, molecular typing and automated sequencing techniques have led to significant accomplishments in diagnostics and biotechnology. NGS technologies offer subtyping data to improve programs based on risk-based sampling algorithms with rapidity, simplicity and at a low cost. Platforms based on sequencing technologies are progressively reported in the monitoring of poultry production aiming to improve food safety in the market and consequently public health [106]. Additionally, NGS technologies have improved our understanding of the bacterial methylation processthat greatly affects pathogenicity. Such an example for the use of NGS in campylobacters is the application of single molecule real-time (SMRT) sequencing for the detection of methylation patterns in *C. jejuni* [107,108]. Lastly, the notion that NGS offers DNA characterization at large and complex populations paves the way towards an improved experimental procedure in the characterization of multispecies and multi-subspecies populations [109].

It is a fact that the majority of research has focused on evaluating the molecular typing and subtyping methods applied for *C. jejuni* and *C. coli*, which are two genetically diverse species due to their innate property of extracellular DNA uptake from horizontal genetic exchange [110]. The highly variable genome of these *Campylobacter* species has raised concerns regarding the application of typing methodologies based on DNA sequence information such as the MLST, *flaA* SVR, and the MOMP [111,112]. This obstacle paved the way towards combining methodologies for a more accurate *Campylobacter* populations investigation, such as Multiplex Ligation-Dependent Probe

Amplification–Binary Typing [102,113]. Genomic mosaicism can adversely impact the understanding of closely related species and the use of few genetic loci can lead to erroneous results. A promising combination could be the MLST method applied with MCGH offering high discriminatory power even in *Campylobacter* populations with extensive recombination and genomic mosaicism [114].

Another burden in typing is the fact that several molecular techniques, such as the random amplification of polymorphic DNA (RAPD), the arbitrarily primed polymerase chain reaction (AP-PCR), the repetitive-element polymerase chain reaction (rep-PCR), and the variable-number tandem repeat typing (VNTR), can be applied for epidemiological surveillance only at a local level, and the data deriving from the analysis cannot be interchangeable; specifically, for *Campylobacter* typing only a few reports exist for these methodologies [73,75]. Such typing tools possess poor reproducibility and low discriminatory power, despite their rapidity, ease of use and low cost.

4. Conclusions

The engagement of the state-of-the-art typing methods with human campylobacteriosis and environmental reservoirs is the main focus of the study of *C. jejuni* and *C. coli*. Our limited ability to understand the interaction between *Campylobacter* and the host lies in the absence of a systematic effort to monitor, evaluate and compare this bidirectional relationship. Additionally, the absence of a "gold standard" identification method—which is mainly attributed to the high variability and genetic instability of *Campylobacter* spp.—restricts the actual range of isolates. This characteristic inevitably makes laboratory diagnosis difficult, since culture-dependent methodologies are effective only for a small subset of *Campylobacter* species. Considering how many of the *Campylobacter* strains isolated globally have gone under-determined, the idea of an efficient and approved storage and maintenance protocol could significantly offer a great advantage in the study of more *Campylobacter* species by currently applied isolation and typing methods. Moreover, in terms of subtyping, there is the need for the development of assays with the ability to target genetic variation so that we can differentiate the various lineages in the population for epidemiological tracking. The fact that there is not a "gold standard" subtyping methodology is a reflection of the insufficient data on *Campylobacter* population genetics due to the absence in tools for detection/identification either at the microbiological or molecular level.

Polyphasic studies for strain taxonomic position classification involving universally applicable molecular methodologies and enable accurate and safe results at a species and subspecies level, such as MALDI-TOF MS and WGS, could offer a high degree of agreement on epidemiologic surveillance. Reliable molecular typing along with the subsequent phylogenetic analysis of *Campylobacter* strains isolated from both clinical settings and the broader environment would contribute to the epidemiological database indispensable for every laboratory. This database should ideally include all the phenotypic and genotypic features, the demographic and clinical data of the patients when it comes to clinical human isolates as well as information about the natural reservoirs of the *Campylobacter* spp. in both animals and water. Such an accessible and comparable intralaboratory database would significantly enhance epidemiological surveillance on a local and universal scale, and would function as a tool for the control of campylobacteriosis. A consistent surveillance system means more than epidemiological surveillance at a national level; it means (i) better understanding, (ii) closer monitoring, (iii) targeted action design, and (iv) efficient strategy implementation.

Acknowledgments: No funds have been received and no funding sources are disclosed.

Author Contributions: All authors have equally contributed to the conception of the idea and the writing of the manuscript. All authors have read and approved the manuscript in the current form.

References

1.   Bolton, D.J. *Campylobacter* virulence and survival factors. *Food Microbiol.* **2015**, *48*, 99–108. [CrossRef] [PubMed]

2.   Kaakoush, N.O.; Castano-Rodriguez, N.; Mitchell, H.M.; Man, S.M. Global epidemiology of *Campylobacter* infection. *Clin. Microbiol. Rev.* **2015**, *28*, 687–720. [CrossRef] [PubMed]

3.   Allos, B.M. *Campylobacter jejuni* Infections: Update on emerging issues and trends. *Clin. Infect. Dis.* **2001**, *32*, 1201–1206. [PubMed]

4.   Luangtongkum, T.; Jeon, B.; Han, J.; Plummer, P.; Logue, C.M.; Zhang, Q. Antibiotic resistance in *Campylobacter*: Emergence, transmission and persistence. *Future Microbiol.* **2009**, *4*, 189–200. [CrossRef] [PubMed]

5.   Centers for Disease Control and Prevention. *Campylobacter* . Available online: https://www.cdc.gov/foodsafety/diseases/campylobacter/ (accessed on 4 May 2017).

6.   European Food Safety Authority; European Centre for Disease Prevention and Control. The European Union summary report on trends and sources of zoonoses, zoonotic agents and food-borne outbreaks in 2015. *EFSA J.* **2016**, *14*. [CrossRef]

7.   WHO. *Campylobacter* . Available online: http://www.who.int/mediacentre/factsheets/fs255/en/ (accessed on 4 May 2017).

8.   Crim, S.M.; Griffin, P.M.; Tauxe, R.; Marder, E.P.; Gilliss, D.; Cronquist, A.B.; Cartter, M.; Tobin-D'Angelo, M.; Blythe, D.; Smith, K.; et al. Preliminary incidence and trends of infection with pathogens transmitted commonly through food—Foodborne diseases active surveillance network, 10 U.S. sites, 2006–2014. *MMWR Morb. Mortal. Wkly. Rep.* **2015**, *64*, 495–499. [PubMed]

9.   European Food Safety Authority. The European Union summary report on trends and sources of zoonoses, zoonotic agents and food-borne outbreaks in 2013. *EFSA J.* **2015**, *13*, 165. [CrossRef]

10. McCrackin, M.A.; Helke, K.L.; Galloway, A.M.; Poole, A.Z.; Salgado, C.D.; Marriott, B.P. Effect of antimicrobial use in agricultural animals on drug-resistant foodborne campylobacteriosis in humans: A systematic literature review. *Crit. Rev. Food Sci. Nutr.* **2016**, *56*, 2115–2132. [CrossRef] [PubMed]

11. Man, S.M. The clinical importance of emerging *Campylobacter* species. *Nat. Rev. Gastroenterol. Hepatol.* **2011**, *8*, 669–685. [CrossRef] [PubMed]

12. Bojanic, K.; Midwinter, A.C.; Marshall, J.C.; Rogers, L.E.; Biggs, P.J.; Acke, E. Variation in the limit-of-detection of the ProSpecT *Campylobacter* microplate enzyme immunoassay in stools spiked with emerging *Campylobacter* species. *J. Microbiol. Methods* **2016**, *127*, 236–241. [CrossRef] [PubMed]

13. Dasti, J.I.; Tareen, A.M.; Lugert, R.; Zautner, A.E.; Gross, U. *Campylobacter jejuni*: A brief overview on pathogenicity-associated factors and disease-mediating mechanisms. *Int. J. Med. Microbiol.: IJMM* **2010**, *300*, 205–211. [CrossRef] [PubMed]

14. Silva, J.; Leite, D.; Fernandes, M.; Mena, C.; Gibbs, P.A.; Teixeira, P. *Campylobacter* spp. as a foodborne pathogen: A review. *Front. Microbiol.* **2011**, *2*, 200. [CrossRef] [PubMed]

15. Van, T.T.; Elshagmani, E.; Gor, M.C.; Scott, P.C.; Moore, R.J. *Campylobacter hepaticus* sp. nov., isolated from chickens with spotty liver disease. *Int. J. Syst. Evol. Microbiol.* **2016**, *66*, 4518–4524. [PubMed]

16. Vandamme, P.; Falsen, E.; Rossau, R.; Hoste, B.; Segers, P.; Tytgat, R.; De Ley, J. Revision of *Campylobacter*, *Helicobacter*, and *Wolinella* taxonomy: Emendation of generic descriptions and proposal of *Arcobacter* gen. nov. *Int. J. Syst. Bacteriol.* **1991**, *41*, 88–103. [CrossRef] [PubMed]

17. Anderson, K.F.; Kiehlbauch, J.A.; Anderson, D.C.; McClure, H.M.; Wachsmuth, I.K. *Arcobacter* (*Campylobacter*) *butzleri*-associated diarrheal illness in a nonhuman primate population. *Infect. Immun.* **1993**, *61*, 2220–2223. [PubMed]

18. Romaniuk, P.J.; Zoltowska, B.; Trust, T.J.; Lane, D.J.; Olsen, G.J.; Pace, N.R.; Stahl, D.A. *Campylobacter pylori*, the spiral bacterium associated with human gastritis, is not a true *Campylobacter* sp. *J. Bacteriol.* **1987**, *169*, 2137–2141. [CrossRef] [PubMed]

19. Vandamme, P.; Harrington, C.S.; Jalava, K.; On, S.L. Misidentifying helicobacters: The *Helicobacter cinaedi* example. *J. Clin. Microbiol.* **2000**, *38*, 2261–2266. [PubMed]

20. Achtman, M.; Wagner, M. Microbial diversity and the genetic nature of microbial species. *Nat. Rev. Microbiol.* **2008**, *6*, 431–440. [CrossRef] [PubMed]

21. Patton, C.M.; Shaffer, N.; Edmonds, P.; Barrett, T.J.; Lambert, M.A.; Baker, C.; Perlman, D.M.; Brenner, D.J. Human disease associated with "*Campylobacter upsaliensis*" (catalase-negative or weakly positive *Campylobacter* species) in the United States. *J. Clin. Microbiol.* **1989**, *27*, 66–73. [PubMed]

22. Salama, S.M.; Tabor, H.; Richter, M.; Taylor, D.E. Pulsed-field gel electrophoresis for epidemiologic studies of *Campylobacter hyointestinalis* isolates. *J. Clin. Microbiol.* **1992**, *30*, 1982–1984. [PubMed]

23. Lindblom, G.B.; Sjogren, E.; Hansson-Westerberg, J.; Kaijser, B. *Campylobacter upsaliensis, C. sputorum sputorum* and *C. concisus* as common causes of diarrhoea in Swedish children. *Scand. J. Infect. Dis.* **1995**, *27*, 187–188. [CrossRef] [PubMed]

24. Ichiyama, S.; Hirai, S.; Minami, T.; Nishiyama, Y.; Shimizu, S.; Shimokata, K.; Ohta, M. *Campylobacter fetus* subspecies *fetus* cellulitis associated with bacteremia in debilitated hosts. *Clin. Infect. Dis.* **1998**, *27*, 252–255. [CrossRef] [PubMed]

25. On, S.L.; Atabay, H.I.; Corry, J.E.; Harrington, C.S.; Vandamme, P. Emended description of *Campylobacter sputorum* and revision of its infrasubspecific (biovar) divisions, including *C. sputorum* biovar paraureolyticus, a urease-producing variant from cattle and humans. *Int. J. Syst. Bacteriol.* **1998**, *48*, 195–206. [CrossRef] [PubMed]

26. Logan, J.M.; Burnens, A.; Linton, D.; Lawson, A.J.; Stanley, J. *Campylobacter lanienae* sp. *nov.*, a new species isolated from workers in an abattoir. *Int. J. Syst. Evol. Microbiol.* **2000**, *50*, 865–872. [CrossRef] [PubMed]

27. Gorkiewicz, G.; Feierl, G.; Zechner, R.; Zechner, E.L. Transmission of *Campylobacter hyointestinalis* from a pig to a human. *J. Clin. Microbiol.* **2002**, *40*, 2601–2605. [CrossRef] [PubMed]

28. Petersen, R.F.; Harrington, C.S.; Kortegaard, H.E.; On, S.L. A PCR-DGGE method for detection and identification of *Campylobacter, Helicobacter, Arcobacter* and related *Epsilobacteria* and its application to saliva samples from humans and domestic pets. *J. Appl. Microbiol.* **2007**, *103*, 2601–2615. [CrossRef] [PubMed]

29. Debruyne, L.; On, S.L.; De Brandt, E.; Vandamme, P. Novel Campylobacter lari-like bacteria from humans and molluscs: Description of *Campylobacter peloridis* sp. *nov.*, *Campylobacter lari* subsp. *concheus* subsp. *nov.* and *Campylobacter lari* subsp. *lari* subsp. *nov. Int. J. Syst. Evol. Microbiol.* **2009**, *59*, 1126–1132. [CrossRef] [PubMed]

30. Zhang, L.; Man, S.M.; Day, A.S.; Leach, S.T.; Lemberg, D.A.; Dutt, S.; Stormon, M.; Otley, A.; O'Loughlin, E.V.; Magoffin, A.; et al. Detection and isolation of *Campylobacter* species other than *C. jejuni* from children with Crohn's disease. *J. Clin. Microbiol.* **2009**, *47*, 453–455. [CrossRef] [PubMed]

31. Man, S.M.; Kaakoush, N.O.; Octavia, S.; Mitchell, H. The internal transcribed spacer region, a new tool for use in species differentiation and delineation of systematic relationships within the *Campylobacter* genus. *Appl. Environ. Microbiol.* **2010**, *76*, 3071–3081. [CrossRef] [PubMed]

32. Man, S.M.; Zhang, L.; Day, A.S.; Leach, S.T.; Lemberg, D.A.; Mitchell, H. *Campylobacter concisus* and other *Campylobacter* species in children with newly diagnosed Crohn's disease. *Inflamm. Bowel Dis.* **2010**, *16*, 1008–1016. [CrossRef] [PubMed]

33. Inglis, G.D.; Boras, V.F.; Houde, A. Enteric campylobacteria and RNA viruses associated with healthy and diarrheic humans in the Chinook health region of southwestern Alberta, Canada. *J. Clin. Microbiol.* **2011**, *49*, 209–219. [CrossRef] [PubMed]

34. Morris, C.N.; Scully, B.; Garvey, G.J. *Campylobacter lari* associated with permanent pacemaker infection and bacteremia. *Clin. Infect. Dis.* **1998**, *27*, 220–221. [CrossRef] [PubMed]

35. Tee, W.; Luppino, M.; Rambaldo, S. Bacteremia due to *Campylobacter sputorum* biovar *sputorum*. *Clin. Infect. Dis.* **1998**, *27*, 1544–1545. [CrossRef] [PubMed]

36. Linscott, A.J.; Flamholtz, R.B.; Shukla, D.; Song, Y.; Liu, C.; Finegold, S.M. Fatal septicemia due to *Clostridium hathewayi* and *Campylobacter hominis*. *Anaerobe* **2005**, *11*, 97–98. [CrossRef] [PubMed]

37. Louwen, R.; van Baarlen, P.; van Vliet, A.H.; van Belkum, A.; Hays, J.P.; Endtz, H.P. *Campylobacter* bacteremia: A rare and under-reported event? *Eur. J. Microbiol. Immunol.* **2012**, *2*, 76–87. [CrossRef] [PubMed]

38. On, S.L.; Ridgwell, F.; Cryan, B.; Azadian, B.S. Isolation of *Campylobacter sputorum* biovar *sputorum* from an axillary abscess. *J. Infect.* **1992**, *24*, 175–179. [CrossRef]

39. Herve, J.; Aissa, N.; Legrand, P.; Sorkine, M.; Calmette, M.J.; Santin, A.; Roupie, E.; Renaud, B. *Campylobacter fetus* meningitis in a diabetic adult cured by imipenem. *Eur. J. Clin. Microbiol. Infect. Dis.* **2004**, *23*, 722–724. [CrossRef] [PubMed]

40. Wetsch, N.M.; Somani, K.; Tyrrell, G.J.; Gebhart, C.; Bailey, R.J.; Taylor, D.E. *Campylobacter curvus*-associated hepatic abscesses: A case report. *J. Clin. Microbiol.* **2006**, *44*, 1909–1911. [CrossRef] [PubMed]

41. Kanayama, S.; Ohnishi, K.; Yamaura, T.; Katayama, M.; Makino, J.; Takemura, N.; Hamabe, Y. Case of bilateral subdural empyema complicating *Campylobacter fetus* subspecies *fetus* meningitis. *Brain Nerve* **2008**, *60*, 659–662. [PubMed]

42. Shimakha Ia, A.; Pozdeev, O.K.; Ibragimova, A.A.; Minullina, N.K.; Fedorova Zh, P.; Khasanov, A.A.; Il'inskaia, O.N. Isolation of *Campylobacter fetus* from persons with obstetric-gynecological infections. *Zh. Mikrobiol. Epidemiol. Immunobiol.* **2009**, 80–83.

43. Lam, J.Y.; Wu, A.K.; Ngai, D.C.; Teng, J.L.; Wong, E.S.; Lau, S.K.; Lee, R.A.; Woo, P.C. Three cases of severe invasive infections caused by *Campylobacter rectus* and first report of fatal *C. rectus* infection. *J. Clin. Microbiol.* **2011**, *49*, 1687–1691. [CrossRef] [PubMed]

44. Ajene, A.N.; Fischer Walker, C.L.; Black, R.E. Enteric pathogens and reactive arthritis: A systematic review of *Campylobacter*, *Salmonella* and *Shigella*-associated reactive arthritis. *J. Health Popul. Nutr.* **2013**, *31*, 299–307. [CrossRef] [PubMed]

45. De Vries, J.J.; Arents, N.L.; Manson, W.L. *Campylobacter* species isolated from extra-oro-intestinal abscesses: A report of four cases and literature review. *Eur. J. Clin. Microbiol. Infect. Dis.* **2008**, *27*, 1119–1123. [CrossRef] [PubMed]

46. Uotila, T.; Korpela, M.; Vuento, R.; Laine, J.; Lumio, J.; Kuusi, M.; Virtanen, M.J.; Mustonen, J.; Antonen, J.; Pirkanmaa Waterborne Outbreak Study Group. Joint symptoms after a faecal culture positive *Campylobacter* infection associated with a waterborne gastroenteritis outbreak: A questionnaire study. *Scand. J. Rheumatol.* **2014**, *43*, 524–526. [CrossRef] [PubMed]

47. Nishiguchi, S.; Sekine, I.; Kuroda, S.; Sato, M.; Kitagawa, I. Myositis Ossificans of the Hip Due to Pyogenic Arthritis Caused by *Campylobacter fetus* Subspecies *fetus*. *Intern. Med.* **2017**, *56*, 967–972. [CrossRef] [PubMed]

48. Inglis, G.D.; Hoar, B.M.; Whiteside, D.P.; Morck, D.W. *Campylobacter canadensis* sp. nov., from captive whooping cranes in Canada. *Int. J. Syst. Evol. Microbiol.* **2007**, *57*, 2636–2644. [CrossRef] [PubMed]

49. Rossi, M.; Debruyne, L.; Zanoni, R.G.; Manfreda, G.; Revez, J.; Vandamme, P. *Campylobacter avium* sp. nov., a hippurate-positive species isolated from poultry. *Int. J. Syst. Evol. Microbiol.* **2009**, *59*, 2364–2369. [CrossRef] [PubMed]

50. Zanoni, R.G.; Debruyne, L.; Rossi, M.; Revez, J.; Vandamme, P. *Campylobacter cuniculorum* sp. nov., from rabbits. *Int. J. Syst. Evol. Microbiol.* **2009**, *59*, 1666–1671. [CrossRef] [PubMed]

51. Debruyne, L.; Broman, T.; Bergstrom, S.; Olsen, B.; On, S.L.; Vandamme, P. *Campylobacter volucris* sp. nov., isolated from black-headed gulls (*Larus ridibundus*). *Int. J. Syst. Evol. Microbiol.* **2010**, *60*, 1870–1875. [CrossRef] [PubMed]

52. Debruyne, L.; Broman, T.; Bergstrom, S.; Olsen, B.; On, S.L.; Vandamme, P. Campylobacter subantarcticus sp. nov., isolated from birds in the sub-Antarctic region. *Int. J. Syst. Evol. Microbiol.* **2010**, *60*, 815–819. [CrossRef] [PubMed]

53. Kaur, T.; Singh, J.; Huffman, M.A.; Petrzelkova, K.J.; Taylor, N.S.; Xu, S.; Dewhirst, F.E.; Paster, B.J.; Debruyne, L.; Vandamme, P.; et al. *Campylobacter troglodytis* sp. nov., isolated from feces of human-habituated wild chimpanzees (*Pan troglodytes schweinfurthii*) in Tanzania. *Appl. Environ. Microbiol.* **2011**, *77*, 2366–2373. [CrossRef] [PubMed]

54. Platts-Mills, J.A.; Liu, J.; Gratz, J.; Mduma, E.; Amour, C.; Swai, N.; Taniuchi, M.; Begum, S.; Penataro Yori, P.; Tilley, D.H.; et al. Detection of *Campylobacter* in stool and determination of significance by culture, enzyme immunoassay, and PCR in developing countries. *J. Clin. Microbiol.* **2014**, *52*, 1074–1080. [CrossRef] [PubMed]

55. Kweon, O.J.; Lim, Y.K.; Yoo, B.; Kim, H.R.; Kim, T.H.; Lee, M.K. First Case Report of *Campylobacter volucris* Bacteremia in an Immunocompromised Patient. *J. Clin. Microbiol.* **2015**, *53*, 1976–1978. [CrossRef] [PubMed]

56. Llarena, A.K.; Taboada, E.; Rossi, M. Whole-Genome Sequencing in Epidemiology of *Campylobacter jejuni* Infections. *J. Clin. Microbiol.* **2017**, *55*, 1269–1275. [CrossRef] [PubMed]

57. Van Belkum, A.; Tassios, P.T.; Dijkshoorn, L.; Haeggman, S.; Cookson, B.; Fry, N.K.; Fussing, V.; Green, J.; Feil, E.; Gerner-Smidt, P.; et al. Guidelines for the validation and application of typing methods for use in bacterial epidemiology. *Clin. Microbiol. Infect.* **2007**, *13* Suppl. 3, 1–46. [CrossRef] [PubMed]

58. Maziero, M.T.; de Oliveira, T.C. Effect of refrigeration and frozen storage on the *Campylobacter jejuni* recovery from naturally contaminated broiler carcasses. *Braz. J. Microbiol.* **2010**, *41*, 501–505. [CrossRef] [PubMed]

59. Wood, T.K.; Knabel, S.J.; Kwan, B.W. Bacterial persister cell formation and dormancy. *Appl. Environ. Microbiol.* **2013**, *79*, 7116–7121. [CrossRef] [PubMed]

60. Li, L.; Mendis, N.; Trigui, H.; Oliver, J.D.; Faucher, S.P. The importance of the viable but non-culturable state in human bacterial pathogens. *Front. Microbiol.* **2014**, *5*, 258. [CrossRef] [PubMed]

61. Ayrapetyan, M.; Oliver, J.D. The viable but non-culturable state and its relevance in food safety. *Curr. Opin. Food Sci.* **2016**, *8*, 127–133. [CrossRef]

62. Fakruddin, M.; Mannan, K.S.; Andrews, S. Viable but nonculturable bacteria: Food safety and public health perspective. *ISRN Microbiol.* **2013**, *2013*, 703813. [CrossRef] [PubMed]

63. ISO. *Microbiology of Food and Animal Feeding Stuff—Horizontal Method for Detection and Enumeration of Campylobacter* spp. *Part 1: Detection Method*; ISO: Geneva, Switzerland, 2006.

64. ISO. *Microbiology of Food and Animal Feeding Stuff—Horizontal Method for Detection and Enumeration of Campylobacter* spp. *Part 2: Colony Count Technique*; ISO: Geneva, Switzerland, 2006.

65. Linton, D.; Lawson, A.J.; Owen, R.J.; Stanley, J. PCR detection, identification to species level, and fingerprinting of *Campylobacter jejuni* and *Campylobacter coli* direct from diarrheic samples. *J. Clin. Microbiol.* **1997**, *35*, 2568–2572. [PubMed]

66. Iwamoto, M.; Huang, J.Y.; Cronquist, A.B.; Medus, C.; Hurd, S.; Zansky, S.; Dunn, J.; Woron, A.M.; Oosmanally, N.; Griffin, P.M.; et al. Bacterial enteric infections detected by culture-independent diagnostic tests—FoodNet, United States, 2012–2014. *MMWR Morb. Mortal. Wkly. Rep.* **2015**, *64*, 252–257. [PubMed]

67. Maher, M.; Finnegan, C.; Collins, E.; Ward, B.; Carroll, C.; Cormican, M. Evaluation of culture methods and a DNA probe-based PCR assay for detection of *Campylobacter* species in clinical specimens of feces. *J. Clin. Microbiol.* **2003**, *41*, 2980–2986. [CrossRef] [PubMed]

68. Kulkarni, S.P.; Lever, S.; Logan, J.M.; Lawson, A.J.; Stanley, J.; Shafi, M.S. Detection of *Campylobacter* species: A comparison of culture and polymerase chain reaction based methods. *J. Clin. Pathol.* **2002**, *55*, 749–753. [CrossRef] [PubMed]

69. Van Belkum, A.; Chatellier, S.; Girard, V.; Pincus, D.; Deol, P.; Dunne, W.M., Jr. Progress in proteomics for clinical microbiology: MALDI-TOF MS for microbial species identification and more. *Expert Rev. Proteom.* **2015**, *12*, 595–605. [CrossRef] [PubMed]

70. Mandrell, R.E.; Harden, L.A.; Bates, A.; Miller, W.G.; Haddon, W.F.; Fagerquist, C.K. Speciation of *Campylobacter coli, C. jejuni, C. helveticus, C. lari, C. sputorum*, and *C. upsaliensis* by matrix-assisted laser desorption ionization-time of flight mass spectrometry. *Appl. Environ. Microbiol.* **2005**, *71*, 6292–6307. [CrossRef] [PubMed]

71. Clark, A.E.; Kaleta, E.J.; Arora, A.; Wolk, D.M. Matrix-assisted laser desorption ionization-time of flight mass spectrometry: A fundamental shift in the routine practice of clinical microbiology. *Clin. Microbiol. Rev.* **2013**, *26*, 547–603. [CrossRef] [PubMed]

72. Fitzgerald, C.; Tu, Z.C.; Patrick, M.; Stiles, T.; Lawson, A.J.; Santovenia, M.; Gilbert, M.J.; van Bergen, M.; Joyce, K.; Pruckler, J.; et al. *Campylobacter fetus* subsp. *testudinum* subsp. *nov.*, isolated from humans and reptiles. *Int. J. Syst. Evol. Microbiol.* **2014**, *64*, 2944–2948. [CrossRef] [PubMed]

73. Boccia, S.; Pasquarella, C.; Colotto, M.; Barchitta, M.; Quattrocchi, A.; Agodi, A.; the Public Health Genomics and GISIO Working Groups of the Italian Society of Hygiene, Preventive Medicine and Public Health (SItI). Molecular epidemiology tools in the management of healthcare-associated infections: Towards the definition of recommendations. *Epidemiol. Prev.* **2015**, *39*, 21–26. [PubMed]

74. Mossong, J.; Mughini-Gras, L.; Penny, C.; Devaux, A.; Olinger, C.; Losch, S.; Cauchie, H.M.; van Pelt, W.; Ragimbeau, C. Human campylobacteriosis in Luxembourg, 2010–2013: A case-control study combined with multilocus sequence typing for source attribution and risk factor analysis. *Sci. Rep.* **2016**, *6*, 20939. [CrossRef] [PubMed]

75. Sabat, A.J.; Budimir, A.; Nashev, D.; Sa-Leao, R.; van Dijl, J.; Laurent, F.; Grundmann, H.; Friedrich, A.W.; Markers, E.S.G.o.E. Overview of molecular typing methods for outbreak detection and epidemiological surveillance. *Euro Surveill.* **2013**, *18*, 20380. [PubMed]

76. Taboada, E.N.; Clark, C.G.; Sproston, E.L.; Carrillo, C.D. Current methods for molecular typing of *Campylobacter* species. *J. Microbiol. Methods.* **2013**, *95*, 24–31. [CrossRef] [PubMed]

77. Newell, D.G.; Fearnley, C. Sources of *Campylobacter* colonization in broiler chickens. *Appl. Environ. Microbiol.* **2003**, *69*, 4343–4351. [CrossRef] [PubMed]

78. Colles, F.M.; Maiden, M.C. *Campylobacter* sequence typing databases: Applications and future prospects. *Microbiology* **2012**, *158*, 2695–2709. [CrossRef] [PubMed]

79. Struelens, M.J. Consensus guidelines for appropriate use and evaluation of microbial epidemiologic typing systems. *Clin. Microbiol. Infect.* **1996**, *2*, 2–11. [CrossRef] [PubMed]

80. Tenover, F.C.; Arbeit, R.D.; Goering, R.V.; Mickelsen, P.A.; Murray, B.E.; Persing, D.H.; Swaminathan, B. Interpreting chromosomal DNA restriction patterns produced by pulsed-field gel electrophoresis: Criteria for bacterial strain typing. *J. Clin. Microbiol.* **1995**, *33*, 2233–2239. [PubMed]

81. Swaminathan, B.; Barrett, T.J.; Hunter, S.B.; Tauxe, R.V.; CDC PulseNet Task Force. PulseNet: The molecular subtyping network for foodborne bacterial disease surveillance, United States. *Emerg. Infect. Dis.* **2001**, *7*, 382–389. [CrossRef] [PubMed]

82. Lajhar, S.A.; Jennison, A.V.; Patel, B.; Duffy, L.L. Comparison of epidemiologically linked *Campylobacter jejuni* isolated from human and poultry sources. *Epidemiol. Infect.* **2015**, *143*, 3498–3509. [CrossRef] [PubMed]

83. Nielsen, E.M.; Engberg, J.; Fussing, V.; Petersen, L.; Brogren, C.H.; On, S.L. Evaluation of phenotypic and genotypic methods for subtyping *Campylobacter jejuni* isolates from humans, poultry, and cattle. *J. Clin. Microbiol.* **2000**, *38*, 3800–3810. [PubMed]

84. Nachamkin, I.; Bohachick, K.; Patton, C.M. Flagellin gene typing of *Campylobacter jejuni* by restriction fragment length polymorphism analysis. *J. Clin. Microbiol.* **1993**, *31*, 1531–1536. [PubMed]

85. Meinersmann, R.J.; Helsel, L.O.; Fields, P.I.; Hiett, K.L. Discrimination of *Campylobacter jejuni* isolates by *fla* gene sequencing. *J. Clin. Microbiol.* **1997**, *35*, 2810–2814. [PubMed]

86. Wang, Y.; Taylor, D.E. Natural transformation in *Campylobacter* species. *J. Bacteriol.* **1990**, *172*, 949–955. [CrossRef] [PubMed]

87. Dingle, K.E.; Colles, F.M.; Falush, D.; Maiden, M.C. Sequence typing and comparison of population biology of *Campylobacter coli* and *Campylobacter jejuni*. *J. Clin. Microbiol.* **2005**, *43*, 340–347. [CrossRef] [PubMed]

88. Dingle, K.E.; Colles, F.M.; Wareing, D.R.; Ure, R.; Fox, A.J.; Bolton, F.E.; Bootsma, H.J.; Willems, R.J.; Urwin, R.; Maiden, M.C. Multilocus sequence typing system for *Campylobacter jejuni*. *J. Clin. Microbiol.* **2001**, *39*, 14–23. [CrossRef] [PubMed]

89. Dingle, K.E.; Colles, F.M.; Ure, R.; Wagenaar, J.A.; Duim, B.; Bolton, F.J.; Fox, A.J.; Wareing, D.R.; Maiden, M.C. Molecular characterization of *Campylobacter jejuni* clones: A basis for epidemiologic investigation. *Emerg. Infect. Dis.* **2002**, *8*, 949–955. [CrossRef] [PubMed]

90. Miller, W.G.; On, S.L.; Wang, G.; Fontanoz, S.; Lastovica, A.J.; Mandrell, R.E. Extended multilocus sequence typing system for *Campylobacter coli*, *C. lari*, *C. upsaliensis*, and *C. helveticus*. *J. Clin. Microbiol.* **2005**, *43*, 2315–2329. [CrossRef] [PubMed]

91. Jolley, K.A.; Bliss, C.M.; Bennett, J.S.; Bratcher, H.B.; Brehony, C.; Colles, F.M.; Wimalarathna, H.; Harrison, O.B.; Sheppard, S.K.; Cody, A.J.; et al. Ribosomal multilocus sequence typing: Universal characterization of bacteria from domain to strain. *Microbiology* **2012**, *158*, 1005–1015. [CrossRef] [PubMed]

92. Feil, E.J.; Li, B.C.; Aanensen, D.M.; Hanage, W.P.; Spratt, B.G. eBURST: Inferring patterns of evolutionary descent among clusters of related bacterial genotypes from multilocus sequence typing data. *J. Bacteriol.* **2004**, *186*, 1518–1530. [CrossRef] [PubMed]

93. Francisco, A.P.; Bugalho, M.; Ramirez, M.; Carrico, J.A. Global optimal eBURST analysis of multilocus typing data using a graphic matroid approach. *BMC Bioinform.* **2009**, *10*, 152. [CrossRef] [PubMed]

94. Cody, A.J.; Colles, F.M.; Sheppard, S.K.; Maiden, M.C. Where does *Campylobacter* come from? A molecular odyssey. *Adv. Exp. Med. Biol.* **2010**, *659*, 47–56. [PubMed]

95. El-Adawy, H.; Hotzel, H.; Tomaso, H.; Neubauer, H.; Taboada, E.N.; Ehricht, R.; Hafez, H.M. Detection of genetic diversity in *Campylobacter jejuni* isolated from a commercial turkey flock using *fla*A typing, MLST analysis and microarray assay. *PLoS ONE* **2013**, *8*, e51582. [CrossRef] [PubMed]

96. Ioannidou, V.; Ioannidis, A.; Magiorkinis, E.; Bagos, P.; Nicolaou, C.; Legakis, N.; Chatzipanagiotou, S. Multilocus sequence typing (and phylogenetic analysis) of *Campylobacter jejuni* and *Campylobacter coli* strains isolated from clinical cases in Greece. *BMC Res. Notes* **2013**, *6*, 359. [CrossRef] [PubMed]

97. Escher, R.; Brunner, C.; von Steiger, N.; Brodard, I.; Droz, S.; Abril, C.; Kuhnert, P. Clinical and epidemiological analysis of *Campylobacter fetus* subsp. *fetus* infections in humans and comparative genetic analysis with strains isolated from cattle. *BMC Infect. Dis.* **2016**, *16*, 198. [CrossRef] [PubMed]

98. Cody, A.J.; Maiden, M.J.; Dingle, K.E. Genetic diversity and stability of the *porA* allele as a genetic marker in human *Campylobacter* infection. *Microbiology* **2009**, *155*, 4145–4154. [CrossRef] [PubMed]

99. Jay-Russell, M.T.; Mandrell, R.E.; Yuan, J.; Bates, A.; Manalac, R.; Mohle-Boetani, J.; Kimura, A.; Lidgard, J.; Miller, W.G. Using major outer membrane protein typing as an epidemiological tool to investigate outbreaks caused by milk-borne *Campylobacter jejuni* isolates in California. *J. Clin. Microbiol.* **2013**, *51*, 195–201. [CrossRef] [PubMed]

100. Huang, S.; Luangtongkum, T.; Morishita, T.Y.; Zhang, Q. Molecular typing of *Campylobacter* strains using the cmp gene encoding the major outer membrane protein. *Foodborne Pathog. Dis.* **2005**, *2*, 12–23. [CrossRef] [PubMed]

101. Schleihauf, E.; Mutschall, S.; Billard, B.; Taboada, E.N.; Haldane, D. Comparative genomic fingerprinting of *Campylobacter*: Application in routine public health surveillance and epidemiological investigations. *Epidemiol. Infect.* **2017**, *145*, 299–309. [CrossRef] [PubMed]

102. Clark, C.G.; Taboada, E.; Grant, C.C.; Blakeston, C.; Pollari, F.; Marshall, B.; Rahn, K.; Mackinnon, J.; Daignault, D.; Pillai, D.; et al. Comparison of molecular typing methods useful for detecting clusters of *Campylobacter jejuni* and *C. coli* isolates through routine surveillance. *J. Clin. Microbiol.* **2012**, *50*, 798–809. [CrossRef] [PubMed]

103. Maiden, M.C.; Jansen van Rensburg, M.J.; Bray, J.E.; Earle, S.G.; Ford, S.A.; Jolley, K.A.; McCarthy, N.D. MLST revisited: The gene-by-gene approach to bacterial genomics. *Nat. Rev. Microbiol.* **2013**, *11*, 728–736. [CrossRef] [PubMed]

104. Carleton, H.A.; Gerner-Smidt, P. Whole-genome sequencing is taking over foodborne disease surveillance. *Microbe* **2016**, *11*, 311–317.

105. Koser, C.U.; Ellington, M.J.; Cartwright, E.J.; Gillespie, S.H.; Brown, N.M.; Farrington, M.; Holden, M.T.; Dougan, G.; Bentley, S.D.; Parkhill, J.; et al. Routine use of microbial whole genome sequencing in diagnostic and public health microbiology. *PLoS Pathog.* **2012**, *8*, e1002824. [CrossRef] [PubMed]

106. Diaz-Sanchez, S.; Hanning, I.; Pendleton, S.; D'Souza, D. Next-generation sequencing: The future of molecular genetics in poultry production and food safety. *Poult. Sci.* **2013**, *92*, 562–572. [CrossRef] [PubMed]

107. Mou, K.T.; Clark, T.A.; Muppirala, U.K.; Severin, A.J.; Plummer, P.J. Methods for genome-wide methylome profiling of *Campylobacter jejuni*. *Methods Mol. Biol.* **2017**, *1512*, 199–210. [PubMed]

108. O'Loughlin, J.L.; Eucker, T.P.; Chavez, J.D.; Samuelson, D.R.; Neal-McKinney, J.; Gourley, C.R.; Bruce, J.E.; Konkel, M.E. Analysis of the *Campylobacter jejuni* genome by SMRT DNA sequencing identifies restriction-modification motifs. *PLoS ONE* **2015**, *10*, e0118533. [CrossRef] [PubMed]

109. Johnson, J.G.; DiRita, V.J. Generation and screening of an insertion sequencing-compatible mutant library of *Campylobacter jejuni*. *Methods Mol. Med.* **2017**, *1512*, 257–272.

110. Didelot, X.; Maiden, M.C. Impact of recombination on bacterial evolution. *Trends Microbiol.* **2010**, *18*, 315–322. [CrossRef] [PubMed]

111. Schouls, L.M.; Reulen, S.; Duim, B.; Wagenaar, J.A.; Willems, R.J.; Dingle, K.E.; Colles, F.M.; Van Embden, J.D. Comparative genotyping of *Campylobacter jejuni* by amplified fragment length polymorphism, multilocus sequence typing, and short repeat sequencing: Strain diversity, host range, and recombination. *J. Clin. Microbiol.* **2003**, *41*, 15–26. [CrossRef] [PubMed]

112. Suerbaum, S.; Lohrengel, M.; Sonnevend, A.; Ruberg, F.; Kist, M. Allelic diversity and recombination in *Campylobacter jejuni*. *J. Bacteriol.* **2001**, *183*, 2553–2559. [CrossRef] [PubMed]

113. Cornelius, A.J.; Vandenberg, O.; Robson, B.; Gilpin, B.J.; Brandt, S.M.; Scholes, P.; Martiny, D.; Carter, P.E.; van Vught, P.; Schouten, J.; et al. Same-day subtyping of *Campylobacter jejuni* and *C. coli* isolates by use of multiplex ligation-dependent probe amplification-binary typing. *J. Clin. Microbiol.* **2014**, *52*, 3345–3350. [CrossRef] [PubMed]

114. Taboada, E.N.; Mackinnon, J.M.; Luebbert, C.C.; Gannon, V.P.; Nash, J.H.; Rahn, K. Comparative genomic assessment of Multi-Locus Sequence Typing: Rapid accumulation of genomic heterogeneity among clonal isolates of *Campylobacter jejuni*. *BMC Evol. Biol.* **2008**, *8*, 229. [CrossRef] [PubMed]

9

Correlation between Preoperative Ultrasonographic Findings and Clinical, Intraoperative, Cytopathological, and Histopathological Diagnosis of Acute Abdomen Syndrome in 50 Dogs and Cats

Ahmed Abdellatif [1,2,*], Martin Kramer [1], Klaus Failing [3] and Kerstin von Pückler [1]

[1] Department of Veterinary Clinical Science, Clinic for Small Animals (Surgery), Justus-Liebig University (JLU), 35392 Gießen, Germany; Martin.Kramer@vetmed.uni-giessen.de (M.K.); Kerstin.H.Pueckler@vetmed.uni-giessen.de (K.v.P.)

[2] Animal Surgery Department, Assiut University, Assiut 71515, Egypt

[3] Unit for Biomathematics and Data Processing, Veterinary Faculty, Justus-Liebig University (JLU), Gießen 35392, Germany; Klaus.Failing@vetmed.uni-giessen.de

* Correspondence: Ahmed.F.Abdellatif@vetmed.uni-giessen.de

Academic Editor: Patrick Butaye

Abstract: Acute abdomen syndrome is an emergency in small animal practice that requires rapid diagnosis to determine the appropriate treatment. No studies have correlated the preoperative abdominal ultrasonography (US) findings with the clinical, surgical, cytopathologic, and histopathologic findings. This retrospective study was designed to evaluate abdominal US in the diagnosis of acute abdomen syndrome using surgery as a "criterion standard". The most frequently misinterpreted lesions with US were also identified. The study included 50 dogs and cats with physical examination, an US diagnosis, US guided fine-needle aspiration cytology, intraoperative findings, and histopathology. Intraoperatively, 49 primary and 43 secondary lesions were identified. The sensitivity, specificity, and positive and negative predictive values for US were calculated. There was a good agreement between the US diagnosis and intraoperative findings of 86.9% (80/92), for both primary and secondary lesions ($p < 0.0001$). Cytology and histopathology examinations corroborated the US in 86.4% ($n = 64/74$) of primary and 66.2% of secondary ($n = 49/79$) lesions. Using US as the "criterion standard", the sensitivity of abdominal palpation for identification of ascites and masses was 32.4% and 43.7%, respectively, while the specificity was 93.7% and 94.4%, respectively. Abdominal US is a useful preoperative modality for diagnosing acute abdominal diseases in dogs and cats. Care should be taken with interpretation of gastrointestinal perforation, omental tumors, and common bile duct rupture, as these lesions are frequently misinterpreted with US.

Keywords: dog; cat; ultrasonography; acute abdomen; laparotomy

---

1. Introduction

Acute abdomen syndrome is a clinical syndrome characterized by the sudden onset of severe abdominal pain accompanied by signs and symptoms of abdominal involvement [1–4]. Acute abdomen syndrome may be associated with a wide variety of disease processes, ranging from self-limiting conditions to surgical emergencies. Disorders of the gastrointestinal, hepatobiliary, or urogenital systems, the spleen, pancreas, and peritoneum have been reported [3–5]. Acute abdomen syndrome requires rapid, careful evaluation, and integration of clinical findings, clinical pathology, and diagnostic imaging to determine the appropriate medical and/or surgical management [4,6,7].

Abdominal ultrasonography (US) is a valuable procedure for the diagnosis of a wide range of acute abdomen diseases [1–4,6,8]. Ultrasound findings of a target-like mass of concentric hyperechoic and hypoechoic rings is diagnostic of intestinal intussusception in dogs and cats [9,10]. Transmural thickening with loss of normal gastrointestinal wall layering and evidence of local lymphadenopathy is indicative of canine and feline intestinal adenocarcinoma [11,12]. Ultrasonographic appearance of an enlarged and hypoechoic pancreas with ascites, hyperechoic peripancreatic tissues, and extrahepatic biliary obstruction is suggestive of pancreatitis [1,13]. In a study of 12 dogs with gallbladder and extrahepatic biliary tract obstruction, US correctly diagnosed obstruction in 10 cases. However, the cause of obstruction could not be determined by abdominal US alone in two cases [14]. In a series of 129 human patients with ovarian cancer, ultrasound had low sensitivity and specificity in patients with lesions less than 2 cm [15].

The purpose of this retrospective study was to evaluate the performance of US as a pre-surgical diagnostic tool in patients with acute abdomen syndrome, and to identify the most frequently misinterpreted lesions. In addition, the ability of abdominal palpation to identify the presence of ascites or masses was evaluated. We hypothesized that abdominal US is useful pre-surgically for the diagnosis of canine and feline acute abdomen disease.

The present study is similar to a previous study that described US features of acute abdomen [1] and a study comparing US and exploratory laparotomy in the dog and cat [16]. However, our study provides cytopathologic and histopathologic identification of lesions. Furthermore, our study compares abdominal palpation with US for the detection of peritoneal effusion and masses.

2. Materials and Methods

This retrospective study was performed at the Clinic for Small Animals Surgery of the Justus Liebig University in Giessen. Surgical and US records of dogs and cats admitted for acute abdomen syndrome were reviewed. Inclusion criteria were: animals with preoperative physical examination, US, US guided fine-needle aspiration cytology, and laparotomy. Clinical records included a complete history, breed, age (months/years), sex (male/female), weight, and duration of clinical signs (hours/days). The patient's general condition was categorized to one of five clinical stages: undisturbed (1); slightly disturbed (2); moderately impaired (3); severely impaired (4); and anesthetized or comatose animals (5).

Abdominal palpation findings were categorized into one of four groups: normal (1); tense abdomen (2); suspicion of ascites (3); and palpable abdominal mass (4).

Records of thoracic and abdominal radiographs were reviewed for evidence of abnormalities involving the parenchymal organs, gastrointestinal tract (GIT), and peritoneal cavity. The US examinations were performed by one of three radiologists, each with more than four years of experience (board-certified radiologists, ECVDI). As a routine procedure in our clinic, the linear transducer (7.5 MHz to 14 MHz) is used to image cats and small dogs (<20 kg); while large dogs (>20 kg) are usually examined with a convex transducer providing greater tissue penetration (5 MHz), typically in combination with a high frequency linear probe (Toshiba, Imaging Systems GmbH, Neuss, Germany).

Each abdominal organ was examined for size, shape, echotexture, and echogenicity. Scanning was performed in dorsal or lateral recumbency. The examination began at the urinary bladder. A standardized template for US was used for all examinations and included any identified abnormalities. Abdominal structures were considered free of abnormalities if no abnormalities were documented in the written US report. To facilitate statistical analysis, the final intraoperative and US diagnoses were recorded in an excel file with a numeric system (1 = intestinal tumor, 2 = stomach tumor, 3 = liver tumor, 4 = splenic tumor, etc.). The numeric system included 20 different diagnoses and one to three diagnoses were listed for each patient. The intraoperative findings were classified according to the anatomical location and gross pathology. The intraoperative reports included the surgeon's remarks and the techniques used. The intraoperative findings were classified as primary or secondary lesions, as designated by the surgeon, and according to the organs involved.

A primary lesion is the main intraoperative finding, while secondary lesions include other associated lesions. For instance, in an animal with a gastrointestinal foreign body, intestinal perforation, and septic peritonitis, the foreign body is the primary lesion, and intestinal perforation, and septic peritonitis the secondary lesions.

Preoperative US guided fine-needle aspiration cytology was performed in 50 patients and postoperative histopathology in 48. Two patients were humanely euthanized during surgery at the owner's request and no histopathology was available. Results from cytology were classified into different categories: ascitic fluid, transudate (1); ascitic fluid, modified transudate (2); ascitic fluid, purulent exudates (3); and hemoperitoneum (4). Cytologic and histopathologic findings of mass lesions were classified into six categories: benign epithelial (1a); malignant epithelial (1b); benign mesenchymal (2a); malignant mesenchymal (2b); lymphatic malignancies (3); neuroendocrine malignancies (4); purulent inflammation (5); and inflammatory or hyperplastic (6).

Statistical analysis was done with the statistical program packages BMDP [17] and BiAS [18] for Windows. For data that met the assumption of normality, mean, minimum, maximum, and standard deviation (SD) were calculated. Fisher's exact test was used to determine the association between preoperative US, intraoperative findings, and abdominal palpation. The sensitivity, specificity, and positive and negative predictive values for US were calculated using the surgical diagnosis as the "criterion standard". To assess the value of abdominal palpation, the sensitivity and specificity were calculated using the US as the "criterion standard". Additionally, the 95% confidence intervals (CI) were calculated. For all tests, a significance level of 0.05 was chosen and a value of $p < 0.05$ was considered statistically significant.

3. Results

Fifty animals met the inclusion criteria. There were 33 dogs (66%) and 17 cats (34%). Thirty-three animals were male (66%) and 17 were female (34%). The mean age of the dogs was 7 ± 4.6 years (range, 3 months to 15 years), and that of the cats was 5.7 ± 4.7 years (range, 7 months to 15 years). The mean weight of dogs was 19.7 ± 13.3 kg (range, 3–50 kg) and that of cats was 4.6 ± 1.5 kg (range, 2.7–7.9 kg). The mean duration of clinical signs prior to presentation was 2.9 ± 1.7 days in dogs (range, 2 h to 5 days), and 4.3 ± 3.7 days (range 2 h to 10 days) in cats. On the day of the first examination, 56% ($n = 28$) had clinical signs for less than three days. In most cases, nonspecific clinical signs including vomiting, abdominal pain, lethargy, anorexia, weight loss, and depression were reported. On physical examination, patients were undisturbed ($n = 11$), slightly disturbed ($n = 12$), moderately impaired ($n = 12$), severely impaired ($n = 13$), and anesthetized ($n = 2$).

Abdominal palpation identified acute abdominal disease in 76% of patients ($n = 38$) and identified an abdominal mass ($n = 14$), ascites ($n = 11$), and tense abdomen ($n = 13$). The abdomen was palpably normal in 10 animals. Ultrasound was used to confirm abdominal palpation of ascites or masses. Palpation of fluid had a sensitivity of 32.4% (CI: 17.4–50.5%) and specificity of 93.7% (CI: 69.7–99.8%) (Figure 1). Palpation of an abdominal mass had a sensitivity of 43.7% (CI: 26.4–62.3%) and a specificity of 94.4% (CI: 72.7–99.9%). There was a significant association between palpation and US diagnosis of ascites ($p < 0.05$), but no significant relationship between palpation and US detection of an abdominal mass ($p > 0.05$).

Ninety-two intraoperative lesions (49 primary and 43 secondary) were documented. The preoperative diagnosis in one case was an intestinal foreign body. However, at surgery, the abdomen was normal. Intraoperative findings are summarized by anatomical location in Table 1. Primary lesions were most frequently located in the gastrointestinal tract (53%, $n = 26$), the peritoneum and peritoneal cavity (14.3%, $n = 7$), and pancreas (12.2%, $n = 6$). Secondary lesions were most commonly located in the peritoneum and peritoneal cavity (60.5%, $n = 26$), gastrointestinal tract (14%, $n = 6$), and spleen (9.3%, $n = 4$).

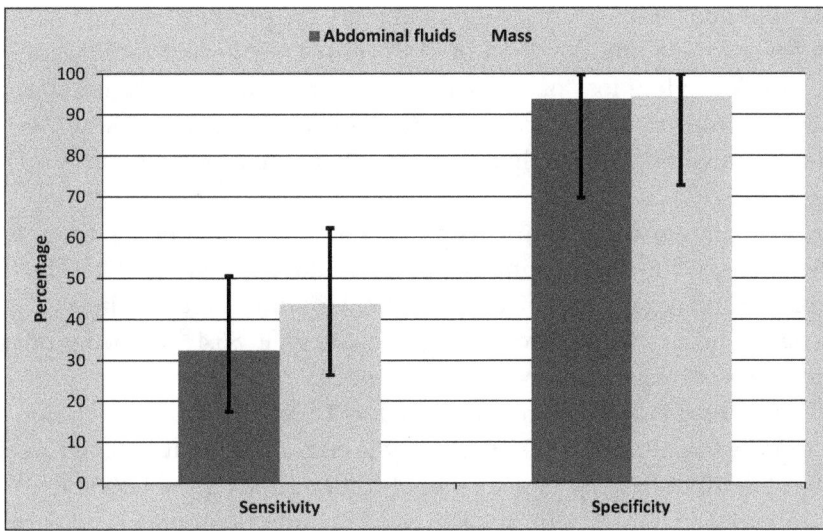

Figure 1. Bar graph showing the sensitivity and specificity of abdominal palpation for the detection of fluid and masses, when compared to ultrasonography. The black error bars denote the 95% confidence intervals.

Table 1. Distribution of intraoperative lesions according to anatomical location.

Surgical Diagnosis				
			Lesion Category	
Surgical Diagnosis	**Dog**	**Cat**	**Primary**	**Secondary**
Gastrointestinal				
Intussusception	6	3	9	0
Intestinal neoplasia	2	5	7	0
Foreign body	4	1	5	0
Perforation	1	3	2	2
Ulcer	2	2	0	4
Stomach neoplasia	3	0	3	0
Peritoneum and peritoneal cavity				
General peritonitis	8	5	4	9
Ascites	7	2	1	8
Focal peritonitis	6	0	0	6
Omental masses	3	2	2	3
Pancreas				
Abscess	5	0	4	1
Neoplasia	2	0	2	0
Liver				
Neoplasia	2	2	1	3
Abscess	1	0	1	0
Bile duct rupture	2	0	2	0
Spleen				
Neoplasia	4	0	0	4
Abscess	1	0	1	0
Abdominal LN ‡				
Enlarged LN	4	2	3	3
Kidney				
Neoplasia	0	1	1	0
Urinoma	0	1	1	0
Total	63	29	49	43

‡ LN: Lymph node.

Thoracic and abdominal radiography did not identify the primary lesion in 71% (35/49) of cases, while secondary lesions were not identified in 41.8% (18/43). Normal radiographic findings were reported in 36% (18/50), while loss of serosal detail was the most common abnormal finding in 32% (16/50). Gastrointestinal obstructions ($n = 8$), splenic tumors ($n = 2$), kidney tumors ($n = 2$), nonspecific intra-abdominal mass ($n = 2$), liver mass ($n = 1$), and intussusception ($n = 1$) were suspected by radiography.

Comparing preoperative abdominal US and intraoperative diagnoses, there was a significant agreement of 86.9% (80/92) for both primary and secondary lesions ($p < 0.0001$). The sensitivity, specificity, and positive and negative predictive values of US with confidence intervals are summarized in Table 2. Ultrasound findings were corroborated by cytology in 86.4% of the lesions ($n = 64/74$) and histopathology in 66.2% of the lesions ($n = 49/74$) (Table 3).

Surgical lesions were not identified not identified by US in 13% (12/92) of lesions. False negative diagnoses were reported in 10.2% (5/49) of primary lesions. This included GIT perforation ($n = 2$), ruptured common bile duct ($n = 2$), and intestinal foreign body ($n = 1$) (Table 4). False positive diagnoses were reported in 14% (7/50) of cases, and included omental tumors ($n = 2$), intestinal neoplasia ($n = 2$), pancreatic tumor ($n = 1$), pancreatic abscess ($n = 1$), and intestinal foreign body ($n = 1$). There was disagreement in the diagnosis of secondary lesions between the US and surgical findings in 16.2% of the secondary lesions ($n = 7/43$). This included omental tumors ($n = 3$), gastrointestinal tract perforation ($n = 2$), generalized peritonitis ($n = 1$), and an intestinal ulcer ($n = 1$). The primary lesions in these cases were correctly diagnosed preoperatively. A false positive diagnosis of the secondary lesions was reported in 9.3% (4/43), and included splenic tumors ($n = 2$), lymphadenopathy ($n = 1$), and pancreatic abscess ($n = 1$).

Lesions of the gastrointestinal tract were reported in 34.8% (32/92); 53% (26/49) were primary and 14% (6/43) were secondary. The pathological conditions included intussusception ($n = 9$), intestinal neoplasia ($n = 7$), foreign body ($n = 5$), perforation ($n = 4$), gastrointestinal ulcer ($n = 4$), and gastric tumor ($n = 3$). Intussusception was accurately diagnosed by US in all cases (9/9). Secondary lesions including omental masses were diagnosed in one case. Intussusceptions were confirmed histologically, with enteritis and lymphadenitis as the most reported findings. Intestinal neoplasia was suspected by US in nine cases and intestinal masses were identified intraoperatively in seven cases (7/9). Histopathology corroborated the US suspicion in five cases (5/9) of lymphoma ($n = 3$) and fibrosarcoma ($n = 2$), while purulent inflammation was documented in four cases. Four of five cases of gastrointestinal foreign body suspected with US were confirmed at surgery. In one case (1/0), a false positive diagnosis was reported by the US. In another case ($n = 1$), the false negative diagnosis was reported by the US. Gastrointestinal perforation location was not detected with abdominal ultrasound (0/4).

Gastrointestinal ulcer was suspected by US and corroborated by histopathology in three cases (3/4). The etiologies were: neoplasia ($n = 3$) and gastric foreign body. Gastric tumors were diagnosed accurately by US in all cases (3/3) and were identified as gastric carcinoma on histopathology. Ulcerative gastritis was reported on histopathology in the case of foreign bodies.

Diseases of the peritoneum and peritoneal cavity were detected in 35.9% ($n = 33/92$) of lesions and included primary (14.3%, 7/49) and secondary (60.5%, 26/43) lesions. Generalized peritonitis ($n = 13$), peritoneal effusion ($n = 9$), focal peritonitis ($n = 6$), and omental masses ($n = 5$) were identified.

Ultrasound correctly identified generalized peritonitis and peritoneal effusions in 12 of 13 cases. A history of previous abdominal surgery was reported in two animals. Purulent exudate was reported in all cases and purulent inflammation was diagnosed in the omentum, liver, and stomach. Ultrasound accurately diagnosed peritoneal effusion as a primary lesion ($n = 1$) and a secondary lesion ($n = 8$). Cytological examination indicated a modified transudate ($n = 7$) and purulent exudate ($n = 2$). Focal peritonitis as a secondary lesion was suspected by US and confirmed intraoperatively in six cases. Cytopathology was available in one case and reported chronic necrotizing peritonitis and omentitis.

Table 2. Preoperative abdominal ultrasound and intraoperative diagnoses of the primary and secondary lesions based on anatomic location. Sensitivities and specificities (with confidence intervals) of ultrasonography are presented for both primary and secondary lesions identified at surgery. The surgical diagnosis was the "criterion standard".

Surgical Diagnosis	Ultrasonographic Findings							
	Primary Lesions				Secondary Lesions			
Diseases	Sensitivity (CI *)	Specificity (CI *)	PPV *	NPV *	Sensitivity (CI *)	Specificity (CI *)	PPV *	NPV *
Gastrointestinal								
Intussusception	100% CI: 72-100	100% CI: 97-100	100%	100%	-	-	-	-
Intestinal neoplasia	100% CI: 60-100	95% CI: 84-99	77%	100%	-	-	-	-
Foreign body	80% CI: 34-98	97.7% CI: 96-99	80%	98%	-	-	-	-
Perforation	0	0	0	100%	0	0	0	100%
Ulcer	-	-	-	-	100% CI: 34-100	98% CI: 34-98	75%	100%
Stomach neoplasia	100% CI: 72-100	100% CI: 97-100	100%	100%	-	-	-	-
Peritoneum and peritoneal cavity								
General Peritonitis								
Ascites	100% CI: 47-100	100% CI: 95-100	100%	100%	89% CI: 60-89	100% CI: 92-100	100%	97%
Focal peritonitis	100% CI: 5.7-100	100% CI: 95-100	100%	100%	100% CI: 68-100	90% CI: 90-97	100%	97%
Omental masses	0	95% CI: 86-99	0	100%	100% CI: 61-100	100% CI: 93-100	0	100%
Pancreas								
Abscess	100% CI: 47-100	97% CI: 84-99	80%	100%	100% CI: 2.5-100	97% CI: 87-99	50%	100%
Neoplasia	100% CI: 56-100	97% CI: 97-98	50%	100%	-	-	-	100%
Liver								
Neoplasia	100% CI: 47-100	100% CI: 97-100	100%	100%	-	-	-	100%
Abscess	100% CI: 57-100	100% CI: 97-100	100%	100%	-	-	-	100%
Bile duct rupture	0	0	0	100%	-	-	-	100%
Spleen								
Neoplasia	-	-	-	-	100% CI: 39-100	94% CI: 82-99	66%	100%
Abscess	100% CI: 57-100	100% CI: 57-100	100%	100%	-	-	-	100%
Abdominal LN ‡								
Enlarged lymph nodes	100% CI: 59-100	100% CI: 96-100	100%	100%	100% CI: 35-100	97% CI: 92-97	75%	100%
Kidney								
Neoplasia	100% CI: 57-100	100% CI: 97-100	100%	100%	-	-	-	-
Urinoma	100% CI: 57-100	100% CI: 97-100	100%	100%	-	-	-	-

* CI: Confidence intervals 95%; ‡ LN: Lymph node.

Table 3. Comparison of ultrasonographic findings with cytopathologic and histopathologic findings. Agreement between the tests is presented as a percentage (%) and number (*n*) of reported ultrasonographic lesions with cytologic or histopathologic confirmation.

Ultrasonography		Preoperative Cytology and Postoperative Histopathology		
		Agreement with US		
Findings	**(*n*)**	**Cytology**	**Histopathology**	**Findings**
		% (*n*)	**% (*n*)**	
GIT diseases				
Intussusception	9	100% (9)	100% (9)	Enteritis and lymphadenitis
Intestinal neoplasia	9	55.5% (5)	55.5% (5)	Lymphoma (3) and fibrosarcoma (2)
Ulcer	3	100% (3)	100% (3)	Ulcerative gastritis duo to carcinoma (3)
Stomach neoplasia	3	100% (3)	100% (3)	Carcinoma
Peritoneum and peritoneal cavity				
Peritonitis				
Ascites				
	13	100% (13)	100% (13)	Purulent inflammation (6) and chronic necrotizing peritonitis and omentitis (7)
	9	100% (9)	-	Modified transudate (7) and purulent exudate (2)
Pancreas				
Abscess	7	100% (7)	57% (4)	Purulent inflammation
Neoplasia	1	100% (1)	0	Chronic purulent pancreatitis
Liver				
Neoplasia	1	100% (1)	0	Lymphoma
Nodular hyperplasia	3	100% (3)	100% (3)	Nodular hyperplasia
Abscess	1	100% (1)	0	Purulent hepatitis
Spleen				
Neoplasia	6	0	0	Extra-medullary hematopoiesis (3), regenerating nodules and hyperplasia (3)
				Purulent splenitis
Abscess	1	100% (1)	100% (1)	
Lymph nodes				
Enlarged lymph nodes	6	100% (6)	100% (6)	Purulent lymphadenitis (3), lymphosarcoma (2) and undifferentiated blastoma (1)
Kidney				
Neoplasia	1	100% (1)	100% (1)	Malignant renal epithelial tumor
Urinoma	1	100% (1)	100% (1)	Proteinaceous granulomatous inflammatory effusion
Total	74	86.4% (64)	66.2% (49)	

Table 4. Lesions misinterpreted by pre-operative abdominal ultrasound, using surgery as "criterion standard".

Intraoperative Lesion(s)	Primary Lesions		Secondary Lesions	
	False Negative	False Positive	False Negative	False Positive
Omental mass	-	2	3	-
GIT perforation	2		2	-
Intestinal neoplasia		2		-
Common bile duct rupture	2	-	-	-
Splenic neoplasia	-	-	-	2
Pancreatic abscess	-	1	-	1
Pancreatic tumor	-	1		-
Intestinal foreign body	1	1	-	-
Peritonitis			1	-
GIT ulcer	-	-	1	-
Lymphadenopathy	-	-	-	1

Five omental masses were diagnosed. The masses measured approximately 1 cm ($n = 3$), 3 cm ($n = 1$), and 15 cm ($n = 1$). However, only the large (3 cm and 15 cm) omental masses were detected by US and were classified as lymphadenopathy and a splenic tumor (false positive diagnosis). The masses were identified as benign hyperplasia (3/5), omental fibrosarcoma (1/5), and lymphoma (1/5).

Pancreatic disease represented 7.6% (7/92) of all lesions including primary (12.2%, 6/49) and secondary (2.3%, 1/43) lesions. Pancreatic abscess ($n = 5$) and neoplasia ($n = 2$) were diagnosed. Ultrasound identified pancreatic abscess in seven cases (7/5), four of which were confirmed by histopathology (4/7). In three cases, the pancreas was normal. Pancreatic neoplasia was suspected by US in three cases (3/2) but was not corroborated by histopathology.

Hepatic lesions were identified in 7.6% (7/92) of lesions as primary (8.2%, 4/49) and secondary (7%, 3/43) lesions. Hepatic masses ($n = 5$) and ruptured common bile duct ($n = 2$) were diagnosed. Based on US, nodular hyperplasia ($n = 3$), neoplastic infiltration ($n = 1$), and abscessation ($n = 1$) were suspected. Fine needle aspiration and postoperative pathology diagnosed extra medullary hematopoiesis in three cases, while hepatic neoplasia and hepatic abscess were confirmed with cytology (2/2). The bile duct lesions were not diagnosed by US (0/2), but cholangitis, pericholecystic echogenic reaction, and duct obstruction were identified.

Splenic masses represented 5.4% (5/92) of lesions as primary (2%, 1/49) and secondary (9.3%, 4/43) lesions. With US, malignant splenic neoplasia was suspected in six cases and confirmed in four cases (4/6). A large mass in the omentum (1/6) and normal spleen (1/6) were reported in the other two cases. Extra-medullary hematopoiesis ($n = 3$), regenerating nodules and nodular hyperplasia ($n = 2$), and omental fibrosarcoma ($n = 1$) were diagnosed by histology. Splenic abscessation was diagnosed preoperatively in one case (1/5) and was confirmed with histopathology.

Lymph node disease was reported in 6.5% (6/92) as primary (6%, 3/49) and secondary (7%, 3/43) lesions. Ultrasound correctly identified all cases (6/6); in three cases, purulent lymphadenitis was the primary US differential diagnosis, followed by neoplasia; the opposite was reported in the other three cases. Histopathology confirmed the US diagnosis as purulent lymphadenitis (3/6), malignant lymphosarcoma (2/6), and undifferentiated blastoma (1/6). A false positive US diagnosis of lymphadenopathy (1/0) was diagnosed intraoperatively as an omental tumor and corroborated by histology as nodular hyperplasia of the omentum.

Kidney lesions were detected in 2.1% (2/92) as primary lesions (4%, 2/49). Ultrasound accurately diagnosed renal neoplasia ($n = 1$) and urinoma ($n = 1$); all were accurately diagnosed by abdominal ultrasound. With histological examination, a malignant renal epithelial tumor was diagnosed in one case, and a proteinaceous granulomatous inflammatory effusion was aspirated in the case of urinoma.

4. Discussion

Although the diagnosis and management of acute abdomen has been reviewed, there is a lack of information correlating the US findings with the clinical, intraoperative, and histopathologic findings.

There are few studies that provide details on the species, sex, predisposition, duration of signs before presentation, and general condition of patients presenting with acute abdomen syndrome. Our study had more dogs (66%, $n = 33$) than cats (34%, $n = 17$), and male animals were more commonly affected (66%, $n = 33$) than the female animals (34%, $n = 17$). Our results are consistent with a large cohort study which reported that three times more dogs ($n = 942$) were affected than cats ($n = 309$), and that male animals were represented 63.1% ($n = 790$) of the cases [19]. The maximum duration of signs prior to presentation was 10 days in cats and 15 days in dogs [19]. In our study, the mean duration in cats was 4.4 days (ranging 2 h to 10 days) and 2.9 days in dogs (ranging 2 h to 5 days).

The physical examination was used to triage patients with acute abdomen syndrome [6]. In our study, 74% of patients ($n = 37/50$) were classified as mildly to severely impaired at presentation, and two were comatose.

Abdominal palpation is a component in the diagnosis of acute abdominal syndrome [20]. Detection of peritoneal effusion by palpation was confirmed by identification of ascites by US with a sensitivity of 32.4% and a specificity of 93.7%. Abdominal palpation of masses had a sensitivity of 43.7% and a specificity of 94.4%. There was no clinical description of the volume of peritoneal effusion or the size of abdominal masses, thus further studies may be required to show the accuracy of the abdominal palpation. Despite poor performance of abdominal palpation, abdominal palpation may guide clinicians to choose the next diagnostic procedure. Protective abdominal muscle spasms in response to pain may hinder abdominal palpation [21], this may explain the inconclusive palpation findings in 10 animals in the present study.

Survey abdominal radiography did not identify abnormalities in 71% of cases. In patients with peritoneal fluid or peritonitis, loss of intra-abdominal detail makes abdominal radiography less useful for diagnosis of acute abdomen [2]. In a prospective study of human patients with abdominal pain, radiographic diagnosis was correct in 50% of patients [22]. Veterinary studies also describe poor performance of plain abdominal radiography for the diagnosis of abdominal lesions [23–26]. There is no information about the accuracy of the abdominal radiography in clinical trials of patients with acute abdomen syndrome of different etiologies. Abdominal radiography can guide abdominal US diagnosis and provide information about the advisability of surgical intervention [4].

The present study showed good agreement (86.9%) between US and intraoperative lesions. This is higher than the 64% agreement reported in a study of 100 dogs and cats [16] where diagnosis was confirmed by gross intraoperative observations [16]. In the present study, US was confirmed with cytology (81%) and histopathology (63.3%) [16]. Surgical lesions were not identified by US in 13% ($n = 12/92$) of lesions. The false positive diagnosis by US was reported in 11 lesions (seven primary and four secondary). A higher rate of misdiagnosis (25%) has been reported and gastrointestinal tract ulcerations and perforations were the most commonly misdiagnosed (16). The experience of the examiner and the quality of the machine are important in the interpretation of US findings, as ultrasonography is highly operator and equipment-dependent [27].

Omental tumors were the most commonly misinterpreted lesions including two primary (false positive diagnosis) and three secondary (false negative diagnosis) lesions. The poor sensitivity of abdominal ultrasound for small lesions has been previously reported in human medicine. Macroscopic peritoneal lesions of less than 2 cm are difficult to identify with US and US had a low sensitivity and specificity. Ultrasound cannot replace exploratory laparotomy for the detection of small lesions [15].

Perforation of the GIT was not identified (false negative) by US in two primary and two secondary lesions. Peritoneal effusion is a principal finding in patients with GIT perforation [16]. Ultrasound correctly identified generalized septic peritonitis and ascites. A low sensitivity for US for the identification of GIT perforation has been reported [28,29]. Ultrasound correctly diagnosed spontaneous gastroduodenal perforation in only 1 of 11 dogs [29]. Strong indicators of perforation are free abdominal gas or a combination of local hyperechoic fat and local effusion. In a descriptive retrospective study, GI perforation was listed as a differential diagnosis in 14/19 cases. [28].

One case of GIT foreign body was not detected by US, resulting in a sensitivity of 80%. A prospective study that assessed small intestinal obstruction using specific ultrasonographic criteria correctly diagnosed obstruction in 11 of 13 dogs [30]. Our results suggest that the low number of patients with foreign bodies may have influenced the sensitivity of the US.

Bile duct rupture was not identified (false negative) as primary lesions in two dogs. Although signs of peritonitis, cholangitis, and pericholecystic echogenic reaction were detected by abdominal ultrasound, duct rupture was not listed in the differential diagnosis, suggesting that identifying pericholecystic reaction, and localized or generalized echogenic peritoneal fluid are suspicious for bile duct rupture [31].

Pancreatic neoplasia was documented as the primary lesion intraoperatively in two cases. Abdominal ultrasound indicated the neoplasia preoperatively ($n = 2$). However, the false positive diagnosis was reported in one case; lymph node neoplasia with pancreatitis and general peritonitis were the reported diagnoses in this case. A neoplastic pancreas may appear normal with US or may mimic or be associated with abscessation, pancreatic necrosis, or pancreatitis [32].

In this study, US findings correlated with surgical findings in all primary lesions of the liver, splenic, lymph nodes, and kidney. Although US is regarded as a useful diagnostic modality to recognize abnormalities in these organs, correlation with intraoperative, cytopathologic, and histopathologic findings was not performed [33,34].

Our study is limited by the small sample size, which resulted in some conditions being represented by only one case. A second limitation is that, in several cases, radiographs were obtained prior to US, which may have resulted in preselection of the cases. Also, preoperative knowledge of the US may have influenced the surgical results.

5. Conclusions

In conclusion, the study confirmed that abdominal ultrasound is a useful preoperative modality for the diagnosis of acute abdominal disease. Care should be taken with interpretation of US images in animals with gastrointestinal perforation, common bile duct rupture, omental neoplasia, pancreatic neoplasia, and a gastrointestinal foreign body, as these lesions were most commonly misinterpreted with US. Cytology and histopathology confirmed the ultrasound diagnosis in 86.4% of primary and 66.2% of secondary lesions. To determine the correct diagnosis and prognosis, the diagnostic assessment of acute abdomen should combine physical examination (including general condition and abdominal palpation); abdominal imaging (e.g., radiography and ultrasound); and cytopathological analysis.

Author Contributions: Ahmed Abdellatif performed ultrasound examinations, collected data, wrote the manuscript, and drafted the figures and tables. Martin Kramer revised the manuscript. Klaus Failing performed the statistical measures. Kerstin von Pückler did the second check of the US examinations and reviewed the manuscript.

References

1. Cruz-Arámbulo, R.; Wrigley, R. Ultrasonography of the acute abdomen. *Clin. Tech. Small Anim. Pract.* **2003**, *18*, 20–31. [CrossRef]
2. Boag, A.; Hughes, D. Emergency management of the acute abdomen in dogs and cats 1. Investigation and initial stabilisation. *Practice* **2004**, *26*, 476–483. [CrossRef]
3. Mazzei, M.A.; Guerrini, S.; Cioffi Squitieri, N.; Cagini, L.; Macarini, L.; Coppolino, F.; Giganti, M.; Volterrani, L. The role of US examination in the management of acute abdomen. *Crit. Ultrasound J.* **2013**, *5*, S6. [CrossRef] [PubMed]

4. Heeren, V.; Edwards, L.; Mazzaferro, E. Acute Abdomen: Diagnosis. *Compend. Cont. Educ. Pract. Vet.* **2004**, *26*, 350–363.

5. Saxon, W.D. The acute abdomen. *Vet. Clin. N. Am. Small Anim. Pract.* **1994**, *24*, 1207–1224. [CrossRef]

6. Walters, P.C. Approach to the acute abdomen. *Clin. Tech. Small Anim. Pract.* **2000**, *15*, 63–69. [CrossRef] [PubMed]

7. Yool, D.A. Peritonitis management and the acute abdomen. In *Small Animal Soft Tissue Surgery*; CAB International: Wallingford, UK, 2012; pp. 205–220, ISBN 9781845938215.

8. Mazzaferro, E.M. Triage and approach to the acute abdomen. *Clin. Tech. Small Anim. Pract.* **2003**, *18*, 1–6. [CrossRef]

9. Lamb, C.R.; Mantis, P. Ultrasonographic features of intestinal intussusception in 10 dogs. *J. Small Anim. Pract.* **1998**, *39*, 437–441. [CrossRef] [PubMed]

10. Patsikas, M.N.; Papazoglou, L.G.; Papaioannou, N.G.; Savvas, I.; Kazakos, G.M.; Dessiris, A.K. Ultrasonographic findings of intestinal intussusception in seven cats. *J. Feline Med. Surg.* **2003**, *5*, 335–343. [CrossRef]

11. Rivers, B.J.; Walter, P.A.; Feeney, D.A.; Johnston, G.R. Ultrasonographic features of intestinal adenocarcinoma in five cats. *Vet. Radiol. Ultrasound* **1997**, *38*, 300–306. [CrossRef] [PubMed]

12. Penninck, D.G. Characterization of gastrointestinal tumors. *Vet. Clin. N. Am. Small Anim. Pract.* **1998**, *28*, 777–797. [CrossRef]

13. Hess, R.S.; Saunders, H.M.; Van Winkle, T.J.; Shofer, F.S.; Washabau, R.J. Clinical, clinicopathologic, radiographic, and ultrasonographic abnormalities in dogs with fatal acute pancreatitis: 70 cases (1986–1995). *J. Am. Vet. Med. Assoc.* **1998**, *213*, 665–670. [PubMed]

14. Vörös, K.; Németh, T.; Vrabély, T.; Manczur, F.; Tóth, J.; Magdus, M.; Perge, E. Ultrasonography and surgery of canine biliary diseases. *Acta Vet. Hung.* **2001**, *49*, 141–154. [CrossRef] [PubMed]

15. Murolo, C.; Costantini, S.; Foglia, G.; Guido, T.; Odicino, F.; Pace, M.; Parodi, S.; Pino, G.; Ragni, N.; Repetto, L. Ultrasound examination in ovarian cancer patients. A comparison with second look laparotomy. *J. Ultrasound Med.* **1989**, *8*, 441–443. [CrossRef] [PubMed]

16. Pastore, G.E.; Lamb, C.R.; Lipscomb, V. Comparison of the results of abdominal ultrasonography and exploratory laparotomy in the dog and cat. *J. Am. Anim. Hosp. Assoc.* **2007**, *43*, 264–269. [CrossRef] [PubMed]

17. Dixon, W.J. *BMDP Statistical Software Manual*; University of California Press: Berkeley, CA, USA, 1993; Volumes 1–2.

18. Ackermann, H. *BiAS. Für Windows–Biometrische Analyse von Stichproben*, Version 11.0 (Software); Epsilon-Verlag: Darmstadt, Germany, 2010; c1989–c2015.

19. Günther, C.S. *Das Akute Abdomen Beim Kleintier aus Chirurgischer Sicht: Eine Retrospektive Studie von 2000–2005*; Edition Scientifique; Laufersweiler: Gießen, Germany, 2011; ISBN 9783835957763.

20. Dye, T. The acute abdomen: A surgeon's approach to diagnosis and treatment. *Clin. Tech. Small Anim. Pract.* **2003**, *18*, 53–65. [CrossRef]

21. Burrows, C. The acute abdomen. In *Röntgendiagnostik des Digestionstraktes und des Abdomen/Roentgen Diagnosis of the Digestive Tract and Abdomen*; Speringer: Lima, Peru, 2010.

22. Van Randen, A.; Laméris, W.; Luitse, J.S.K.; Gorzeman, M.; Hesselink, E.J.; Dolmans, D.E.J.G.J.; Peringa, J.; van Geloven, A.A.W.; Bossuyt, P.M.; Stoker, J.; et al. The role of plain radiographs in patients with acute abdominal pain at the ED. *Am. J. Emerg. Med.* **2011**, *29*, 582–589. [CrossRef] [PubMed]

23. Saunders, H.M.; Neath, P.J.; Brockman, D.J. B-mode and Doppler ultrasound imaging of the spleen with canine splenic torsion: A retrospective evaluation. *Vet. Radiol. Ultrasound* **1998**, *39*, 349–353. [CrossRef] [PubMed]

24. Sharma, A.; Thompson, M.S.; Scrivani, P.V.; Dykes, N.L.; Yeager, A.E.; Freer, S.R.; Erb, H.N. Comparison of radiography and ultrasonography for diagnosing small-intestinal mechanical obstruction in vomiting dogs. *Vet. Radiol. Ultrasound* **2011**, *52*, 248–255. [CrossRef] [PubMed]

25. Levitt, L.; Bauer, M.S. Intussusception in dogs and cats: A review of 36 cases. *Can. Vet. J.* **1992**, *33*, 660–664. [PubMed]

26. Kumar, V.; Kumar, A.; Varshney, A.C.; Tyagi, S.P.; Kanwar, M.S.; Sharma, S.K. Diagnostic imaging of canine hepatobiliary affections: A review. *Vet. Med. Int.* **2012**, *2012*, 672107. [CrossRef] [PubMed]

27. Kralik, R.; Trnovsky, P.; Kopáčová, M. Transabdominal ultrasonography of the small bowel. *Gastroenterol. Res. Pract.* **2013**, *2013*, 896704. [CrossRef] [PubMed]

28. Boysen, D.R.; Tidwell, A.S.; Penninck, D.G. Ultrasonographic findings in dogs and cats with gastrointestinal perforation. *Vet. Radiol.* **2003**, *44*, 556–564. [CrossRef]

29. Hinton, L.E.; McLoughlin, M.A.; Johnson, S.E.; Weisbrode, S.E. Spontaneous gastroduodenal perforation in 16 dogs and seven cats (1982–1999). *J. Am. Anim. Hosp. Assoc.* **2002**, *38*, 176–187. [CrossRef] [PubMed]

30. Manczur, F.; Vörös, K.; Vrabély, T.; Wladár, S.; Németh, T.; Fenyves, B. Sonographic diagnosis of intestinal obstruction in the dog. *Acta Vet. Hung.* **1998**, *46*, 35–45. [PubMed]

31. Crews, L.J.; Feeney, D.A.; Jessen, C.R.; Rose, N.D.; Matise, I. Clinical, ultrasonographic, and laboratory findings associated with gallbladder disease and rupture in dogs: 45 cases (1997–2007). *J. Am. Vet. Med. Assoc.* **2009**, *234*, 359–366. [CrossRef] [PubMed]

32. Hecht, S.; Henry, G. Sonographic evaluation of the normal and abnormal pancreas. *Clin. Tech. Small Anim. Pract.* **2007**, *22*, 115–121. [CrossRef] [PubMed]

33. Liptak, J.M.J.; Dernell, W.; Withrow, S. Liver tumors in cats and dogs. *Compend. Contin. Educ. Pract. Vet.* **2004**, *26*, 50–57.

34. Bryan, J.N.; Henry, C.J.; Turnquist, S.E.; Tyler, J.W.; Liptak, J.M.; Rizzo, S.A.; Sfiligoi, G.; Steinberg, S.J.; Smith, A.N.; Jackson, T. Primary renal neoplasia of dogs. *J. Vet. Intern. Med.* **2006**, *20*, 1155–1160. [CrossRef] [PubMed]

10

Pathogen and Host Response Dynamics in a Mouse Model of *Borrelia hermsii* Relapsing Fever

Christopher D. Crowder, Arash Ghalyanchi Langeroudi, Azadeh Shojaee Estabragh, Eric R. G. Lewis, Renee A. Marcsisin and Alan G. Barbour *

Departments of Microbiology & Molecular Genetics and Medicine, University of California Irvine, Irvine, CA 92697, USA; ccrowder@gmail.com (C.D.C.); arashghalyanchi@gmail.com (A.G.L.); ashojaiestabragh@gmail.com (A.S.E.); erlewis@utmb.edu (E.R.G.L.); reneemarcsisin@gmail.com (R.A.M.)
* Correspondence: abarbour@uci.edu

Academic Editor: Ulrike Munderloh

Abstract: Most *Borrelia* species that cause tick-borne relapsing fever utilize rodents as their natural reservoirs, and for decades laboratory-bred rodents have served as informative experimental models for the disease. However, while there has much progress in understanding the pathogenetic mechanisms, including antigenic variation, of the pathogen, the host side of the equation has been neglected. Using different approaches, we studied, in immunocompetent inbred mice, the dynamics of infection with and host responses to North American relapsing fever agent *B. hermsii*. The spirochete's generation time in blood of infected mice was between 4–5 h and, after a delay, was matched in rate by the increase of specific agglutinating antibodies in response to the infection. After initiating serotype cells were cleared by antibodies, the surviving spirochetes were a different serotype and, as a population, grew more slowly. The retardation was attributable to the host response and not an inherently slower growth rate. The innate responses at infection peak and immediate aftermath were characterized by elevations of both pro-inflammatory and anti-inflammatory cytokines and chemokines. Immunodeficient mice had higher spirochete burdens and severe anemia, which was accounted for by aggregation of erythrocytes by spirochetes and their partially reversible sequestration in greatly enlarged spleens and elsewhere.

Keywords: tick-borne disease; zoonosis; spirochete; antigenic variation; *Ornithodoros*; *Mus musculus*

---

1. Introduction

1.1. Early Animal Experiments

Relapsing fever was one of the first diseases for which the cause, the etiology, was identified. In 1868 Otto Obermeier, a junior-level physician at a Berlin hospital, observed thin "threads" with "corkscrew"-like shapes and undulating and "locomotive" movements in the blood of several patients with relapsing fever during an epidemic. The motile organisms were among the blood "corpuscles" at the times of fever in the patients but were consistently undetectable during remission. This observation and his subsequent studies were published by Obermeier in 1873 in a German medical journal [1], and then reported by Fitz in digest form in English later that year [2]. Obermeier also carried out the first experimental animal studies of relapsing fever. He injected the blood of patients into dogs, guinea pigs, and rabbits, but was not able to reproduce the infection in any of these species. This is likely because his patients had epidemic or louse-borne relapsing fever and were thus infected with *Borrelia recurrentis*, whose host range in nature is effectively restricted to humans [3]. Motschutkoffsky could experimentally reproduce the illness and Obermeier's microbiological findings but only by injecting healthy individuals and himself with blood from patients with relapsing fever [4].

If Obermier's relapsing fever cases were tick instead of louse in origin, his attempts to infect adult non-primate animals with a *Borrelia* species probably would have succeeded. However, it would be another three decades before "tick fever" in central Africa was attributed to a similar but distinct organism from the "*Spirillum obermeieri*" (*B. recurrentis*) which was causing relapsing fever in its epidemic form in Europe and Asia at the time. The disease in sub-Saharan Africa, as it was described in a tropical disease textbook of the time [5], featured recurrent febrile episodes, and it was associated with the bites of the soft tick *Ornithodoros moubata* [6]. Ross and Milne [7] and Dutton and Todd [8] independently demonstrated that "tick fever" was caused by "spirilla" in the blood. Dutton and Todd were able to "uniformly" infect *Cercopithecus* sp. monkeys but inconsistently guinea pigs. This host range profile for the "spirillum" is consistent with adaptation of what was likely *Borrelia duttonii* for exploitation of humans as a major if not sole reservoir host [9]. Contemporary studies by Robert Koch demonstrated transovarial transmission of the organisms in the tick vector [10].

In the year following publications of these seminal studies in Africa, Robert Carlisle in New York City reported a case of relapsing fever and the isolation of spirochetes, which had been observed in the patient's blood smear, by inoculation of a blood sample into a Rhesus macaque [11]. From Carlisle's history of the case, the patient likely acquired the infection in Texas in North America, not in Africa, Europe, or Asia. Breinl reported that this North American agent of "tick fever" was serologically distinguishable from the African variety [12].

Norris et al. in turn used this isolate and confirmed the susceptibility of macaques and replicated the relapsing course under experimental conditions [13]. Norris et al. also carried out experiments with large numbers of white rats, which routinely had "spirillosis" of the blood within one to five days of subcutaneous inoculation of infected macaque blood. A characteristic feature of the infected rats was splenomegaly. The authors also successfully infected "white mice" and some rabbits but not guinea pigs. In both macaques and rats, previous infection conferred immunity to challenge with the same isolate.

Novy and Knapp in Michigan also obtained Carlisle's isolate and carried out an extensive and well-documented series of experiments with animals [14]. Rats and mice were highly susceptible to infection, but rabbits and guinea pigs were relatively or absolutely resistant, a host range profile compatible with *Borrelia turicatae* [15,16]. The identity of "Spirochaeta novyi" with *B. turicatae* was confirmed by Brumpt [17].

Once these researchers in the early 1900s demonstrated experimental models of relapsing fever in standard laboratory animals, such as mice and rats, as well as primates, hundreds of published studies on this subject in several languages followed over the succeeding decades. Many of these were reviewed in one or more of References [18–26]. Here, we focus on one of the *Borrelia* species that cause tick-borne relapsing fever: *B. hermsii*. One justification for this emphasis is the arguably greater cumulative knowledge about this species in the laboratory up to this point.

1.2. The North American Species B. hermsii

In the 1930s *B. hermsii* and the tick *Ornothodoros hermsi* were identified as, respectively, the cause and arthropod vector of cases of relapsing fever in California [27,28]. *B. hermsii* is also found in mountains and foothills elsewhere in western North America, from British Columbia in the north, through the Great Basin region and the Rocky Mountains, and south into Arizona and New Mexico [29]. Reports of *B. hermsii* relapsing fever have included cases among residents and visitors of the Sierra Nevada mountains of California since 1922 [30] and of the Grand Canyon National Park in Arizona [31]. The usual reservoir hosts for *B. hermsii* are chipmunks and squirrels [32,33], but can also include *Peromyscus* spp., such as the deer mouse [34].

On the basis of whole-genome as well as shorter sequences, *B. hermsii*, together with *B. turicatae*, *B. parkeri*, and *B. coriaceae*, constitute a North American or "New World" clade [35]. Another set of species, including *B. duttonii*, *B. crocidurae*, *B. hispanica*, and *B. persica*, in Africa and Eurasia coherently constitute an "Old World" taxonomic clade [36]. The sole louse-borne relapsing fever agent, *B. recurrentis*, has a reduced genome and is a close derivative of *B. duttonii* [37]. There are other species (e.g., *B. miyamotoi*) in the combined relapsing fever group in the genus *Borrelia* that are carried hard ticks, such as *Ixodes scapularis*, instead of soft ticks, and are found in North America as well as Eurasia [35], but these are not further considered here. *B. anserina* is another species in the relapsing fever group and is transmitted by soft ticks of the genus *Argas*, but its host range is largely restricted to birds, and recurrences of the bacteremia have not been observed [38].

Following *B. hermsii*'s identification in California, this organism and other relapsing fever agents were studied by Gordon Davis and Willy Burgdorfer at the National Institutes of Health's Rocky Mountain Laboratory (RML) (e.g., [39,40]), by Dorthy Beck in California [41], and later by Coffey and Eveland in California [42,43]. Richard Kelly's breakthrough in cultivating a relapsing fever agent in the laboratory was achieved with *B. hermsii* [44]. Herbert Stoenner at the RML improved Kelly's medium [45] and used a strain, now named HS1, which was originally isolated in mice by Willy Burgdorfer from ticks collected at the site of an outbreak of relapsing fever in eastern Washington in 1968 [46]. Stoenner and Barbour used clonal populations of strain HS1 and variant-specific antibodies in their studies of antigenic variation during relapsing fever [47,48]. Schwan and his colleagues in their in-depth studies of the biology of *B. hermsii* at the RML used isolate HS1 through 1998 [49], but since 2000 they have primarily used isolate DAH, which has a different origin than HS1 [50]. However, the DAH and HS1 isolates are near-identical in sequence and essentially are the same strain [51,52]. In one study DAH and HS1 isolates reached the same peak densities in the blood of infected mice [53].

1.3. Overview

Two major aims of the paper are, first, to report on a series of experiments we have carried out that further define the biology of *B. hermsii* infection of *Mus musculus* in the laboratory, and, second, to put these findings in the context of previous work, with an emphasis, as for this introduction, on early investigations that have stood up over time. Inclusion of all pertinent studies of relapsing fever in animal models—a century-long, global endeavor—was beyond the scope of our more limited ambition. Many exemplary articles of our predecessors and contemporaries in the field could not be included. Mechanisms of disease are not neglected, but attention is focused primarily on the dynamics of growth and responses and the variances for the dynamics. Another objective is the provision of empirical data for those who would build deterministic or agent-based models of relapsing fever that incorporate both pathogen and host parameters. Although most of the space is devoted to experiments in laboratory animals and most other references are to human infection, there is increasing recognition of the occurrence of tick-borne relapsing fever in dogs and cats [54–57]. The studies of experimental animal models of relapsing fever likely provide insights for research on and clinical management of relapsing fever in domestic and companion animals.

2. Materials and Methods

2.1. Animals

The vertebrate animals protocol was approved by the Institutional Animal Care and Utilization Committee of the University of California Irvine (Approval code: 2080-1999). Inbred *Mus musculus* mice were strain BALB/c (Charles Rivers Laboratories) and two strains congenic with BALB/c with the severe combined immunodeficiency phenotype (SCID) and mutation (*scid*): CBySmn.CB17-*Prkdc*^{scid}/J from Jackson Laboratory (BALB/c *scid*) and CB17/lcr-*Prkdc*^{scid}/IcrlcoCrl from Charles River Laboratories (C.B-17 *scid*). Other mice were Nu/J nude mice from Jackson Laboratory. Immunodeficient mice were housed in isolator cages under ABSL2 containment in an ALAAC-approved facility, provided with autoclaved bedding and food (Harlan Teklad Global Soy Protein-Free Rodent Diet), were kept on a 12 h light-dark cycle, and received autoclaved distilled water ad libitum. During experiments mice were examined and weighed daily. Blood was collected from either the tail (10–25 µL) or the saphenous vein (50 µL) in lithium-heparin coated Microvette CB300 collection tubes (Sarstedt). Terminal exsanguination and euthanasia under isoflurane or CO_2 anesthesia was performed by cardiac puncture and collection of the blood into either a heparinized syringe or heparinized tubes (Becton-Dickinson Microcontainer #365965).

2.2. Bacterial Strains and Culture Conditions

The Browne Mountain isolate of the type strain HS1 of *B. hermsii* (ATCC 35209; BioSample SAMN04481062) was used [46,52]. Original frozen stocks of mouse plasma with either 25% glycerol or 10% dimethyl sulfoxide were ≥98% pure in serotype identity by immunoflourescence assay with serotype-specific antisera [47]. For the present study, serotype 7 from these stocks was cloned again by limiting dilution in C.B-17 *scid* mice. The serotype of a relapse population was identified by PCR amplification and sequence of the expression site for the variable major proteins, as described [58,59]. Two other serotypes of strain HS1 used in the study were serotype 19 and serotype 33. The second *B. hermsii* strain was CC1 serotype 1 (BioSample SAMN03408291) [59,60], which was first passed into C.B-17 *scid* mice from frozen stocks before inoculation of the freshly-obtained plasma into other sets for mice for experiments. *B. hermsii* cells were cultivated in BSK II medium with 12% rabbit serum at 34 °C unless otherwise stated [61]. Bacteria were harvested from cultures and then washed as described [59]. Spirochetes in plasma or culture medium were counted in duplicate by phase microscopy on an Olympus BX40 microscope using a Petroff-Hausser counting chamber with a depth of 0.02 mm and 400× magnification. A volume of 4.5 µL was placed into the chamber and spirochetes in its 400 squares (1 mm^2 total area) were counted.

2.3. Mouse Infections

Mice were inoculated intraperitoneally with 1–10 *B. hermsii* cells in 100 µL of phosphate-buffered saline, pH 7.4 (PBS), with 5 mM $MgCl_2$ (PBS-Mg) by intraperitoneal injection, unless otherwise noted. The innoculum cell count was determined either by limiting dilution for frozen stock of known viability or microscopic quantitation of cultures as described above. A rotation of one or two members of each group of inoculated mice was monitored daily for the presence and density of spirochetes by phase-contrast microscopy of a wet mount of blood obtained from the tail vein. Infected plasma was obtained from blood anti-coagulated with heparin or sodium citrate by centrifugation at 100× *g* for 3 min. Cell-free plasma was obtained by centrifugation of the infected plasma at 9500× *g* for 5 min for the aggregation experiment and at 16,000× *g* for 10 min for antibody experiments. At the time terminal anesthesia, the mice were weighed, and whole spleens were dissected and weighed. Spleens of some mice were fixed in 10% buffered formalin for histopathology processing at University of California Davis' Comparative Pathology Laboratory (Davis, CA, USA). Mice that were treated with an antibiotic received ceftriaxone (Sigma-Aldrich) at a dose of 25 µg per gm of body weight and administered subcutaneously every 12 h for 3 d, as described [62]. The hematocrit, percentage of packed red blood cells, was determined with heparinized microhematocrit capillary tubes (Fisher Scientific) with Critoseal caps (Oxford Labware, St. Louis, MO, USA) and centrifugation for 5 min on a ZIPocrit microhematocrit centrifuge (LW Scientific, Lawrenceville, GA, USA).

2.4. Antibody Agglutination Assays

The macro-agglutination and micro-agglutination assays were performed in 96-well, round-bottom, polystyrene 96-well microtiter plates. To each of the wells, which contained 25 µL of PBS-Mg with 5% bovine serum albumin (BSA) and 10^7 in vitro—cultivated or plasma-borne bacteria, was added an equal volume of mouse plasma serially two-fold diluted in the same buffer. Reactions were shaken at 200 rpm and incubated at 37 °C for 2 h. The highest dilution in which there was cell pellet surrounded by clear liquid rather than a homogeneous haze was recorded as the titer of the assay. For the micro-agglutination assay 12.5 µL of plasma serially-diluted in BSK II medium were added to 12.5 µL of a suspension of bacteria at a concentration of 5×10^7 per mL of medium. The suspension was incubated at 37 °C for 2 h on a shaker at 200 rpm. A 5 μL volume was examined under a cover slip by phase microscopy at 400× magnification. Agglutination was scored positive if >50% of the spirochetes were in clumps of ≥5 cells. A positive control for the micro-agglutination was a mouse monoclonal antibody H7-7 to serotype 7 with documented agglutinating capacity [63].

2.5. Growth Inhibition Assay

The growth inhibition assay for *B. hermsii* HS1 serotype 33 was performed in 200 μL reaction volumes in a 96-well microtiter plate as described [63]. A two-fold dilution series was made for both *B. hermsii* serotype 33 cells in BSKII media and monoclonal antibody H4825 diluted in BSK II media, IgG2a antibody specific for the Vtp protein of serotype 33 [64]. Each reaction well consisted of 195 μL of *B. hermsii* cell dilution and 5 μL of antibody dilution in a checkerboard fashion. Guinea pig complement (Diamedix) at two units per mL was added to some wells. The plate was then sealed and incubated at 34 °C for two weeks. The plate was monitored daily for growth of *B. hermsii* cells as indicated by a change in media color from pink to yellow. Wells were considered positive for growth inhibition if the media remained pink.

2.6. Indirect Immunofluorescence Assay (IFA)

Methanol-fixed thin smears of blood from mice infected with *B. hermsii* were incubated with mouse plasma diluted 1:10 in PBS at 37 °C for 1 h. The slides were washed with PBS for twice for 10 min each, and then incubated with fluorescein-labeled goat anti-mouse IgM antibody (Kierkegaard & Perry Laboratory, Gaithersburg, MD, USA) at 1:1000 dilution at 37 °C for 1 h. After washing again with PBS, buffered-glycerol and a cover slip were applied, and the slides were examined by UV microscopy.

2.7. Enzyme-Linked Immunosorbent (ELISA) Assay for IgM Antibodies

To wells of a 96-well flat-bottom polystyrene microtiter plate were added 10^8 washed bacteria suspended in 50 μL of 50 mM sodium carbonate, pH 9.6 buffer. Plate were centrifuged at 700× *g* for 30 min, buffer was removed by aspiration, wells were washed with 50 μL of PBS-Mg, and plates were centrifuged again at 700× *g* for 30 min. Wells were blocked with 200 μL blocking 50 mM Tris, pH 8.0-140 mM NaCl-1% BSA for 30 min. This solution was removed and the wells were washed three times with 50 mM Tris-140 mM NaCl, pH 8.0-0.05% Tween 20 (wash solution). Serial two-fold dilutions of the mouse plasma were made in the wash solution and added in 100 μL volumes to the wells of the plates, which were then incubated at 22 °C for 1 h. The wells were aspirated of their contents and then washed five times with the wash solution. Volumes of 100 μL of horse radish peroxidase-conjugated goat antibody for murine IgM (Bethyl Laboratories) at a 1:100,000 dilution in wash solution were then added to wells and incubation at 22 °C for 1 h was carried out. After the wells were aspirated, they were washed five times with wash solution. The reaction was developed with 3,3′, 5,5′-tetramethylbenzidine (TMB) of the ELISA Starter Accessory Kit (Bethyl Labs), and optical densities of the colorimetric reactions were read at 450 nm. The cutoff value for a positive titer was defined as >3 standard deviations above the mean of 16 plasma samples from uninfected mice.

2.8. Assays for Cytokines, Chemokines, and Other Serum Components

Samples of freshly-obtained heparinized mouse blood were centrifuged at 13× *g* for 10 min. The plasma was then drawn off and snap-frozen at −80 °C. The samples were then shipped on dry ice to Myriad RBM (Austin, TX, USA) for performance of the bead-based quantitaive immunoassay for 68 analytes of the RodentMAP v. 1.0 panel (Supplementary Table S1). For samples in which the analyte in question was below the laboratory's lower threshold for accurate measurement (or, as it was termed, the "least detectable dose") and was reported as "low", we substituted a dummy value of 50% of the lower threshold value. For instance, if the reported least detectable dose was 68 and a particular result interpretation was "low", we substituted "34" (i.e., half the least detectable dose) for this particular analyte for that sample.

2.9. Iron Assay

The quantity of ferrous and ferric ions in the spleen was determined colorimetrically at optical density 593 nm with Ferene S of Biovision kit K390-100 (Biovision, Milpitas, CA, USA). Results were expressed as nmol iron per g of spleen mass.

2.10. In Vitro Blood Cell Aggregation Assay

In wells of round-bottomed 96-well polystyrene microtiter plates 5 µL volumes of heparinized blood from uninfected mice were mixed with equal volumes of plasma from infected mice taken on day 5 after i.p. inoculation on day 0. Bacterial densities in the plasma were determined by phase microscopy, as described above, and quantitative PCR, as described below. The infected plasma was either untreated, centrifuged at $9500\times g$ for 5 min at 22 °C, or centrifuged and then heated in a water bath at 56 °C for 30 min to inactivate complement. The plates were covered and then incubated at 37 °C for 1 h. The plates were then placed at 4 °C for 12 h. The plates were backlit on a light table and digital pictures were taken with a Nikon D5000 and AF-S Micro Nikor 60 mm lens. TIFF-format photo files were subjected to image analysis with ImageJ v. 1.34 software (National Institutes of Health). Dispersion of the blood cells in the well was measured as the area under the curve of the histogram of values above the background. Samples from wells were examined by phase microscopy at 400× magnification, and pictures were taken with QImaging's (Surrey, BC, Canada) QIClick CCD camera.

2.11. Nucleic Acid Extraction and cDNA Synthesis

DNA was extracted from 20 µL of whole blood with Qiagen's QIAmp DNA micro kit or DNeasy Blood and Tissue kit. DNA was extracted from 100 mg spleen with the DNeasy kit. In some experiments the DNA Clean & Concentrator kit (Zymo Research) was used to remove inhibitors from the DNA sample per manufacturer's recommendations. The DNA standard for quantitative PCR was total genomic DNA extracted from culture-grown strain HS1 using a phenol-chloroform protocol as described (58). Total RNA was isolated from whole blood with TriReagent BD (Molecular Research Center) according to the manufacturer's instructions. Nucleic acid concentrations were measured with a NanoDrop™ 1000 spectrophotometer (Thermo Scientific). RNA extracts were treated with RNase-free DNase I (Ambion) according to the manufacturer's instructions. Reverse transcription reactions were carried out in reactions containing 2.5 µM of random hexamers (New England Biolabs), two units of Moloney Murine Leukemia Virus reverse transcriptase (New England Biolabs) per µL, 0.5 mM dNTPs, and 2 units of RNase inhibitor (Roche Applied Science) per µL in the following buffer: 5 mM Tris HCl, pH 8.3-7.5 mM KCl-0.3 mM $MgCl_2$-2.1 mM dithiothreitol. Reactions were serially incubated in water baths at 25°C for 10 min, 37 °C for 3 h, and 100 °C for 5 min, and then immediately frozen at −80 °C. Reactions without the reverse transcriptase were carried out in parallel.

2.12. Quantitative PCR (qPCR)

The primers and probe targeted the single copy 16S ribosomal RNA (rrs) gene of B. hermsii and other relapsing fever group species as described [65,66]. The master mix was from Eurogentec (San Diego, CA, USA), and the reactions were run on either an iCycler (Bio-Rad Laboratories, Richmond, CA, USA) or a Rotor Gene 3000 (Corbett Research, Australia). By both methods the sensitivity was two to four gene copies; the coefficient of determination (R^2) for replicate qPCR assays of the same samples was ≥ 0.90. One copy of a complete genome is equivalent to one copy of the rrs gene (Genbank CP000048). Quantitation of cDNA of transcripts of the flaB flagellin gene used the forward and reverse primers 5′-GTTGATTTCATCTGTAAGTTGCTCAATT-3′ and 5′-ACTTGCTGTTCAATCTGGTAATGG-3′, respectively, and the minor groove binding probe 6FAM-5′AACCTCTGTCTGCATC3′.

2.13. Growth Rate Determinations

The generation time in hours based on change in measurements of numbers (N) in genome copies between two time points, 0 and t, for the same mouse was calculated with this formula: $\ln(2)*(t-0)/\ln(N_t/N_0)$. The generation time in hours based on change in measurements of numbers in genome or RNA copies for groups of mice sampled at times into the infection was determined by linear regression of log-transformed data.

2.14. Statistics

Standard statistical tests were carried out with the SYSTAT v. 13 suite of programs (Systat Software, Inc., Chicago, IL, USA) and with Confidence Interval Analysis v. 2.1.2 (CIA Software, University of Southampton, Southampton, UK). Mean values and differences in means are presented with 95% confidence intervals (CIs). Parametric (t test) and non-parametric (Mann-Whitney rank sum) significance tests were carried out for continuous data and were two-tailed. Fisher's exact test was used for categorical data in a 2×2 contingency table and was two-tailed. Linear regression was by the least-squares method, and 95% confidence interval for the slope was calculated. Z scores were the number of standard deviations above or below the mean of the control group values. Euclidean distance cluster analysis was performed and a two-color graphic display (heat map) of multiplex continuous data was generated using the MultiExperiment Viewer v 4.0 software (The Institute for Genomic Research, Baltimore, MD, USA) [67].

3. Results and Discussion

3.1. Growth of B. hermsii in the Blood

3.1.1. Background

Novy and Knapp in their 1906 article noted "rapid multiplication" of what was likely *B. turicatae* in rats and mice and that the organism reached its maximum in the blood within three days after passage [14]. They wrote that "white mice are very susceptible" to infection, had up to four relapses, and "so regularly do [the relapses] return that one can quite accurately predict when this will occur". They observed further that " . . . the number of spirilla which appear in the blood during a relapse is much less than in the first attack, which clearly indicates the existence of a partial immunity". From the results provided in the article for the amount of spirochetes in the blood, the generation or doubling time for this *Borrelia* species in a rat was between 4 and 8 h.

Helen Russell reported in 1931 that there were lower numbers of spirochetes in the blood in relapses than the initial bacteremia in the Gambian giant pouched rat (*Cricetomys gambianus*) and that the blood was infectious for other rodents when not detectable microscopically [68]. Eidmann et al. estimated a generation time of 6 h for *B. crocidurae* in the blood of white mice [69]. Coffey and Eveland passed a *B. hermsii* isolate from the Sierra Nevada Mountains in outbred mice every 48 h before injection into Sprague-Dawley rats for their experiments [42,43]. In the rats the generation time was estimated as ~6 h. Stoenner et al. counted spirochetes under the microscope and reported a generation or doubling time for *B. hermsii* in the blood of about 3 h [47]. The doubling time of *B. turicatae* was between 6 and 7 h in mice [70] and ~7 h in vitro [71]. The doubling time was found to be similar regardless of whether mice were examined individually or if all the mice were grouped together as a whole.

The ability to use a group of mice and consider them as a single animal for data analysis allows for more flexibility in experimental design since the researcher is not necessarily limited by the amount of blood in a single animal. However, counts based on microscopy are limited by the sensitivity that can be achieved with a phase or dark field microscope and a counting chamber. In our hands the detection limit for counts that use the entire counting area of the chamber is a density of ~10^4 cells per milliliter. Benoit et al. sampled small volumes of blood and diluted it 10-fold before counting and reported a limit of detection of 10^5 bacteria/mL [72]. Counts of replicate samplings of the same population at the extreme of sensitivity approximate a Poisson distribution, and the coefficient of variation increases as the mean approaches zero. For the present study the lower limit of measurements that provided reproducible growth rate determinations by microscopy was ~5 × 10^4 cells/mL (Figure 1), which is what Coffey and Eveland reported for their studies of infections in rats [42].

For studies of many types of bacteria, an alternative to microscopic counts of cells is plating of non-aggregated cells on solid media and the subsequent enumeration of colonies. While this is possible with some strains of *B. burgdorferi* [73], colony formation has yet to be achieved with wild-type *B. hermsii* (unpublished findings). In addition, the practical limit for counting by plating is 10–100 colony-forming units per milliliter, depending on the number of plates used.

3.1.2. PCR Quantitation of Bacteria in the Blood

Quantitative PCR was the means to estimate cells numbers at low densities in the blood and thereby to measure growth of the population over a greater range. Using as a standard the total DNA extracted from a known number of cells, we reproducibly detected two to four genome copies in a PCR reaction. Given a genome copy number in the range of 10–20 per cell of *B. hermsii* [74] and the sampling volume of 20 µL of blood, the lower limit of detection of the qPCR assay used in this study was approximately five spirochetes per milliliter of blood. Figure 2 shows the results of two experiments that compared the cell counts as determined by microscopy with genome counts as determined by qPCR over a range of ~50,000 to 2,000,000 bacteria per milliliter. There were, as expected [74], 10–20 genomes measured by PCR for every cell counted by microscopy.

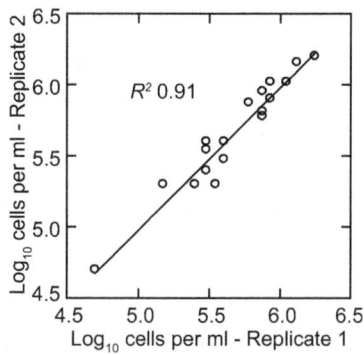

Figure 1. Scatter plot of replicate log-transformed counts of *Borrelia hermsii* cells in plasma samples from infected mice by phase microscopy and counting chamber. The linear regression and coefficient of determination (R^2) are shown.

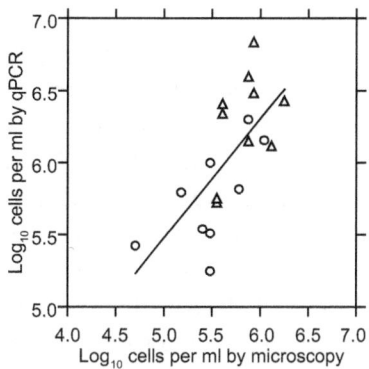

Figure 2. Scatter plot with linear regression of log-transformed counts of *B. hermsii* cells in plasma by phase microscopy and counting chamber (*x*-axis) and quantitative PCR (qPCR; *y*-axis). Circles and triangles denote samples of blood taken at hours 94.5 or 102 from immunocompetent BALB/c mice infected at hour 0, as described in the text. The slope (95% confidence interval) for the least-squares regression was 0.85 (0.4–1.3), and the combined R^2 was 0.46 ($p < 0.001$).

With this qPCR assay, we assessed the growth rate of serotype 7 of *B. hermsii* HS1 in the *M. musculus* host. We used BALB/c mice and their congenic SCID varieties, because of the long history of studies with this strain [75], and our experience that mice of the C57BL/6 lineage were more resistant to initial infection with *B. hermsii* than BALB/c mice (Alan G. Barbour, unpublished findings). For the experiment, 95 adult BALB/c mice were infected with one to 10 spirochetes in cohorts of 50 and 45 animals, the second cohort being inoculated 11.5 h after the first. Starting 12 h post-inoculation, a sample of blood was collected from the saphenous vein and a second sample was collected 7.5 h later. A new mouse was successively processed in this fashion every 3 h. Each mouse was bled no more than two times. DNA was extracted from each sample, quantitated, and then subjected to qPCR.

Spirochete genomes were first detected in the blood 54 h post-inoculation and thereafter displayed steady growth up to around 120 h, at which time spirochete genome densities were as high as 1.2×10^8 per milliliter (Figure 3). This density corresponded to ~10^7 cells per milliliter at the peak in these immunocompetent mice. In comparison, for three BALB/c SCID mice infected with the same serotype, the mean peak density was six-fold higher, at 7.5 (4.7–10.0) $\times 10^8$ genomes per milliliter of blood.

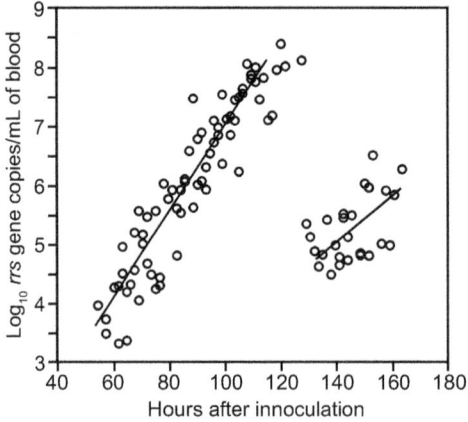

Figure 3. Proliferation and decline of *B. hermsii* HS1 cells in the blood of infected immunocompetent mice over time. The graph is a scatter plot of collected data on gene copies of 16S ribosomal RNA (*rrs*) of *B. hermsii* by qPCR (*y*-axis) against time in hours (*x*-axis) after inoculation of 95 BALB/c mice with serotype 7 of strain HS1. Samples were collected every 3 h beginning 12 h after inoculation; second samples were obtained from each mouse 7.5 h after the first. Each data point is a sampling from a single mouse. Linear regression determinations were made separately for hours 50–120 ($R^2 = 0.86$) and >120.

The means and 95% confidence intervals for the doubling time of genomes by linear regression for each of the two cohorts were calculated separately to stratify for possible diurnal differences in in vivo growth. The first and second inoculation cohorts had generation times of 4.5 (4.0–5.1) h and 4.1 (3.6–4.8) h, respectively, for the period when *B. hermsii* DNA was first detected to peak. We also calculated generation times separately for measurements of first samplings and second samplings to assess possible effects of a prior bleeding of the mouse. The mean generation times for these two sets were similar: 4.5 (4.0–5.1) h and 4.2 (3.7–4.9) h, respectively. The overall genome doubling time for 69 samples obtained from hours 54 to 120 was 4.1 (3.9–4.6) h with an R^2 value of 0.86 (Figure 3). A second estimate of the growth rate was obtained by averaging generation times individually calculated from pairs of counts for 23 mice that were sampled between hours 70 and 110 of infection. There was greater variance in the estimate based on pairs, but the generation time of 4.8 (3.8–6.6) h was similar to that estimated by linear regression for the mice as a group. The increase in copies of DNA in the blood was paralleled by the increase in the mRNA for the *flaB* flagellin gene, which is constitutively expressed in vivo and in vitro [76] (Figure 4). The doubling rate for *flaB* mRNAs at 5.1 (3.8–7.7) h was similar to that of the DNA.

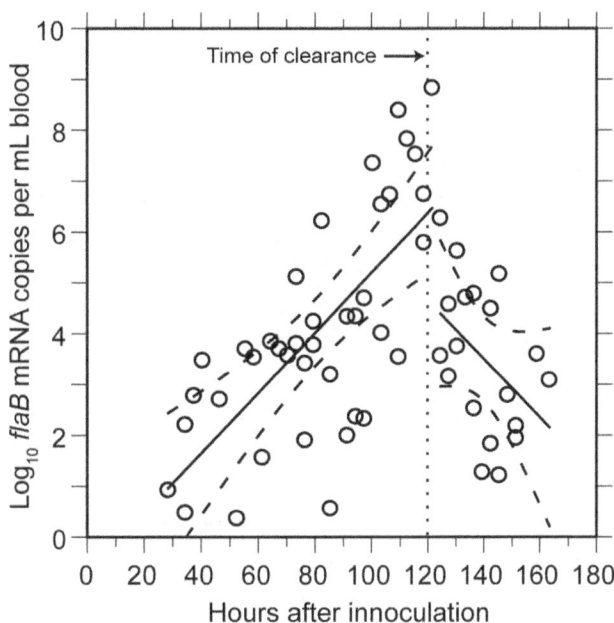

Figure 4. Rise and decline in mRNA for FlaB flagellin of *B. hermsii* in blood of infected mice. The experiment and sampling protocol were the same as described for Figure 3. The *flaB* transcripts were estimated by qPCR of cDNA produced with random hexamers. Each data point is a sampling from a single mouse. Linear regression determinations (with 95% confidence intervals denoted by dashed lines) were made separately for time points up to hour 120 and after hour 120. The time of clearance indicated is the approximate time point that genome counts began to decline (Figure 3).

3.1.3. Clearance of Bacteria from Blood

Beginning around hour 120 (or after five days), there was a steep decline in the genome density in the blood over a period of 6 h (Figure 3). At the nadir there were 2.5×10^4 genomes, or about 1300–2500 bacterial cells, per milliliter of blood. This was below the usual threshold for detection of cells by microscopy of unconcentrated blood. The decline had an estimated half-life of 1.4 h for the collective samples, but for individual mice the clearance of 99% or more of the cells from the blood could have occurred more rapidly. A slower decline in concentration was noted for the *flaB* transcripts in the whole blood (Figure 4).

3.1.4. Relapse of Bacteria in the Blood

From this nadir in *B. hermsii* genomes, the counts rose again logarithmically during what we designated as the relapse. This relapse population was identified by the sequence of the expressed gene for a variable major protein which as predominantly serotype 26, which was previously noted to commonly follow serotype 7 in infections of mice [77]. The generation time for the relapse population, as determined by overall linear regression was 7.6 (4.6–22) h, slower than that for infecting serotype 7.

In a previous study we had not observed a difference in growth rates in vivo between two serotypes, 7 and 19 [78]. So, the slower growth rate of serotype 26 in the relapse population than serotype 7 in the original infecting population was unexpected. To determine whether serotypes 7 and 26 inherently grow at different rates, serotype 26 of this specific relapse was first obtained in a pure population by cloning by limiting dilution in mice. This clonal population was then in turn compared with serotype 7 in naïve mice. Groups of eight six-week-old female BALB/c mice were infected with one to five cells of either serotype 7 or 26 from the plasma of infected SCID mice. Blood samples that were taken from each of the mice 57 and 74 h after inoculation were subjected to DNA extractions and qPCR for quantitation of genome copies. The growth rates were calculated for each of the mice from pairs of data. Serotype 7 in this set of mice had a mean genome generation time of 4.4 (3.8–5.3) h. Serotype 26 in naïve mice had a generation time of 5.3 (4.5–6.5) h. This was not significantly different from that of serotype 7 ($p = 0.4$), but was faster than what was observed for the relapse population.

3.1.5. Comments

An advantage of qPCR over microscopy for measuring growth is its sensitivity for low numbers of gene copies in the reaction. A drawback of qPCR is its endpoint of genomes of cells and not cells per se. *Borrelia* cells with their filamentous shapes have multiple genomes per individual cell [74]. Equating genomes with cells gives unrealistically high estimates of cell densities in the blood [79]. As the stationary phase is approached, the lengths of cells increase, and there may be correspondingly more genomes per cell, thus confounding inferences of cell numbers from genome quantities. This may occur in SCID mice if the stationary phase of growth is reached for the bacteria in the absence of immunity. However, we found that the peak densities in immunocompetent mice before clearance were five- to 10-fold lower than what we observed in the SCID mice here and what others reported for immunodeficient mice [79,80]. Thus, it is likely that the spirochetes were in the log-phase of growth in the blood of BALB/c mice until antibody-mediated clearance began on day 5.

Benoit et al. in their study of three different inbred strains of mice reported that juvenile BALB/c mice were more "resistant" to *B. hermsii* infection than either C57BL/6 or C3H/HeJ mice were [72]. This conclusion was based on their observation of a four- to six-fold difference between the strains in peak spirochete counts in the blood of the mice. In the experiment they used an inoculum of 10^5 bacteria from a broth culture and delivered it intravenously. Our experience is that rodents can be infected routinely with one to five organisms [47,78,81], as has been similarly found by investigators of *B. duttonii* [82] and *B. turicatae* [83]. In the Benoit et al. report, the peak of spirochetemia occurred on day 3, which would be unexpected for an infection initiated by a tick bite or a much lower needle inoculum [72]. There was not a significant difference between the three strains in their counts on day 2. The relatively depressed spirochete count in BALB/c mice on day 3 was as plausibly attributable to an earlier antibody response in this strain as to a difference in innate immunity.

In the experiment with 95 mice, following the clearance event during day 5, an estimated 1000 spirochetes per mL of blood remained. This is consistent with previous reports of persistent infectiousness of blood between relapses [14,68,84]. Assuming an antigen switching rate of ~10^{-4} per cell per generation for strain HS1 [47], we would expect a relapse population size of ~3000 spirochetes by the time the total bacterial density reached 10^7 per milliliter of blood. So, our experimental finding was about what we anticipated.

During the period of relapse, the overall population increased at a slower rate than did the infecting serotype 7 during its run-up in the blood. However, in immunologically naïve mice, serotype 26, which was the predominant serotype of the relapse population, had a similar growth rate to that of serotype 7. This finding is consistent with Coffey and Eveland's observation that each relapse had successively lower peak densities in their rats infected with *B. hermsii*, while in naïve animals the different serotypes of relapses grew just as fast as the initiating serotype [42]. In trypanosomes, another blood-borne pathogen that undergoes antigenic variation, the expressed antigenic protein does not appear to be a major determinant of the growth rate of the organism [85].

3.2. Innate Host Responses to B. hermsii Infection

3.2.1. Background

The last experiment's results and our review of the literature indicated that the slower growth rate of the relapse population was attributable to host factors and not to inherent differences between serotypes in growth rates. Since the proliferating relapse population presumably was unaffected by the circulating antibodies that were specific for serotype 7 cells [42,47], the slower growth rate and lower peak densities plausibly were attributable to non-adaptive, or innate, host responses to the infection. Benoit et al. observed a temporary decline in the numbers of spirochetes after the initial peak in the blood of B cell-deficient $rag2^{-/-}$ mice, a finding which was interpreted as evidence of a role of innate immunity in reducing the bacterial burden [72].

Taken together, these findings indicate that innate immunity, as it develops in response to the infection, can restrain spirochete proliferation. However, by what mechanism(s) does this occur? Innate immunity during relapsing fever remains poorly understood. Perhaps the best known manifestation of these responses and the one with major clinical significance is the Jarisch-Herxheimer (J-H) reaction, the shock-like state that occurs within a few hours of the initiation of antibiotic therapy of patients [86]. This state is associated with marked elevations of pro-inflammatory cytokines [87]. At one time this phenomenon was attributed to an "endotoxin" released by the dying spirochetes [88]. Neither *Borrelia* spp. nor *Treponema pallidum*, another agent associated with the J-H reaction, have lipopolysaccharides with endotoxin-like activity [89,90]. More likely, the so-called "cytokine storm" is in response to the release from distressed or autolyzing cells of large numbers of membrane blebs bearing abundant lipoproteins [91]. The bacterial lipoproteins are recognized by Toll-like receptors (TLR), principally TLR2, and a signaling cascade leading to the release of pro-inflammatory cytokines and chemokines follow [92]. This in turn elicits an anti-inflammatory counter-reaction, which is exemplified by the rise in cytokine IL-10 levels [93,94].

3.2.2. Analysis of Proteins in Plasma during Experimental Infection

To begin to identify innate mechanisms for the restraint on spirochete growth by day 5 of infection, we examined the concentrations of various cytokines, chemokines, acute phase reactants, or other serum components at different stages of infection and compared those values to those of uninfected controls measured at the same time. To this end, 15 BALB/c mice were inoculated with an estimated one to two spirochetes of serotype 7 of strain HS1, and five mice were inoculated with the same volume of PBS as non-infected controls. The mice were then monitored for the presence and density of spirochetes by microscopic examination of tail blood. Of the 15 inoculated mice, 12 became infected, and these mice were the source of the plasma for the subsequent studies. At the peak of bacteremia on day 4, anti-coagulated blood was collected from six mice by terminal exsanguination under anesthesia. On day 5 there were no microscopically detectable spirochetes in the blood of the remaining six infected mice, and anticoagulated blood was collected by terminal exsanguination from these six mice. The three inoculated but uninfected mice and the five control mice were likewise terminally exsanguinated on day 5.

Individual plasma samples were analyzed for a concentration of 68 different proteins in the blood by immunoassay with specific antibodies (Table S1). A preliminary analysis of the data showed no significant difference between the three inoculated but uninfected mice and the five mice injected with buffer alone, so these were combined into a group of eight that was categorized as the control of "uninfected". The other two groups for the analysis were "peak" of infection (day 4), and "clearance" of infection (day 5). At the time of the peak, the mice typically had ruffled fur and reduced locomotor activity in comparison to uninfected animals. There was no evidence of the neurologic disorders we had noted in mice infected with *B. turicatae* [71].

Figure 5 is a two-color graphical representation in heat map format of the results of the analysis with the 68 analytes and the three groups of samples: uninfected (designated as "1" in the figure), peak ("2"), and clearance ("3"). The data were normalized across the different analytes as Z scores, which were within a range of −3 to +6 and corresponded to numbers of standard deviations below or above the mean of the controls. The heat map is structured horizontally by experimental group and vertically by similarities in profiles. Three general patterns of analyte results across the three groups are apparent: similar analyte levels for all conditions, elevated values during the peak of infection and a decline with clearance, and elevated values over the controls during both the peak and clearance. The 28 analytes of Table S1 that did not significantly vary at the 0.05 level by either parametric or non-parametric tests between the three conditions were the following: apoliprotein A1, calbindin, CD40, CD40 ligand, cystatin, eotaxin, Factor VII, Fibroblast Growth Factor (FGF)-9, FGF-2, the chemokine

Granulocyte Chemotactic Protein-2 (CXCL6), Granulocyte Macrophage-Colony Stimulating Factor, glutathione *S*-transferase, Interferon (IFN)-γ, Interleukin (IL)-1α, immunoglobulin A, IL-2, IL-3, IL-4, IL-12, IL-17, leptin, Leukemia Inhibitory Factor, myoglobin, lipocalin-2, RANTES, Tissue Factor, thrombopoietin, and von Willebrand Factor.

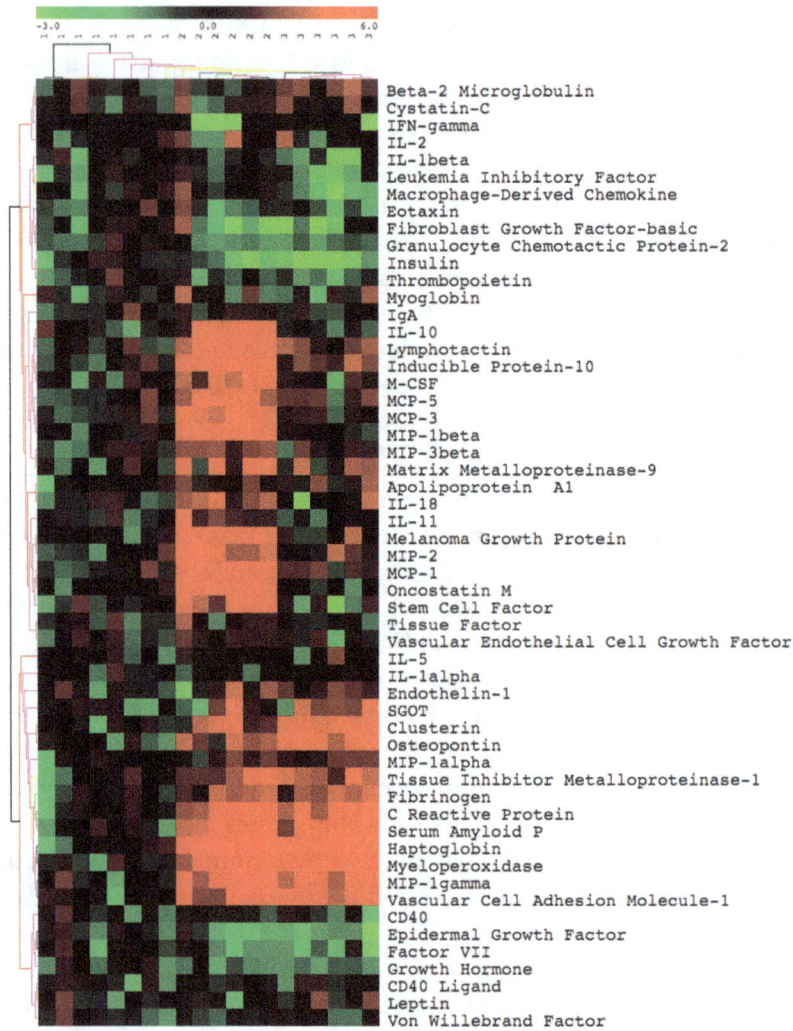

Figure 5. Cytokines, chemokines, acute-phase reactant, and selected other serum proteins in plasma of BALB/c mice before (group 1), at the peak of spirochetemia (group 2), and after clearance (group 3) of infection with *B. hermsii*. The figure is a two-color display and gradient heat map of values (normalized across the individual assays by *Z* scores) ranging from −3 (green) to +6 (red) for 20 plasma samples and 68 analytes, which were assayed by bead-based immunoassays, as described in the text. The analytes and their abbreviations and alternative names are listed in Table S1. Differences in means between time points and conditions 1, 2, and 3 for 39 analytes are given in Table 1.

These three patterns were also observed when differences in means between the pairings of the three different conditions, e.g., peak vs. uninfected, etc., were calculated (Table 1). In addition, two other patterns were noted among the group of analytes that were not elevated at the peak of spirochete density: first, elevation of an analyte only at the time of clearance of infected mice, and, second, reduced concentrations of a serum protein in the infected mice, either at the peak or clearance. Table 1 lists 39 analytes that differed between at least two of the conditions, as well as, for comparison, three other analytes (IFN-γ, IL-1α, and IL-2) that showed no discernible difference from uninfected controls.

Table 1. Changes in selected proteins in blood of BALB/c mice during course of experimental relapsing fever.

Analyte	Unit [a]	Difference in Means (Lower, Upper 95% Confidence Limits)			Change [b]
		Peak vs. Uninfected	Clearance vs. Uninfected	Clearance vs. Peak	
β-2 Microglobulin	μg	+0.1 (−0.2, +0.3)	+0.4 (+0.2, +0.6) [c]	+0.3 (+0.1, +0.5)	C
Clusterin	μg	+62 (+19, +106)	+131 (+91, +171)	+69 (+7, +130)	P,C
C-reactive protein	μg	+3.8 (+2.5, +5.0)	+3.6 (+2.3, +4.8)	0.2 (−2.0, +1.6)	P,C
EGF [d]	pg	−3.6 (−8.0, +0.7)	−6.5 (−10.8, −2.3)	−2.9 (−8.0, +2.2)	(P,C)
Endothelin-1	pg	+5.5 (−9.6, +20.5)	+11.2 (+3.3, +19.2)	+5.8 (−10.9, +22.4)	C
Fibrinogen	μg	+3421 (+1710, +5131)	+3703 (+2135, +5269)	+282 (−1643, +2207)	P,C
Growth hormone	ng	−15.8 (−28.2, −3.4)	−14.3 (−26.5, −2.0)	+1.5 (−3.2, +6.2)	(P,C)
Haptoglobin	μg	+88 (+70, +105)	+112 (+103, +121)	+25 (+1.7, +48)	P,C
IP-10 (CXCL10) [e]	pg	+151 (+108, +195)	+29 (+13, +45)	−122 (−173, −71)	P
Interferon-γ	pg	+6.0 (-0.5, +12.6)	+1.3 (−1.1, +3.6)	−4.8 (−13.0, +3.5)	
IL-1α	pg	−26 (−62, +9)	−28 (−64, +7.9)	1.4 (−4.2, +1.4)	
IL-1β	pg	+120 (−670, +910)	−900 (−1810, +10)	−1020 (−1690, −350)	(C)
IL-2	pg	+7.0 (−8.6, +23)	+0.4 (−14.4, +15.2)	−6.7 (−27.9, +14.5)	
IL-6	pg	+14.4 (+6.0, +22.9)	+1.3 (−0.2, +2.7)	−13.2 (−23.4, −3.0)	P
IL-7	pg	+60 (+40, +70)	+10 (0, +30)	−50 (−70, −20)	P
IL-10	pg	+378 (+237, +520)	−38 (−103, +28)	−416 (−581, −251)	P
IL-11	pg	+64 (+2.0, +126)	6.5 (−25.0, +12.1)	71 (−143, +2.0)	P
IL-18	pg	+520 (+300, +740)	−50 (−520, +430)	−570 (−1130, −10)	P
Insulin	μIU	−0.7 (−1.1, −0.2)	−1.1 (−1.5, −0.7)	−0.5 (−1.0, +0.1)	(P,C)
KC/GROα (CXCL1)	pg	+680 (+460, +890)	+40 (+40, +120)	−640 (−900, −370)	P
Lymphotactin (XCL1)	pg	+144 (+101, +188)	+41 (+15, +68)	−103 (−154, −51)	P
MCP-1 (CCL2)	pg	+700 (+563, +837)	+65 (+5.9, +124)	−635 (−796, −474)	P
MCP-3 (CCL7)	pg	+550 (+396, +703)	+78 (−45, +201)	−472 (−635, −310)	P
MCP-5 (CCL12)	pg	+145 (+190, +100)	+46 (+90, +2.8)	−99 (−44, −153)	P
M-CSF	pg	+1180 (+780, +1590)	+180 (−220, +580)	−1000 (−1460, −540)	P
MDC (CCL22)	pg	+29 (−44, +102)	−97 (−166, −28)	−126 (−207, −45)	(C)
MIP-1α (CCL3)	pg	+90 (+20, +200)	+120 (+30, +220)	+30 (−50, +110)	P,C
MIP-1β (CCL4)	pg	+216 (+180, +253)	+15 (−13, +44)	−201 (−240, −163)	P
MIP-1γ (CCL9)	pg	+7420 (+4980, +9860)	+7230 (+4540, +10,010)	−180 (−4100, +3730)	P,C
MIP-2 (CXL1)	pg	+11.3 (+5.7, +16.9)	+2.3 (+0.7, +5.3)	+9.0 (+15.8, +2.2)	P,C
MIP-3β (CCL19)	pg	+210 (+120, +310)	+80 (−40, +190)	−140 (−240, −40)	P
MMP-9	ng	+37 (+14, +60)	+12 (−1.3, +25)	−25 (−54, +4.1)	P
Myeloperoxidase	ng	+93 (+62, +123)	+118 (+102, +135)	+25 (−14, +65)	P,C
Oncostatin M	pg	+100 (+70, +150)	−10 (−20, +10)	−120 (−160, −70)	P
Osteopontin	pg	+22.9 (+8.8, +37.0)	+81 (+52, +109)	+58 (+23, +93)	P,C
Serum Amyloid P	μg	+15.4 (+10.1, +20.6)	+14.0 (+9.5, +18.5)	−1.4 (−8.5, +5.8)	P,C
SGOT	μg	+5.6 (−4.9, +16.1)	+13.7 (+2.8, +24.6)	+8.1 (−8.2, +24.4)	C
Stem Cell Factor	pg	+68 (+39, +97)	−6.3 (−32, +19.5)	−74 (−115, −34)	P
TIMP-1	pg	+940 (+480, +1,400)	+980 (+630, +1,330)	+50 (−460, +560)	P,C
TNF-α	pg	+20 (0, +40)	0 (−10, 0)	−20 (−50, 0)	P
VCAM-1	ng	+405 (+257, +552)	+540 (+395, +685)	+135 (−67, +337)	P,C
VEGF	pg	+49 (+8.5, +90)	+6.6 (−44, +57)	−43 (−88, +2.9)	P

[a] Measurement unit per milliliter of plasma; IU, International Unit; [b] P, increase during peak; C, increase during clearance; (P), decrease during peak; (C), decrease during clearance; [c] Italics, $p < 0.01$ by two-tailed T-test; [d] Abbreviations defined in Table S1; [e] (CXCL10), standardized chemokine designation.

The serum proteins that were significantly elevated at the peak but had declined by the time of clearance were following: (i) the cytokines IL-6, IL-7, IL-10, IL-11, IL-18, Macrophage-Colony Stimulating Factor (M-CSF), Oncostatin M, Stem Cell Factor, and Tumor Necrosis Factor-α (TNF-α); (ii) the chemokines Inducible Protein-10 (CXCL10), KC/GROα (CXCL1), lymphotactin (XCL1), Monocyte Chemoattractant Protein (MCP)-1 (CCL2), MCP-3 (CCL7), MCP-5 (CCL12), Macrophage Inflammatory Protein (MIP)-1β (CCL4), and MIP-3 β (CCL19); (iii) the enzyme Matrix Metalloproteinase-9 (MMP-9), and (iv) the growth factor Vascular Endothelial Cell Growth Factor (VEGF).

The serum proteins that were significantly elevated at the peak and remained so after clearance were the following: (i) the chemokines MIP-1α (CCL3) and MIP-2 (CXCL1); (ii) the acute-phase proteins C-reactive Protein (CRP), fibrinogen, haptoglobin, and Serum Amyloid P (SAP); and (iii) clusterin, myeloperoxidase, osteopontin, Tissue Inhibitor of Metalloproteinase-1 (TIMP-1), and Vascular Cell Adhesion Molecule-1 (VCAM-1).

Analytes that were higher at the clearance sampling but not at the peak were the vasoconstrictor endothelin-1, the MHC class I component β-2 microglobulin, and the liver enzyme serum glutamic-oxaloacetic transaminase (SGOT). Significantly lower concentrations at either the peak or clearance samplings than in uninfected mice were observed for Epidermal Growth Factor (EGF), the cytokine IL-1β, Macrophage-Derived Chemokine (CCL22), and the hormones insulin and growth hormone.

The profiles of these analytes in the infected immunocompetent mice were similar to what we observed with SCID mice of the same genetic background infected with the CC1 strain instead of the HS1 strain [95]. Infected mice at peak spirochete densities had 10- to 20-fold higher concentrations in comparison to uninfected mice of both the pro-inflammatory cytokine IL-6 and the anti-inflammatory cytokine IL-10, as well as the inflammation chemokines MIP-1α (CCL3), MIP-1β (CCL4), MIP-2 (CXCL1), MCP-1 (CCL2), MCP-3 (CCL7), and MCP-5 (CCL12). Other serum components that were elevated in both infected SCID and infected immunocompetent mice were the acute-phase proteins CRP, haptoglobin, and SAP, as well as endothelin-1, myeloperoxidase, MMP-9, TIMP-1, and chemokine MCP-5 (CCL12). As we observed with infected immunocompetent mice, there were no discernible elevations of either cytokine IFN-γ nor IL-1β in the infected SCID mice [95].

3.2.3. Comments

Overall, the profile of the analyte changes in the infected immunocompetent mice corresponds to a marked systemic inflammatory response and an accompanying modulation of those pro-inflammatory cytokines and chemokines by anti-inflammatory cytokines, such as IL-10. There were several similarities to and some differences from the early responses of mice to injections of E. coli lipopolysaccharide (LPS) [96]. More specifically, 4 h after injection the LPS-treated mice showed marked elevations of both IL-6 and IL-10, and while IL-6 had declined toward normal by 24 h after injection, IL-10 remained elevated. The concentration of chemokines MIP-1β, MIP-2, MCP-1, MCP-3, and MCP-5 at 4 h after LPS injection were comparable to those of B. hermsii-infected mice. A limitation of the study was the absence of the B cell chemokine CXCL13 from the analyte panel. Gelderblom et al. reported high CXCL13 concentrations in the blood of B cell-deficient C57BL/6-$Igh6^{-/-}$ mice infected with B. turicatae [97].

3.3. Antibody Responses to B. hermsii Infection

3.3.1. Background

In 1896 Gabritchewsky reported that serum from a recovering relapsing fever patient lysed the etiologic spirochetes when they were mixed together in the laboratory [98]. In 1906 Novy and Knapp showed that once infected animals had recovered, they were immune to challenge by the same organism and, in addition, that anti-serum obtained from the immune mice provided passive protection for other animals against infection [14]. Novy and Knapp noted that the antibodies were both agglutinating and bactericidal. Stoenner et al. and Barbour et al. working with the *B. hermsii* model of mice demonstrated that anti-serum to a specific serotype would clear the blood of that particular serotype but not other serotypes [47,99]. Newman and Johnson found that neither T cells nor the terminal components of complement were necessary for clearance of *B. turicatae* from the blood of mice [100,101]. IgM antibody is sufficient for clearance from the blood [99,102]. Some of the antibodies elicited by infection or immunization are bactericidal in the absence of a complement [99,103,104].

3.3.2. Agglutination Assays

Assays for antibody function, such as agglutination, neutralization, or growth inhibition, are more predictive of protection against infectious challenge by *Borrelia* spp. than matrix-based assays, such as ELISA or Western blot [105,106]. Accordingly, we examined by macro-agglutination assay the plasma collected during the course of the growth experiment with 95 mice that is described in Section 3.1.2. The antibody to serotype 7 was first detected by agglutination at about the same time as the sharp decline in spirochetes in the blood began at hour 120 (Figure 6). The agglutinating antibody concentration doubled every 4.3 (3.6–5.3) h for the duration of the experiment. This rate was similar to the genome doubling rate for *B. hermsii* in the blood.

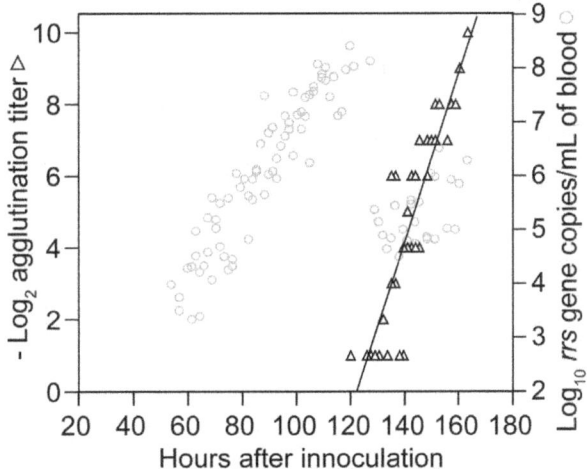

Figure 6. Rise in agglutinating antibodies to *B. hermsii* during infection. The graph superimposes a scatter plot of log-transformed reciprocal titers of antibody to serotype 7 of *B. hermsii* by a macro-agglutination assay (black triangles) on to the values for *B. hermsii* growth in the blood (gray circles) of Figure 3. The samples were drawn from the same group of mice described for Figures 3 and 4 (Section 3.1.2). Each data point is a sampling from a single mouse.

To assess the specificity of these agglutinating antibodies, on day 0 we infected groups of five BALB/c mice with an estimated one to two spirochetes of either serotype 7 or serotype 19, which had been propagated in SCID mice. On day 5 anti-coagulated blood was obtained from all mice by terminal exsanguination. Whole blood was subjected to qPCR: four of five serotype 7-injected mice were positive, and three of five serotype 19-injected mice were positive. The genome count per milliliter of blood in the infected mice ranged between 138 and 16,600 with a mean of 3811, approximately the same genome density observed at the time of clearance in Section 3.1.2. For the micro-agglutination assay, cell-free plasma from each mouse was then mixed 1:1 with SCID mouse plasma containing either serotype 7 or 19. All four BALB/c mice who had been infected with serotype 7 had agglutinating antibodies against serotype 7 cells but not to serotype 19 on day 5. In contrast, on day 5 all three BALB/c mice infected with serotype 19 had agglutinating antibodies to serotype 19 but not serotype 7 ($p = 0.03$). The three uninfected mice did not have detectable agglutinating antibodies to either serotype 7 or 19 cells. This experiment indicated that these early-appearing antibodies were serotype-specific, and thus permissive of the growth of other serotypes.

3.3.3. Antibody Response Detected by ELISA and IFA

While matrix-based assays such as ELISA have lower predictive value for assessing immunity status [99,107], they often have the advantage of greater sensitivity for detection of antibodies to a given pathogen. Accordingly, we examined the antibody response to infection with serotype 7 strain HS1 using a whole-cell ELISA. Mouse serum samples collected from the 95-mouse experiment of Section 3.1.2 were assayed for the presence of antibody to serotype 7 cells. Anti-*B. hermsii* antibodies were detectable in the blood at a reciprocal titer of ≥ 20 at hour 99 post-infection, which was about 20 h before clearance was underway and agglutinating antibodies were first detected (Figure 7, panel A). The amount of antibodies reacting with cells in the wells increased over time with a doubling time of 9.8 (7.9–11.6) h and an R^2 of 0.78. By hour 120 post-infection, antibody levels were at reciprocal titers between 40 and 80.

There were nine mice for which there were pairs of ELISA results, with the first bleeding beginning at hour 100 post-infection and then with a second bleeding 7.5 h later (Figure 7, panel B). From hour 110 onwards, the anti-*B. hermsii* antibody levels approximately doubled during the testing interval, a result consistent with the doubling rate calculated by linear regression from the collected individual values of the entire group. These findings indicated that production of anti-*B. hermsii* antibodies began no later than day 4 of an infection started from fewer than 10 spirochetes. The total number of antibodies reactive against antigens displayed on the matrix increased at a rate one-half of that noted for agglutinating antibodies against live bacteria.

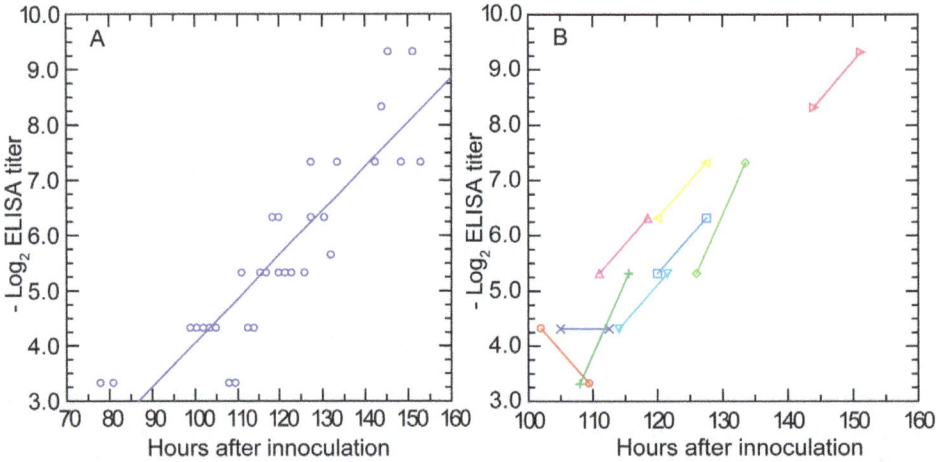

Figure 7. Serum antibody to whole cells of *B. hermsii* by enzyme-linked immunosorbent assay (ELISA) over time in infected mice. The experiment and blood collection protocol are the same as described for Figure 3. Panel (**A**) is a scatter plot of log-transformed reciprocal titer values for individual mice against time in hours after inoculation; Panel (**B**) shows pairs of values for nine individual mice obtained 7.5 h apart and denoted by different colors and symbols as given in the figure.

The early appearance and then increase of antibodies while the spirochetes were still multiplying in the blood was further documented by IFA for IgM antibodies. Five plasma samples from each of the time points at hours 66, 72, 78, 84, 94.5, 100.5, 106.5, and 112.5 into the infection were examined at a dilution of 1:10 for the first appearance of reactivity to either serotype 7 or serotype 19 in thin blood smears. No reactivity to either serotype was detected in the samples from hours 66 to 84. However, at hour 94.5, one (20%) of the five mice sampled at that time had antibodies to serotype 7 cells by IFA. The proportions of the mice with antibodies to serotype 7 thereafter increased from two (40%) of five at hour 100.5 to three (60%) of five at hour 106.5 and then to four (80%) of five at hour 112.5. No mouse had detectable antibodies to serotype 19 or any shared antigens between serotype 19 and serotype 7 before clearance had occurred.

3.3.4. Antibody Response in Nude Mice

Newman and Johnson demonstrated that nude mice deficient in T cell-mediated immunity cleared *B. turicatae* from the blood as well as congenic immunocompetent ones and within the same time [101]. We subsequently confirmed this with nude mice infected with *B. hermsii* [99]. Here we report the timing of antibodies to the infecting strain in nude mice. Five five-week-old female homozygous nude mice and three five-week-old female BALB/c mice were injected with ~10^4 serotype 7 cells from an infected mouse on day 0. Five other nude mice were injected with buffer alone. On days 2 or 3 spirochetes were observed in tail vein blood of all the mice injected with *B. hermsii*. On day 4 no spirochetes were noted in the blood of any of the mice, and the mice were exsanguinated on that day. By IFA with sera serially diluted two-fold beginning with 1:2, we observed reciprocal titers of 16, 128, and 256 for the BALB/c mice and reciprocal titers of 16, 32, 64, 64, and 64 for the five nude mice on the same day on which clearance was first recorded ($p = 0.4$ for log-transformed data).

3.3.5. In Vitro Neutralization with a Monoclonal Antibody

The simultaneous presence of the *B. hermsii* cells and antibodies to *B. hermsii* in the blood before final clearance occurred raises the question about the relationship between densities of the spirochetes and concentrations of the antibody. The in vivo findings suggested that there may be, for both cells and antibodies, critical threshold densities and concentrations, only above which the functional effect, such as agglutination or growth inhibition, manifests. We investigated this using a growth inhibition assay, which had been shown to correlate better with protective immunity for both vaccinated mice and humans than matrix-based immunoassays, such as ELISA [105,106]. The assay usually provides an unambiguous distinction between wells in which there is unimpeded growth and those with inhibition. Different concentrations of serotype 33 cells and antibody to serotype 33 were distributed in microtiter plates in a checkerboard format [63]. The antibody was a monoclonal antibody that had both agglutinating and growth-inhibiting properties [63]. The study was carried out in the presence and absence of complement.

Figure 8 shows plots of the densities of bacteria and concentrations of antibody at which growth inhibition occurred and below which there was no discernible effect. The same ratio of antibodies to bacteria for achieving inhibition roughly held over the entire range. For a given density of cells, ~50% less antibody was required for growth inhibition when complement was included.

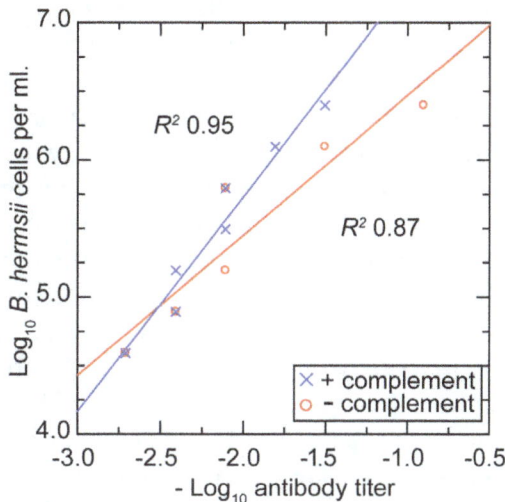

Figure 8. Scatter plot of in vitro growth inhibition assay titers at different densities (log-transformed) of *B. hermsii* cells and different titers (log-transformed) of a monoclonal antibody to *B. hermsii* and in presence or absence of complement. Linear regression for each of the two conditions and corresponding coefficients of determination (R^2) are shown.

3.3.6. Comments

Returning again to the pioneering study of Novy and Knapp [14], we noted in their rat model experiments an interval of about two days between the first detection of spirochetes in the blood and their clearance. If we assume that there were $\sim 10^5$ bacteria per mL at detection and $\sim 10^7$ per mL at clearance, then these kinetics of antibody production would be similar to what be observed in mice infected with *B. hermsii*. Coffey and Eveland observed the specific antibody to the infecting serotype as detected by immunofluorescence assay appeared within five days of injection of the rats [42].

Our results and those of the aforementioned studies suggest to us the following account for the simultaneous presence of both antibodies and spirochetes in the blood: Until the concentration of antibodies reaches a critical threshold, at which complete or near-complete neutralization of the targeted cells ensues, the majority of spirochetes are not affected and continue to replicate. Plausibly this is because when there are few antibodies binding to the spirochetes, they can be shed through a patching phenomenon and the release of membrane blebs or vesicles [108]. The findings suggest that the threshold for an antibody effect varies directly with the density of bacteria. The similarity in doubling rates for the spirochetes and for the agglutinating antibodies against them is noteworthy. It suggests that the head start of three days or so afforded to the pathogen over the adaptive immune response can be sustained for a few days more, until the carrying capacity of the host is reached and the rising antibody concentration finally passes the threshold.

3.4. Anemia during Infection

3.4.1. Background

Anemia during relapsing fever occurs in human cases of the disease [109]. Anemia was noted in two of three dogs infected with *B. turicatae* [55] and in the majority of cases of *B. persica* infections in dogs and cats in Israel [57]. Anemia has also been noted in experimental infections, including *B. crocidurae* [110]. In our preliminary studies with strain CC1 of *B. hermsii* we observed decreased hematocrit values with splenomegaly in SCID mice (unpublished findings). This phenomenon was further investigated in the present study.

3.4.2. Changes in Hematocrit during Infection and after Antibiotic Treatment

In the first experiment 15 eight- to 10-week-old male C.B-17 SCID mice weighing between 19 and 23 g were inoculated on day 0 with $\sim 10^3$ strain CC1 bacteria in freshly obtained infected mouse plasma. On day 3, infection was confirmed in all mice by phase microscopy of tail vein blood. On day 5, eight infected mice were weighed, euthanized, terminally exsanguinated, and dissected with removal of the spleen for weighing and histopathology. The seven remaining infected mice were administered ceftriaxone for three days before euthanasia and processing on day 8. At that time, four uninfected SCID mice of the same sex and age were similarly euthanized and processed.

Figure 9 summarizes the results. Panel A shows the profound anemia of infected mice and the near-complete restoration of the erythrocyte count with three days of antibiotic treatment. The means (95% CI) for the hematocrits (%) of uninfected, infected, and antibiotic-treated mice were 49.5 (48.5–50.5), 10.9 (7.9–13.8), and 40.1 (39.3–41.0), respectively. The short course of antibiotics was effective in reducing the bacterial count in the blood by $\sim 99.99\%$ (panel B). However, while the red blood cell count increased with a decrease in the number of bacteria in the blood (panels A and B), the spleens remained enlarged (panel C). The mean percentage ratios (95% CI) of spleen weight-to-body weight for uninfected, infected, and antibiotic-treated mice were 0.24 (0.20–0.28), 2.2 (1.9–2.5), and 1.5 (1.1–1.9), respectively. The continued elevated iron content of the spleen after treatment (panel D) was an indication that the enlarged spleen was attributable to retained erythrocytes or their debris inside the spleen. The constitutional effects of the infection on the mice were seen in the weight loss displayed by the infected mice, even those who had received the antibiotic (panel E).

The relationship between the hematocrit and relative spleen weight in the infected mice and the corresponding discordance in those parameters in the treated mice are shown in panel F.

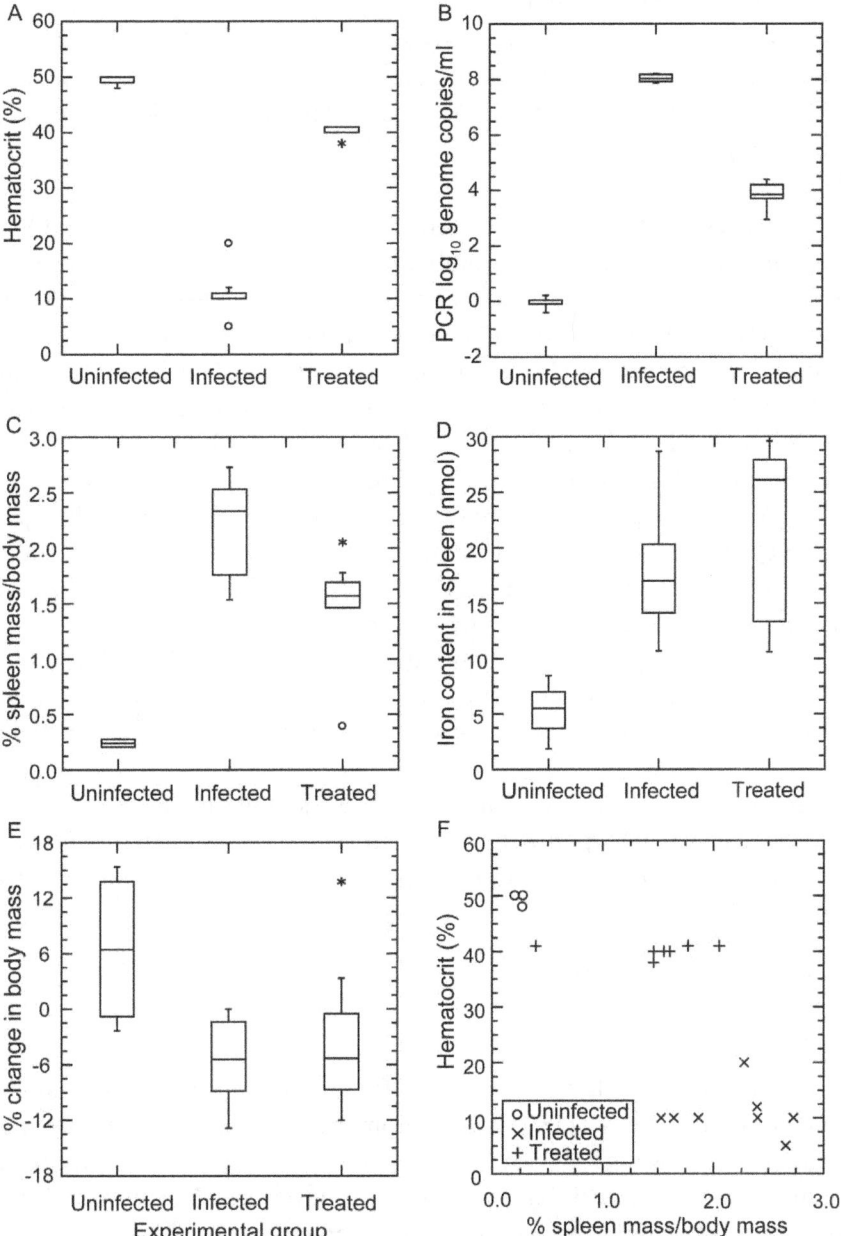

Figure 9. Severe anemia in BALB/c mice with severe combined immunodeficiency (SCID) and infected with strain CC1 of *B. hermsii*. The experiment is described in the accompanying text. Panels (**A–E**) are box-whisker plots in which each horizontal box indicates the first and third quartiles, and the indentation inside the box is the median. * The 1.5× interquartile range is indicated by the horizontal line (whiskers) bisecting the box, and values outside this range are indicated by asterisks and circles. The three conditions were uninfected (*n* = 4 mice), infected without antibiotics (*n* = 8), and infected with antibiotics (*n* = 7). Panel (**A**) is of the hematocrit values for the whole blood from the mice. Panel (**B**) is of the spirochete burdens in the groups of mice as estimated by qPCR as described for Figure 3; Panel (**C**) displays the ratios in percentages of the spleen weight to total body weight after euthanasia; Panel (**D**) shows the iron content in the spleen in nmol per gram of spleen; Panel (**E**) shows the net change in body mass in percentage between initial measurement and measurement at time of euthanasia; Panel (**F**) is a scatter plot of hematocrit values against ratio of spleen weight to body weight for individual mice in each group.

3.4.3. Histopathology

Microscopic examination of thin sections of fixed spleens from four infected mice and one uninfected mouse revealed sinusoids that were heavily congested with erythrocytes in the infected mice. There was erythrophagocytosis and marked vasculitis with neutrophils in the walls of arteries and arterioles. Hematopoietic units, with their tell-tale megakaryocytes, were present in the congested spleens of infected mice and were evidence of extramedullary hematopoiesis.

3.4.4. Comments

Benoit et al. observed that the B cell-deficient $rag2^{-/-}$ mutants of strains BALB/c, C57BL/6, and C3H/HeN became anemic as well as thrombocytopenic with infection of strain DAH *B. hermsii* of an unreported serotype [72]. On day 5 of infection, the erythrocyte counts were about 40% lower than what they were on day 0 [72]. The drop in red blood cells and platelets inversely correlated with spirochete burden and with spleen and liver weights, as noted here (Figure 9). Histopathologic studies by Benoit et al. revealed inflammatory cells, marked erythrophagocytosis, and extramedullary hematapoiesis in spleens of the infected immunodeficient animals [72].

The role of the spleen in limiting pathogen burden during spirochetemia was recognized as early as 1928, when Meleney reported a more severe course of relapsing fever in squirrels that been splenectomized [111]. This was confirmed in subsequent studies by, among others, Baltazard in 1937 [112] and Alugupalli et al. more recently [113]. While splenectomy could also affect the adaptive immune response, the greater deficiency during relapsing fever appears to result in loss of the spleen's filtering function for spirochetes, either in aggregates with blood cells, with antibodies, or both. The release back into the circulation of most of erythrocytes with antibiotic therapy in the present study indicates that much of the erythrocyte sequestration, whether in the spleen, liver, or elsewhere, is reversible.

Moderate to severe anemia also occurs in mice experimentally infected with *Trypanosoma brucei*, another blood-borne, extracellular pathogen that features antigenic variation [114]. This has been attributed to sensitization to IgM-antigen complexes [115], inflammatory cytokines such as TNF-α [116], and erythrophagocytosis [117].

3.5. Erythrocyte Aggregation during Infection

3.5.1. Background

The adhesiveness of relapsing fever *Borrelia* cells for erythrocytes in the blood of infected patients was noted by Cook as early as 1904 [118]. This phenomenon of erythrocyte rossetting was explored in depth by Bergström and colleagues with the "Old World" species *B. crocidurae* of Africa [110,119]. Although an in vitro interaction of *B. hermsii* cells with human erythrocytes had been noted [120], this species has drawn most scientific interest for its cells' interactions with platelets and the consequent thrombocytopenia [53].

3.5.2. In Vitro Aggregation Experiment

The foregoing study of experimental infection suggested that the anemia was attributable in part to sequestration of the erythrocytes and, furthermore, that much of this was reversible with timely antibiotic therapy. The antibiotic presumably had this salutary effect by killing or disarming spirochetes, thereby releasing whatever blood cells had been removed from the circulation of blood. However, not all was reversible; the hematocrits rose, but not back to normal. The post-therapy persistence of splenomegaly and elevated iron in the spleen indicated that erythrocytes or their debris remained in the spleen. Since this occurred in animals lacking adaptive immunity, antibodies binding to erythrocyte-borne spirochetes in a complex could not be evoked as an explanation.

However, it was not clear whether the sequestration was attributable to direct effects of the spirochetes, such as was noted for *B. crocidurae* and erythrocytes, or consequences of the host response.

To begin to investigate this, we infected 12 adult female C.B-17 SCID mice and BALB/c mice with 10^3 cells of strain CC1 on day 0. Infection was monitored by microscopy of tail vein blood. At or near of the peak of spirochetemia on day 5, the blood was obtained at the time of euthanasia. The pooled plasma from the infected mice was compared with pooled plasma from uninfected mice of the same strain for their aggregation effects when mixed with an equal volume of heparinized whole blood from uninfected mice of the same strain. The blood was subjected to low-speed centrifugation, brief enough to sediment blood cells but not spirochetes in the suspension. This provided infected plasma. Samples of the infected plasma were also subjected to high-speed centrifugation to pellet the spirochetes present. Some of the latter supernatants were also heated under conditions that would inactivate complement. These preparations from infected mice were compared with plasma from uninfected mice in 1:1 mixtures with heparinized whole blood from uninfected mice.

Figure 10 shows representative photomicrographs of the mixtures of these plasma preparations after incubation with whole blood. There was little or no aggregation or clumping of the blood cells in the mixture of uninfected plasma with the whole blood. In the mixture of red cells with infected plasma, which contained an estimated 5×10^6 spirochetes per milliliter, there were large clumps of erythrocytes with numerous spirochetes attached on the periphery. With the centrifuged plasma the spirochetes were absent. Aggregates of erythrocytes were noted, but these were characterized as rouleaux, with the red blood cells in stacks rather than a more disordered clump.

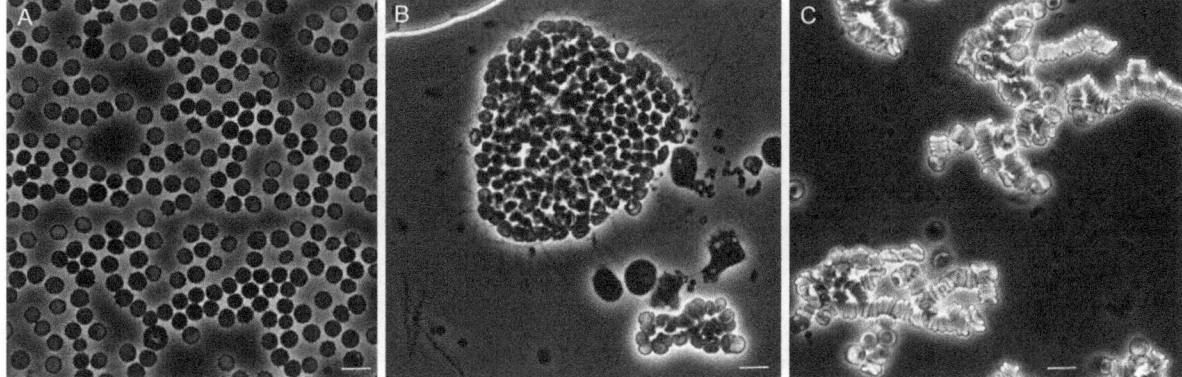

Figure 10. Phase photomicrographs of uninfected mouse blood mixed with equal volumes of plasma from uninfected SCID mice (panel **A**); plasma from *B. hermsii*-infected BALB/c mice (panel **B**); and plasma from infected mice that had been centrifuged (panel **C**). In panel B numerous spirochetes are seen singly, in clumps, and adhered to the aggregate of blood cells. Panel C is an example of rouleaux formation. The size marker in each panel is 10 μm.

These effects of the different plasma preparations in the mixtures with blood cells could also be quantitated by measuring the dispersion of cells in microtiter plates after incubation. The more disperse the cells in the wells, the wider the area of opacity. This can be seen in panel A of Figure 11. The resultant image analysis values are summarized in panel B. The samples from 12 infected SCID mice were divided into two groups by the densities of the spirochetes in the blood at the time of collection. Eight SCID mice had bacteria densities of ~10^7 cells/mL, and in the four others the densities were ~10^6/mL. The third group for the experiment was the immunocompetent five BALB/c mice, which averaged ~10^7 spirochetes per milliliter. The greatest amount of aggregation was observed with infected plasma of the more heavily infected SCID mice and BALB/c mice. Centrifugation and centrifugation followed by heating reduced the aggregation, as measured by this method, but did not return the values to that of the uninfected sera. The continuing presence of rouleaux in the heated plasma was confirmed by microscopy.

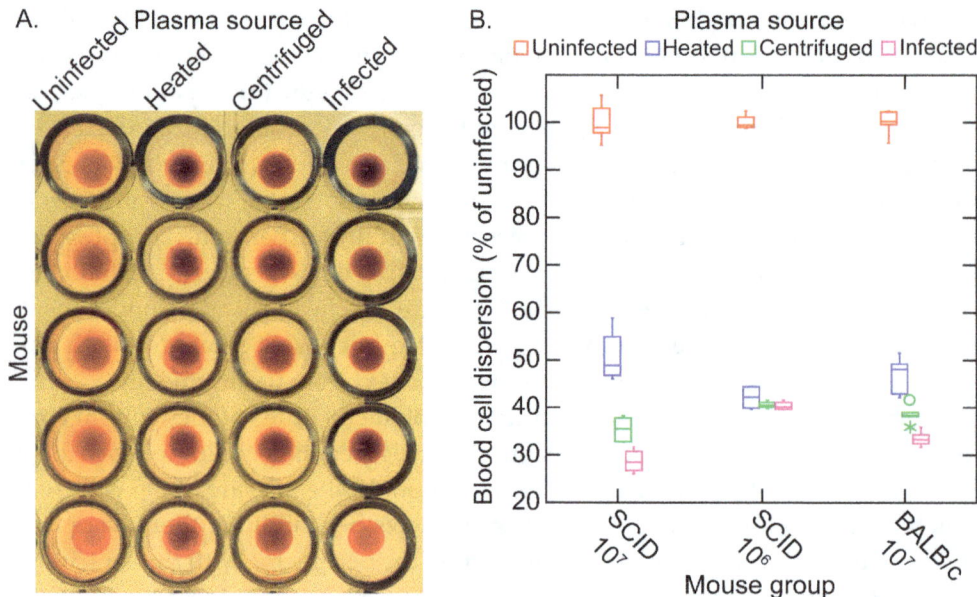

Figure 11. In vitro erythrocyte aggregation assay of uninfected blood mixed with plasma from uninfected mice and plasma from infected mice that was unaltered (infected), centrifuged, or centrifuged and heated. The assay method is described in the text. (**A**) Panel A shows a microtiter plate for which the source of plasma was from immunocompetent BALB/c mice (five uninfected or five infected); (**B**) Panel B is a box-whisker graph of the blood cell dispersion as estimated by image analysis and expressed as the percentage of each of four experimental conditions' values to the mean of the uninfected values. The 12 infected SCID mice were divided into a group of eight with a high spirochete burden (10^7 cells/mL) and a group of four with a moderate spirochete burden (10^6 cells/mL) in the plasma. There were five infected BALB/c mice.

3.5.3. Comments

The occurrence of the aggregation with the blood of both immunocompetent and SCID blood argues against a role of antibodies. The results indicate there may be at least two components to the erythrocyte aggregation phenomenon in these in vitro assays. The first is the rouleaux formation that is commonly noted during acute infections and is attributable to acute-phase proteins, particularly fibrinogen [121]. We observed high concentrations of fibrinogen and other acute-phase proteins in the blood of infected mice and their persistence even during clearance (Table 1).

The second component appears to be the binding of the spirochetes to erythrocytes and then a secondary clumping together of smaller aggregates into the larger ones that can be seen in Figure 10. This effect may be rapidly reversible with antibiotics, especially those with bactericidal activity, such as ceftriaxone [62,122]. It conceivably could also be reversed with the rise of antibodies that have bactericidal activity [103].

The degree of anemia observed in our experiments with the CC1 strain in the SCID mice was more severe, to the point of being life-threatening, than Benoit et al. reported for their *rag2*$^{-/-}$ mice infected with the DAH strain of unreported serotype [72]. This suggests to us that strains or serotypes within a strain differ in their capacities to mediate the aggregation phenomenon. The molecular phenotype that this corresponds to remains to be determined.

4. Conclusions

One caveat for our and most other contemporary animal models of relapsing fever is their dependence on either the house mouse *M. musculus* or the brown rat *Rattus rattus*. Neither of these murids are a natural reservoir of a relapsing fever *Borrelia* sp. With the exceptions of *B. recurrentis* and *B. duttonii*, humans are not natural reservoirs for relapsing fever agents either. In North America humans, like dogs, cats, and some other domestic animals, are inadvertent hosts and probably evolutionary dead-ends for these zoonotic pathogens. In that light, the *M. musculus* experimental model can be justified for the insights it provides for understanding pathogenesis and immunity of relevance for human disease. However, for a more comprehensive appreciation of the ecology of these zoonoses, a case can be made for a return to experimental studies with reservoir hosts that share evolutionary histories with a *Borrelia* sp.

In the case of *B. hermsii* in western North America, suitable alternatives to *M. musculus* among natural hosts are chipmunks or squirrels [40]. However, these species are not routinely available as laboratory-reared specimens from a breeding facility. Field capture of a sufficient number of animals for experiments that include terminal exsanguination, such as those presented here, would have been prohibitive in cost and difficult to justify on an animal welfare basis. To more fully represent the diversity of host populations, there is an argument for using outbred mice, as was routinely done before the 1980s. Inbred strains are more stereotypical in their responses and only narrowly capture the diversity of wild populations. However, more heterogeneous populations, with their greater variances of values for a variable, usually call for larger sample sizes for experiments with either a continuous or categorical endpoint.

For the nearer term, the question of whether BALB/c mice or some other strain, such as C57BL/6, is the preferred lineage to use with respect to either pathogenesis or immunity of relapsing fever in a *M. musculus* model remains unresolved. With the exception of one limited study [72], there has not been a comprehensive investigation of different inbred strains of *M. musculus* infected with *B. hermsii* or other relapsing fever to the extent to which there has been for the Lyme disease agent *B. burgdorferi* [123–125].

Another possible limitation of the present study was infection by needle inoculation rather than tick bite. The mice in most of the experiments were infected with low doses of organisms that were comparable to those delivered by a feeding tick. The source was fresh blood of an infected mouse, so the phenotype of infecting bacteria was that expressed in the mammal [49]. However, some of the key early events of natural infections, such as at that tick bite site, were not captured by the experiments as designed. Tick transmission of infection is a more demanding experimental design and requires a functioning breeding colony of *Ornithodoros* sp. ticks, but it still is possible, as Schwan and Lopez and their colleagues have shown [126–128].

Recognition of both the limitations and the achievements of these studies and those of other investigations informs our following views for research priorities for animal models of relapsing fever: (1) assess the growth and immune response dynamics of a relapsing fever agent in a natural host. This may be most feasible for species in North America with *P. maniculatus*, which is a reservoir host for some strains of *B. hermsii* and which has a long history of successful breeding and maintenance of colonies in captivity; (2) Keeping within the *M. musuculus* model, evaluate the diversity of host responses to infection by using a mixed-stock population (e.g., Collaborative Cross mice [129,130]) that more closely approximates the diversity of wild populations. Highly multiplexed arrays and low-cost whole-genome sequencing allow stratification by genotype; (3) Initiate more experimental infections by transmission from *Ornithodoros* sp. ticks, preferably first with an inbred strain of mouse to minimize host heterogeneity, and compare them with needle inoculations; (4) Identify the factor(s) that confer(s) partial resistance to *B. hermsii*, as evidenced by the slower growth rates and lower peak densities during relapses, before neutralizing antibodies come to the fore; (5) Further characterize the overlooked phenomenon of erythrocyte aggregation by a "New World" relapsing fever *Borrelia* sp.

Acknowledgments: The work was supported by National Institutes of Health grants AI-24424 and AI-065359. We thank Qiyuan Dia, April Phillips, and Adrienne Puteet-Driver for their valued contributions to the extended time course experiment presented here and Fong Hue for technical assistance.

Author Contributions: Christopher D. Crowder, Arash Ghalyanchi Langeroudi, Azadeh Shojaee Estabragh, Eric R. G. Lewis, Renee A. Marcsisin and Alan G. Barbour conceived and designed the experiments, performed the experiments, and analyzed the data; Christopher D. Crowder and Alan G. Barbour wrote the paper.

Abbreviations

The following abbreviations are used in this manuscript:

J-H	Jarisch-Herxheimer
IFA	indirect immunofluorescence assay
PBS	phosphate-buffered saline
qPCR	quantitative polymerase chain reaction
SCID	severe combined immunodeficient
TLR	Toll-like receptor

References

1. Obermeier, O. Vorkommen feinster, eine eigenbewegung zeigender fäden im Blute von recurrenskranken, vorläufige mittheilung. *Centrablatt Med. Wiss.* **1873**, *10*, 145–147. (In German)
2. Fitz, R.H. Report on pathology and pathological anatomy. *Boston Med. Surg. J.* **1873**, *88*, 393–397. [CrossRef]
3. Cutler, S.J.; Abdissa, A.; Trape, J.F. New concepts for the old challenge of African relapsing fever borreliosis. *Clin. Microbiol. Infect.* **2009**, *15*, 400–406. [CrossRef] [PubMed]
4. Motschutkoffsky, D. Experimentelle studien iiber die impfbarkeit typhoser fieber. *Zentralbl. Med. Wissensch* **1876**, *14*, 193–197. (In German)
5. Manson, P. *Tropical Diseases, a Manual of the Diseases of the Warm Climate*; Cassell and Co.: London, UK, 1898.
6. Christy, C. *Ornithodoros moubata* and tick fever in man. *Br. Med. J.* **1903**, *2*, 652–653.
7. Ross, P.H.; Milne, A.D. Tick fever. *Br. Med. J.* **1904**, *2*, 1453–1454. [CrossRef] [PubMed]
8. Dutton, J.E.; Todd, J.L. The nature of tick fever in the eastern part of the Congo Free State. *Br. Med. J.* **1905**, *2*, 1259–1260.
9. Davis, G.E.; Burgdorfer, W. On the susceptibility of the guinea pig to the relapsing fever spirochete *Borrelia duttonii*. *Bull. Soc. Pathol. Exot. Filiales* **1954**, *47*, 498–501. [PubMed]
10. Koch, R. Vorläufige mitteilungen über die ergebnisse einer forschungsreise nach Ostafrika. *Dtsch. Med. Wochenschr.* **1905**, *31*, 1865–1869. (In German) [CrossRef]
11. Carlisle, R.J. Two cases of relapsing fever; with notes on the occurrence of this disease throughout the world at the present day. *J. Infect. Dis.* **1906**, *3*, 233–265. [CrossRef]
12. Breinl, A. On the specific anture of the spirochaeta of the African tick fever. *Lancet* **1906**, *167*, 1690–1691. [CrossRef]
13. Norris, C.; Pappenheimer, A.M.; Flournoy, T. Study of a spirochete obtained from a case of relapsing fever in man, with notes on morphology, animal reactions, and attempts at cultivation. *J. Infect. Dis.* **1906**, *3*, 266–290.
14. Novy, F.G.; Knapp, R.E. Studies on *Spirillum obermeieri* and related organisms. *J. Infect. Dis.* **1906**, *3*, 291–293. [CrossRef]
15. Kemp, H.; Moursund, W.; Wright, H. Relapsing fever in Texas. III. Some notes on the biological characteristics of the causative organism. *Am. J. Trop. Med.* **1934**, *14*, 163–169.
16. Baltazard, M.; Bahmanyar, M.; Chamsa, M. Sur l'usage du cobaye pour la differenciation des spirochetes recurrents. *Bull. Soc. Pathol. Exot.* **1954**, *47*, 864–877. (In French)
17. Brumpt, E. Etude de la fievre recurrente sporadique des etats-unis, transmise dans la nature par *Ornithodoros turicata*. *C. R. Soc. Biol.* **1933**, *113*, 1366–1369. (In French)
18. Davis, G.E. The spirochetes. *Ann. Rev. Microbiol.* **1948**, *2*, 305–334. [CrossRef] [PubMed]
19. Felsenfeld, O. Borrelia, human relapsing fever, and parasite-vector-host relationships. *Bacteriol. Rev.* **1965**, *29*, 46–74. [PubMed]
20. Southern, P.M.; Sanford, J.P. Relapsing fever: A clinical and microbiological review. *Medicine* **1969**, *48*, 129–150. [CrossRef]

21. Felsenfeld, O. *Borrelia. Strains, Vectors, Human and Animal Borreliosis*; Warren H. Greene, Inc.: St. Louis, MO, USA, 1971; p. 180.

22. Goubau, P.F. Relapsing fevers. A review. *Ann. Soc. Belg. Med. Trop.* **1984**, *64*, 335–364. [PubMed]

23. Barbour, A.G.; Hayes, S.F. Biology of Borrelia species. *Microbiol. Rev.* **1986**, *50*, 381–400. [PubMed]

24. Barbour, A.G. Immunobiology of relapsing fever. *Contrib. Microbiol. Immunol.* **1987**, *8*, 125–137. [PubMed]

25. Cadavid, D.; Barbour, A.G. Neuroborreliosis during relapsing fever: Review of the clinical manifestations, pathology, and treatment of infections in humans and experimental animals. *Clin. Infect. Dis.* **1998**, *26*, 151–164. [CrossRef] [PubMed]

26. Barthold, S.W.; Cadavid, D.; Phillip, M.T. Animal models of borreliosis. In *Borrelia: Molecular Biology, Host Interaction, and Pathogenesis*; Radolf, J.D., Samuels, D.S., Eds.; Caister Academic Press: Norfolk, UK, 2010; pp. 359–412.

27. Wheeler, C.; Herms, W.; Meyer, K. A new tick vector of relapsing fever in California. *Proc. Soc. Exp. Biol. Med.* **1935**, *32*, 1290–1292. [CrossRef]

28. Wheeler, C.M. Relapsing fever in California. Attempts to transmit spirochaetes of california relapsing fever to human subjects by means of the bite of the vector *Ornithodoros hermsi. Am. J. Trop. Med.* **1938**, *18*, 641–657.

29. Barbour, A. Relapsing fever. In *Tick-Borne Diseases of Humans*; Dennis, D.T., Goodman, J.L., Sonenshine, D.E., Eds.; ASM Press: Washington, DC, USA, 2005; pp. 220–236.

30. Briggs, L.H. Relapsing fever in California. *JAMA* **1922**, *79*, 941–944. [CrossRef]

31. Boyer, K.M.; Munford, R.S.; Maupin, G.O.; Pattison, C.P.; Fox, M.D.; Barnes, A.M.; Jones, W.L.; Maynard, J.E. Tick-borne relapsing fever: An interstate outbreak originating at Grand Canyon National Park. *Am. J. Epidemiol.* **1977**, *105*, 469–479. [PubMed]

32. Fritz, C.L.; Payne, J.R.; Schwan, T.G. Serologic evidence for *Borrelia hermsii* infection in rodents on federally owned recreational areas in california. *Vector Borne Zoonotic Dis.* **2013**, *13*, 376–381. [CrossRef] [PubMed]

33. Nieto, N.C.; Teglas, M.B. Relapsing fever group Borrelia in Southern California rodents. *J. Med. Entomol.* **2014**, *51*, 1029–1034. [CrossRef] [PubMed]

34. Schwan, T.G.; Raffel, S.J.; Schrumpf, M.E.; Schrumpf, M.E.; Webster, L.S.; Marques, A.R.; Spano, R.; Rood, M.; Burns, J.; Hu, R. Tick-borne relapsing fever and *Borrelia hermsii*, Los Angeles County, California, USA. *Emerg. Infect. Dis.* **2009**, *15*, 1026–1031. [CrossRef] [PubMed]

35. Barbour, A.G. Phylogeny of a relapsing fever Borrelia species transmitted by the hard tick *Ixodes scapularis. Infect. Genet. Evol.* **2014**, *27*, 551–558. [CrossRef] [PubMed]

36. Elbir, H.; Abi-Rached, L.; Pontarotti, P.; Yoosuf, N.; Drancourt, M. African relapsing fever borreliae genomospecies revealed by comparative genomics. *Front. Public Health* **2014**, *2*. [CrossRef] [PubMed]

37. Lescot, M.; Audic, S.; Robert, C.; Nguyen, T.T.; Blanc, G.; Cutler, S.J.; Wincker, P.; Couloux, A.; Claverie, J.M.; Raoult, D.; et al. The genome of *Borrelia recurrentis*, the agent of deadly louse-borne relapsing fever, is a degraded subset of tick-borne *Borrelia duttonii. PLoS Genet.* **2008**, *4*, e1000185. [CrossRef] [PubMed]

38. McNeil, E.; Hinshaw, W.R.; Kissling, R.E. A study of *Borrelia anserina* infection (spirochetosis) in turkeys. *J. Bacteriol.* **1949**, *57*, 191–206. [PubMed]

39. Davis, G.E. The relapsing fevers: Tick-spirochete specificity studies. *Exp. Parasitol.* **1952**, *1*, 406–410. [CrossRef]

40. Burgdorfer, W.; Mavros, A.J. Susceptibility of various species of rodents to the relapsing fever spirochete, *Borrelia hermsii. Infect. Immun.* **1970**, *2*, 256–259. [PubMed]

41. Beck, M. California field and laboratory studies on relapsing fever. *J. Infect. Dis.* **1937**, *60*, 64–80. [CrossRef]

42. Coffey, E.M.; Eveland, W.C. Experimental relapsing fever initiated by *Borrelia hermsii*. II. Sequential appearance of major serotypes in the rat. *J. Infect. Dis.* **1967**, *117*, 29–34. [CrossRef] [PubMed]

43. Coffey, E.M.; Eveland, W.C. Experimental relapsing fever initiated by *Borrelia hermsii*. I. Identification of major serotypes by immunofluorescence. *J. Infect. Dis.* **1967**, *117*, 23–28. [CrossRef] [PubMed]

44. Kelly, R. Cultivation of *Borrelia hermsii. Science* **1971**, *173*, 443–444. [CrossRef] [PubMed]

45. Stoenner, H.G. Biology of *Borrelia hermsii* in Kelly's medium. *Appl. Microbiol.* **1974**, *28*, 540–543. [PubMed]

46. Thompson, R.S.; Burgdorfer, W.; Russell, R.; Francis, B.J. Outbreak of tick-borne relapsing fever in Spokane County, Washington. *JAMA* **1969**, *210*, 1045–1050. [CrossRef] [PubMed]

47. Stoenner, H.G.; Dodd, T.; Larsen, C. Antigenic variation of *Borrelia hermsii. J. Exp. Med.* **1982**, *156*, 1297–1311. [CrossRef] [PubMed]

48. Barbour, A.G.; Tessier, S.L.; Stoenner, H.G. Variable major proteins of *Borrelia hermsii. J. Exp. Med.* **1982**, *156*, 1312–1324. [CrossRef] [PubMed]

49. Schwan, T.G.; Hinnebusch, B.J. Bloodstream- versus tick-associated variants of a relapsing fever bacterium. *Science* **1998**, *280*, 1938–1940. [CrossRef] [PubMed]

50. Magoun, L.; Zuckert, W.R.; Robbins, D.; Parveen, N.; Alugupalli, K.R.; Schwan, T.G.; Barbour, A.G.; Leong, J.M. Variable Small Protein (Vsp)-dependent and Vsp-independent pathways for glycosaminoglycan recognition by relapsing fever spirochaetes. *Mol. Microbiol.* **2000**, *36*, 886–897. [CrossRef] [PubMed]

51. Hinnebusch, B.J.; Barbour, A.G.; Restrepo, B.I.; Schwan, T.G. Population structure of the relapsing fever spirochete *Borrelia hermsii* as indicated by polymorphism of two multigene families that encode immunogenic outer surface lipoproteins. *Infect. Immun.* **1998**, *66*, 432–440. [PubMed]

52. Barbour, A.G. The chromosome and plasmids of the tick-borne relapsing fever agent *Borrelia hermsii*. *Genome Announc.* **2016**, *4*, e00528-16. [CrossRef] [PubMed]

53. Alugupalli, K.R.; Michelson, A.D.; Joris, I.; Schwan, T.G.; Hodivala-Dilke, K.; Hynes, R.O.; Leong, J.M. Spirochete-platelet attachment and thrombocytopenia in murine relapsing fever borreliosis. *Blood* **2003**, *102*, 2843–2850. [CrossRef] [PubMed]

54. Breitschwerdt, E.B.; Nicholson, W.L.; Kiehl, A.R.; Steers, C.; Meuten, D.J.; Levine, J.F. Natural infections with *Borrelia* spirochetes in two dogs from Florida. *J. Clin. Microbiol.* **1994**, *32*, 352–357. [PubMed]

55. Whitney, M.S.; Schwan, T.G.; Sultemeier, K.B.; McDonald, P.S.; Brillhart, M.N. Spirochetemia caused by *Borrelia turicatae* infection in 3 dogs in Texas. *Vet. Clin. Pathol.* **2007**, *36*, 212–216. [CrossRef] [PubMed]

56. Kelly, A.L.; Raffel, S.J.; Fischer, R.J.; Bellinghausen, M.; Stevenson, C.; Schwan, T.G. First isolation of the relapsing fever spirochete, *Borrelia hermsii*, from a domestic dog. *Ticks Tick Borne Dis.* **2014**, *5*, 95–99. [CrossRef] [PubMed]

57. Baneth, G.; Nachum-Biala, Y.; Halperin, T.; Hershko, Y.; Kleinerman, G.; Anug, Y.; Abdeen, Z.; Lavy, E.; Aroch, I.; Straubinger, R.K. *Borrelia persica* infection in dogs and cats: Clinical manifestations, clinicopathological findings and genetic characterization. *Parasites Vectors* **2016**. [CrossRef] [PubMed]

58. Restrepo, B.I.; Kitten, T.; Carter, C.J.; Infante, D.; Barbour, A.G. Subtelomeric expression regions of *Borrelia hermsii* linear plasmids are highly polymorphic. *Mol. Microbiol.* **1992**, *6*, 3299–3311. [CrossRef] [PubMed]

59. Dai, Q.; Restrepo, B.I.; Porcella, S.F.; Raffel, S.J.; Schwan, T.G.; Barbour, A.G. Antigenic variation by *Borrelia hermsii* occurs through recombination between extragenic repetitive elements on linear plasmids. *Mol. Microbiol.* **2006**, *60*, 1329–1343. [CrossRef] [PubMed]

60. Marcsisin, R.A.; Lewis, E.R.; Barbour, A.G. Expression of the tick-associated Vtp protein of *Borrelia hermsii* in a murine model of relapsing fever. *PLoS ONE* **2016**, *11*, e0149889.

61. Barbour, A.G. Isolation and cultivation of Lyme disease spirochetes. *Yale J. Biol. Med.* **1984**, *57*, 521–525. [PubMed]

62. Kazragis, R.J.; Dever, L.L.; Jorgensen, J.H.; Barbour, A.G. In vivo activities of ceftriaxone and vancomycin against *Borrelia* spp. In the mouse brain and other sites. *Antimicrob. Agents Chemother.* **1996**, *40*, 2632–2636. [PubMed]

63. Sadziene, A.; Thompson, P.A.; Barbour, A.G. In vitro inhibition of *Borrelia burgdorferi* growth by antibodies. *J. Infect. Dis.* **1993**, *167*, 165–172. [CrossRef] [PubMed]

64. Barbour, A.G.; Tessier, S.L.; Hayes, S.F. Variation in a major surface protein of Lyme disease spirochetes. *Infect. Immun.* **1984**, *45*, 94–100. [PubMed]

65. Tsao, J.I.; Wootton, J.T.; Bunikis, J.; Luna, M.G.; Fish, D.; Barbour, A.G. An ecological approach to preventing human infection: Vaccinating wild mouse reservoirs intervenes in the Lyme disease cycle. *Proc. Natl. Acad. Sci. USA* **2004**, *101*, 18159–18164. [CrossRef] [PubMed]

66. Barbour, A.G.; Bunikis, J.; Travinsky, B.; Hoen, A.G.; Diuk-Wasser, M.A.; Fish, D.; Tsao, J.I. Niche partitioning of *Borrelia burgdorferi* and *Borrelia miyamotoi* in the same tick vector and mammalian reservoir species. *Am. J. Trop. Med. Hyg.* **2009**, *81*, 1120–1131. [CrossRef] [PubMed]

67. Saeed, A.I.; Sharov, V.; White, J.; Li, J.; Liang, W.; Bhagabati, N.; Braisted, J.; Klapa, M.; Currier, T.; Thiagarajan, M.; et al. Tm4: A free, open-source system for microarray data management and analysis. *BioTechniques* **2003**, *34*, 374–378. [PubMed]

68. Russell, H. Human and experimental relapsing fever, Accra, Gold Coast, 1929–1930. *West Afr. Med. J.* **1931**, *4*, 59–66.

69. Eidmann, E.; Lippelt, H.; Poespodihardjo, J. Quantitative Untersuchungen über die Vermehrung von *Borrelia erratici* in der weißen Maus. *Z. Tropenmed. Parasitol.* **1959**, *10*, 339. (In German) [PubMed]

70. Pennington, P.M.; Allred, C.D.; West, C.S.; Alvarez, R.; Barbour, A.G. Arthritis severity and spirochete burden are determined by serotype in the *Borrelia turicatae*-mouse model of Lyme disease. *Infect. Immun.* **1997**, *65*, 285–292. [PubMed]

71. Cadavid, D.; Thomas, D.D.; Crawley, R.; Barbour, A.G. Variability of a bacterial surface protein and disease expression in a possible mouse model of systemic Lyme borreliosis. *J. Exp. Med.* **1994**, *179*, 631–642. [CrossRef] [PubMed]

72. Benoit, V.M.; Petrich, A.; Alugupalli, K.R.; Marty-Roix, R.; Moter, A.; Leong, J.M.; Boyartchuk, V.L. Genetic control of the innate immune response to *Borrelia hermsii* influences the course of relapsing fever in inbred strains of mice. *Infect. Immun.* **2010**, *78*, 586–594. [CrossRef] [PubMed]

73. Sadziene, A.; Barbour, A.G.; Rosa, P.A.; Thomas, D.D. An OspB mutant of *Borrelia burgdorferi* has reduced invasiveness in vitro and reduced infectivity in vivo. *Infect. Immun.* **1993**, *61*, 3590–3596. [PubMed]

74. Kitten, T.; Barbour, A.G. The relapsing fever agent *Borrelia hermsii* has multiple copies of its chromosome and linear plasmids. *Genetics* **1992**, *132*, 311–324. [PubMed]

75. Barbour, A.G. Antigenic variation of a relapsing fever Borrelia species. *Ann. Rev. Microbiol.* **1990**, *44*, 155–171. [CrossRef] [PubMed]

76. Zhong, J.; Barbour, A.G. Cross-species hybridization of a *Borrelia burgdorferi* DNA array reveals infection- and culture-associated genes of the unsequenced genome of the relapsing fever agent *Borrelia hermsii*. *Mol. Microbiol.* **2004**, *51*, 729–748. [CrossRef] [PubMed]

77. Restrepo, B.I.; Carter, C.J.; Barbour, A.G. Activation of a *vmp* pseudogene in *Borrelia hermsii*: An alternate mechanism of antigenic variation during relapsing fever. *Mol. Microbiol.* **1994**, *13*, 287–299. [CrossRef] [PubMed]

78. Barbour, A.G.; Dai, Q.; Restrepo, B.I.; Stoenner, H.G.; Frank, S.A. Pathogen escape from host immunity by a genome program for antigenic variation. *Proc. Natl. Acad. Sci. USA* **2006**, *103*, 18290–18295. [CrossRef] [PubMed]

79. Bolz, D.D.; Sundsbak, R.S.; Ma, Y.; Akira, S.; Weis, J.H.; Schwan, T.G.; Weis, J.J. Dual role of Myd88 in rapid clearance of relapsing fever *Borrelia* spp. *Infect. Immun.* **2006**, *74*, 6750–6760. [CrossRef] [PubMed]

80. Alugupalli, K.R.; Akira, S.; Lien, E.; Leong, J.M. Myd88- and Bruton's tyrosine kinase-mediated signals are essential for T cell-independent pathogen-specific IgM responses. *J. Immunol.* **2007**, *178*, 3740–3749. [CrossRef] [PubMed]

81. Restrepo, B.I.; Barbour, A.G. Antigen diversity in the bacterium *B. hermsii* through "somatic" mutations in rearranged *vmp* genes. *Cell* **1994**, *78*, 867–876. [CrossRef]

82. Geigy, R.; Sarasin, G. Isolatstamme von *Borrelia duttonii* und immunisierungsverhalten gegenuber der weissen maus. *Acta Trop.* **1958**, *15*, 254–258. (In German) [PubMed]

83. Schuhardt, V.T.; Wilkerson, M. Relapse phenomena in rats infected with single spirochetes (*Borrelia recurrentis* var. turicatae). *J. Bacteriol.* **1951**, *62*, 215–219. [PubMed]

84. Cunningham, J.; Fraser, A.G.L. Further observations on Indian relapsing fever. III. Persistence of spirochaetes in the blood and organs of infected animals. *Indian J. Med. Res.* **1937**, *24*, 581–592.

85. Aslam, N.; Turner, C.M. The relationship of variable antigen expression and population growth rates in trypanosoma brucei. *Parasitol. Res.* **1992**, *78*, 661–664. [CrossRef] [PubMed]

86. Bryceson, A. Clinical pathology of the Jarisch-Herxheimer reaction. *J. Infect. Dis.* **1976**, *133*, 696–704. [CrossRef] [PubMed]

87. Negussie, Y.; Remick, D.G.; DeForge, L.E.; Kunkel, S.L.; Eynon, A.; Griffin, G.E. Detection of plasma tumor necrosis factor, interleukins 6, and 8 during the Jarisch-Herxheimer reaction of relapsing fever. *J. Exp. Med.* **1992**, *175*, 1207–1212. [CrossRef] [PubMed]

88. Galloway, R.E.; Levin, J.; Butler, T.; Naff, G.B.; Goldsmith, G.H.; Saito, H.; Awoke, S.; Wallace, C.K. Activation of protein mediators of inflammation and evidence for endotoxemia in *Borrelia recurrentis* infection. *Am. J. Med.* **1977**, *63*, 933–938. [CrossRef]

89. Takayama, K.; Rothenberg, R.J.; Barbour, A.G. Absence of lipopolysaccharide in the Lyme disease spirochete, *Borrelia burgdorferi*. *Infect. Immun.* **1987**, *55*, 2311–2313. [PubMed]

90. Young, E.J.; Weingarten, N.M.; Baughn, R.E.; Duncan, W.C. Studies on the pathogenesis of the Jarisch-Herxheimer reaction: Development of an animal model and evidence against a role for classical endotoxin. *J. Infect. Dis.* **1982**, *146*, 606–615. [CrossRef] [PubMed]

91.   Vidal, V.; Scragg, I.G.; Cutler, S.J.; Rockett, K.A.; Fekade, D.; Warrell, D.A.; Wright, D.J.; Kwiatkowski, D. Variable major lipoprotein is a principal TNF-inducing factor of louse-borne relapsing fever. *Nat. Med.* **1998**, *4*, 1416–1420. [CrossRef] [PubMed]

92.   Wooten, R.M.; Ma, Y.; Yoder, R.A.; Brown, J.P.; Weis, J.H.; Zachary, J.F.; Kirschning, C.J.; Weis, J.J. Toll-like receptor 2 is required for innate, but not acquired, host defense to *Borrelia burgdorferi*. *J. Immunol.* **2002**, *168*, 348–355. [CrossRef] [PubMed]

93.   Londoño, D.; Marques, A.; Hornung, R.L.; Cadavid, D. Relapsing fever borreliosis in IL-10 deficient mice. *Infect. Immun.* **2008**, *76*, 5508–5513. [CrossRef] [PubMed]

94.   Londoño, D.; Marques, A.; Hornung, R.L.; Cadavid, D. IL-10 helps control pathogen load during high-level bacteremia. *J. Immunol.* **2008**, *181*, 2076–2083. [CrossRef] [PubMed]

95.   Barbour, A.G.; Hirsch, C.M.; Ghalyanchi Langeroudi, A.; Meinardi, S.; Lewis, E.R.; Estabragh, A.S.; Blake, D.R. Elevated carbon monoxide in the exhaled breath of mice during a systemic bacterial infection. *PLoS ONE* **2013**, *8*, e69802. [CrossRef] [PubMed]

96.   Langeroudi, A.G.; Hirsch, C.M.; Estabragh, A.S.; Meinardi, S.; Blake, D.R.; Barbour, A.G. Elevated carbon monoxide to carbon dioxide ratio in the exhaled breath of mice treated with a single dose of lipopolysaccharide. *Open Forum Infect. Dis.* **2014**, *1*, ofu085. [CrossRef] [PubMed]

97.   Gelderblom, H.; Londono, D.; Bai, Y.; Cabral, E.S.; Quandt, J.; Hornung, R.; Martin, R.; Marques, A.; Cadavid, D. High production of CXCL13 in blood and brain during persistent infection with the relapsing fever spirochete *Borrelia turicatae*. *J. Neuropathol. Exp. Neurol.* **2007**, *66*, 208–217. [CrossRef] [PubMed]

98.   Gabritchewsky, G.N. Les bases de la sérothérapie de la fievre récurrente. *Ann. Inst. Pasteur* **1896**, *10*, 629–659. (In French)

99.   Barbour, A.G.; Bundoc, V. In vitro and in vivo neutralization of the relapsing fever agent *Borrelia hermsii* with serotype-specific immunoglobulin M antibodies. *Infect. Immun.* **2001**, *69*, 1009–1015. [CrossRef] [PubMed]

100. Newman, K., Jr.; Johnson, R.C. In vivo evidence that an intact lytic complement pathway is not essential for successful removal of circulating *Borrelia turicatae* from mouse blood. *Infect. Immun.* **1981**, *31*, 465–469. [PubMed]

101. Newman, K., Jr.; Johnson, R.C. T-cell-independent elimination of *Borrelia turicatae*. *Infect. Immun.* **1984**, *45*, 572–576. [PubMed]

102. Arimitsu, Y.; Akama, K. Characterization of protective antibodies produced in mice infected with *Borrelia duttonii*. *Jpn. J. Med. Sci. Biol.* **1973**, *26*, 229–237. [CrossRef]

103. Sadziene, A.; Jonsson, M.; Bergström, S.; Bright, R.K.; Kennedy, R.C.; Barbour, A.G. A bactericidal antibody to *Borrelia burgdorferi* is directed against a variable region of the OspB protein. *Infect. Immun.* **1994**, *62*, 2037–2045. [PubMed]

104. Connolly, S.E.; Benach, J.L. Cutting edge: The spirochetemia of murine relapsing fever is cleared by complement-independent bactericidal antibodies. *J. Immunol.* **2001**, *167*, 3029–3032. [CrossRef] [PubMed]

105. Luke, C.J.; Marshall, M.A.; Zahradnik, J.M.; Bybel, M.; Menefee, B.E.; Barbour, A.G. Growth-inhibiting antibody responses of humans vaccinated with recombinant outer surface protein a or infected with *Borrelia burgdorferi* or both. *J. Infect. Dis.* **2000**, *181*, 1062–1068. [CrossRef] [PubMed]

106. Sadziene, A.; Thompson, P.A.; Barbour, A.G. A flagella-less mutant of *Borrelia burgdorferi* as a live attenuated vaccine in the murine model of Lyme disease. *J. Infect. Dis.* **1996**, *173*, 1184–1193. [CrossRef] [PubMed]

107. Brown, G.V.; Anders, R.F.; Knowles, G. Differential effect of immunoglobulin on the in vitro growth of several isolates of *Plasmodium falciparum*. *Infect. Immun.* **1983**, *39*, 1228–1235. [PubMed]

108. Barbour, A.G.; Tessier, S.L.; Todd, W.J. Lyme disease spirochetes and ixodid tick spirochetes share a common surface antigenic determinant defined by a monoclonal antibody. *Infect. Immun.* **1983**, *41*, 795–804. [PubMed]

109. Chung, H.; Chang, F. Relapsing fever; clinical and statistical study of 337 cases. *Chin. Med. J.* **1939**, *55*, 6–33.

110. Burman, N.; Shamaei-Tousi, A.; Bergström, S. The spirochete *Borrelia crocidurae* causes erythrocyte rosetting during relapsing fever. *Infect. Immun.* **1998**, *66*, 815–819. [PubMed]

111. Meleney, H.E. Relapse phenomena of *Spironema recurrentis*. *J. Exp. Med.* **1928**, *48*, 65–82. [CrossRef] [PubMed]

112. Baltzard, M. Identification des spirochètes récurrents. Individualité de l'espèce *Spirochaeta recurrentis*. *Bull. Soc. Pathol. Exot.* **1947**, *40*, 77–81. (In French)

113. Alugupalli, K.R.; Gerstein, R.M.; Chen, J.; Szomolanyi-Tsuda, E.; Woodland, R.T.; Leong, J.M. The resolution of relapsing fever borreliosis requires IgM and is concurrent with expansion of B1b lymphocytes. *J. Immunol.* **2003**, *170*, 3819–3827. [CrossRef] [PubMed]

114. Magez, S.; Schwegmann, A.; Atkinson, R.; Claes, F.; Drennan, M.; de Baetselier, P.; Brombacher, F. The role of B-cells and IgM antibodies in parasitemia, anemia, and VSG switching in *Trypanosoma brucei*-infected mice. *PLoS Pathog.* **2008**, *4*, e1000122. [CrossRef] [PubMed]

115. Amole, B.O.; Clarkson, A.B., Jr.; Shear, H.L. Pathogenesis of anemia in *Trypanosoma brucei*-infected mice. *Infect. Immun.* **1982**, *36*, 1060–1068. [PubMed]

116. Naessens, J.; Kitani, H.; Nakamura, Y.; Yagi, Y.; Sekikawa, K.; Iraqi, F. TNF-alpha mediates the development of anaemia in a murine *Trypanosoma brucei* rhodesiense infection, but not the anaemia associated with a murine *Trypanosoma congolense* infection. *Clin. Exp. Immunol.* **2005**, *139*, 405–410. [CrossRef] [PubMed]

117. Cnops, J.; de Trez, C.; Stijlemans, B.; Keirsse, J.; Kauffmann, F.; Barkhuizen, M.; Keeton, R.; Boon, L.; Brombacher, F.; Magez, S. NK-, NKT- and CD8-derived IFNgamma drives myeloid cell activation and erythrophagocytosis, resulting in trypanosomosis-associated acute anemia. *PLoS Pathog.* **2015**, *11*, e1004964. [CrossRef] [PubMed]

118. Cook, A.R. Relapsing fever in Uganda. *J. Trop. Med.* **1904**, *7*, 24–26.

119. Shamaei-Tousi, A.; Martin, P.; Bergh, A.; Burman, N.; Brannstrom, T.; Bergström, S. Erythrocyte-aggregating relapsing fever spirochete *Borrelia crocidurae* induces formation of microemboli. *J. Infect. Dis.* **1999**, *180*, 1929–1938. [CrossRef]

120. Guyard, C.; Chester, E.M.; Raffel, S.J.; Schrumpf, M.E.; Policastro, P.F.; Porcella, S.F.; Leong, J.M.; Schwan, T.G. Relapsing fever spirochetes contain chromosomal genes with unique direct tandemly repeated sequences. *Infect. Immun.* **2005**, *73*, 3025–3037. [CrossRef] [PubMed]

121. Brust, M.; Aouane, O.; Thiebaud, M.; Flormann, D.; Verdier, C.; Kaestner, L.; Laschke, M.W.; Selmi, H.; Benyoussef, A.; Podgorski, T.; et al. The plasma protein fibrinogen stabilizes clusters of red blood cells in microcapillary flows. *Sci. Rep.* **2014**, *4*, 4348. [CrossRef] [PubMed]

122. Barbour, A.G.; Todd, W.J.; Stoenner, H.G. Action of penicillin on borrelia hermsii. *Antimicrob. Agents Chemother.* **1982**, *21*, 823–829. [CrossRef] [PubMed]

123. Barthold, S.W.; Beck, D.S.; Hansen, G.M.; Terwilliger, G.A.; Moody, K.D. Lyme borreliosis in selected strains and ages of laboratory mice. *J. Infect. Dis.* **1990**, *162*, 133–138. [CrossRef] [PubMed]

124. Barthold, S.W. Infectivity of *Borrelia burgdorferi* relative to route of inoculation and genotype in laboratory mice. *J. Infect. Dis.* **1991**, *163*, 419–420. [CrossRef] [PubMed]

125. Weis, J.J.; McCracken, B.A.; Ma, Y.; Fairbairn, D.; Roper, R.J.; Morrison, T.B.; Weis, J.H.; Zachary, J.F.; Doerge, R.W.; Teuscher, C. Identification of quantitative trait loci governing arthritis severity and humoral responses in the murine model of Lyme disease. *J. Immunol.* **1999**, *162*, 948–956.

126. Lopez, J.E.; McCoy, B.N.; Krajacich, B.J.; Schwan, T.G. Acquisition and subsequent transmission of *Borrelia hermsii* by the soft tick *Ornithodoros hermsi*. *J. Med. Entomol.* **2011**, *48*, 891–895. [CrossRef] [PubMed]

127. Lopez, J.E.; Wilder, H.K.; Hargrove, R.; Brooks, C.P.; Peterson, K.E.; Beare, P.A.; Sturdevant, D.E.; Nagarajan, V.; Raffel, S.J.; Schwan, T.G. Development of genetic system to inactivate a *Borrelia turicatae* surface protein selectively produced within the salivary glands of the arthropod vector. *PLoS Negl. Trop. Dis.* **2013**, *7*, e2514. [CrossRef] [PubMed]

128. Policastro, P.F.; Raffel, S.J.; Schwan, T.G. Cotransmission of divergent relapsing fever spirochetes by artificially infected *Ornithodoros hermsi*. *Appl. Environ. Microbiol.* **2011**, *77*, 8494–8499. [CrossRef] [PubMed]

129. Aylor, D.L.; Valdar, W.; Foulds-Mathes, W.; Buus, R.J.; Verdugo, R.A.; Baric, R.S.; Ferris, M.T.; Frelinger, J.A.; Heise, M.; Frieman, M.B.; et al. Genetic analysis of complex traits in the emerging Collaborative Cross. *Genome Res.* **2011**, *21*, 1213–1222. [CrossRef] [PubMed]

130. Shusterman, A.; Salyma, Y.; Nashef, A.; Soller, M.; Wilensky, A.; Mott, R.; Weiss, E.I.; Houri-Haddad, Y.; Iraqi, F.A. Genotype is an important determinant factor of host susceptibility to periodontitis in the Collaborative Cross and inbred mouse populations. *BMC Genet.* **2013**, *14*. [CrossRef] [PubMed]

11

Establishment and Characterization of New Canine and Feline Osteosarcoma Primary Cell Lines

Florian R. L. Meyer and Ingrid Walter *

Department of Pathobiology, Institute of Anatomy, Histology and Embryology,
University of Veterinary Medicine, Veterinaerplatz 1, Vienna 1210, Austria; florian.r.l.meyer@gmail.com
* Correspondence: Ingrid.Walter@vetmeduni.ac.at

Academic Editors: Duncan C. Ferguson and Margarethe Hoenig

Abstract: Osteosarcomas are the most abundant form of bone malignancies in multiple species. Canine osteosarcomas are considered a valuable model for human osteosarcomas because of their similar features. Feline osteosarcomas, on the other hand, are rarely studied but have interesting characteristics, such as a better survival prognosis than dogs or humans, and less likelihood of metastasis. To enable experimental approaches to study these differences we have established five new canine osteosarcoma cell lines out of three tumors, COS_1186h, COS_1186w, COS_1189, and COS_1220, one osteosarcoma-derived lung metastasis, COS_1033, and two new feline osteosarcoma cell lines, FOS_1077 and FOS_1140. Their osteogenic and neoplastic origin, as well as their potential to produce calcified structures, was determined by the markers osteocalcin, osteonectin, tissue unspecific alkaline phosphatase, p53, cytokeratin, vimentin, and alizarin red. The newly developed cell lines retained most of their markers *in vitro* but only spontaneously formed spheroids produced by COS_1189 showed calcification *in vitro*.

Keywords: osteosarcoma; cell culture; dog; cat

1. Introduction

Tumors are one of the major diseases in both human and companion animals with an annual incidence rate of about 182/100,000 in humans [1] 381/100,000 in dogs and 156/100,000 of cats [2]. When comparing numerical data between human and veterinary patients it has to be considered that a number of unrecorded cases are present in animal patients, in particular in the feline species. It is, therefore, of major clinical importance to investigate issues such as tumor progression and metastasis behavior, the main reason for tumor related death, and to test tumor cells for drug response. For ethical reasons, *in vitro* methods are preferable whenever possible over experiments on living animals. A suitable method for experimental approaches, especially drug tests in cancer research, is the use of cell cultures. Due to of the natural immortality of tumor cells, they retain their *in vivo* features better than normal cells which have to be artificially immortalized to be used for longer periods of time [3–5].

Osteosarcoma is the most common neoplasm of the bone in human patients, cats, and dogs, and it is generally assumed that it derives from osteoblastic cells, but now pluripotent stem cells have also been under discussion as a source of neoplastic cells [6–8]. Due to the many similarities between human and canine osteosarcomas, the latter is considered a valuable model organism for this disease [9,10]. These similarities include the sites most often affected, a predominance of male sex, and the high likelihood of metastasis development, preferably to the lung [10]. Due to the generally late diagnosis of the disease, micrometastases are often already present at the time of diagnosis [11]. However, there are also noteworthy differences between osteosarcomas of the two species, like the age of onset; generally, adolescence in humans—although there is a notable second peak in patients >60 years [12]—and middle-aged to older dogs are affected [13]. It also seems that human osteosarcoma is caused by growth during adolescence [14,15], while the older age of onset in canines has been supposed to be induced by mechanical forces, such as (micro-) fractures [16].

A number of cell lines have successfully been cultivated and characterized from human [11,16–19] and canine [20,21] osteosarcomas. While a large number of human osteosarcoma cell lines are commercially available, like HOS [22], U2 OS [23], Saos-2 [24], or MG-63 [25], only the canine osteosarcoma cell line D-17 (CCL-183) [26] is accessible for scientists. Feline osteosarcomas, on the other hand, were rarely studied, and to our knowledge this work presents the first establishment and description of a feline osteosarcoma cell line. Despite this, we believe feline osteosarcoma to be a valuable model in understanding osteosarcoma tumor mechanisms. While feline osteosarcomas have a strong histological similarity to human and canine osteosarcomas [27], their behavior in tumor progression, especially the much lower rate of metastases [28], stands opposed to their human and canine counterparts.

The aim of the present study was the isolation and cultivation of primary cells from different types of canine and feline osteosarcomas. The cell cultures were tested for bone tumor markers as determined before, such as tissue unspecific alkaline phosphatase [29,30], osteocalcin [31], and osteonectin [19,20,32,33]. The deposition of calcified structures was assessed by alizarin red staining [34]. Cultivated osteosarcoma cells were further characterized immunohistochemically for vimentin [20,32,33] and cytokeratin intermediate filaments [32] and the tumor-suppressor p53 [33]. All of the above-mentioned factors were comparatively stained on formalin-fixed paraffin-embedded (FFPE) sections of the corresponding tumor tissue. Furthermore, the origin of cells from the respective tumor was verified by DNA fingerprinting.

2. Experimental Section

2.1. Animals

Osteosarcoma tumor samples from dogs ($n = 4$) and cats ($n = 2$) were collected after therapeutic limb amputation or euthanasia. The study was approved by the Ethical and Animal Welfare Committee of the University of Veterinary Medicine (15 December 2014) and conducted according to the guidelines of the local ethical committee. Animal data and tumor subtypes are reported in Table 1. Tumor tissues were transferred under sterile conditions to the VetBiobank of the VetCore Facility for Research of the University of Veterinary Medicine, Vienna. Tumors were dissected and aliquots of tumor tissue were formaldehyde-fixed and paraffin-embedded or shock frozen in liquid nitrogen with and without RNAlater (Life Technologies, Vienna, Austria) for RNA and DNA analysis. Before embedding in paraffin, strongly calcified samples were decalcified in 8% EDTA before the embedding process. Further parts of the tumors were used for cell culture experiments.

Table 1. Animals used for the creation of the new cell lines.

Sample	Resulting Cell Line	Species	Sex [a]	Age	Breed	OS Subtype	Location
1033	COS_1033	Dog	F	7y 1m	Boxer	Teleangiectatic OS with giant cell participation	Lung metastasis
1077	FOS_1077	Cat	F	10y	Domestic shorthair	FibroblasticOS	Costa
1140	FOS_1140	Cat	M °	n/s	Domestic shorthair	Osteoblastic OS	Tibia
1186	COS_1186w COS_1186h	Dog	M °	11y 2m	Dachshund	Osteoblastic OS	Scapula
1189	COS_1189	Dog	M °	7y 3m	Mixed breed	Poorly defined OS/ signs of osteo-or synovialsarkom	Humerus
1220	COS_1220	Dog	F °	5y 3m	Boxer	Fibroblastic OS	Radius

[a] F = female, M = male, ° = neutered; n/s = not specified.

2.2. Cell Culture

Pieces of fresh tumor tissue were cut into cubes of about 1 mm^3. The pieces were washed three times in DPBS (Sigma Aldrich, Vienna, Austria) to remove erythrocytes and then transferred to individual wells of a four-well plate (Thermo Fischer Scientific Vienna, Austria) with either DMEM (Sigma Aldrich) or Q286 medium (GE-Healthcare, Munich, Germany), supplemented with 10% fetal calf serum (FCS, Sigma-Aldrich), 625 pg/100 mL Amphotericin B (Bio and Sell, Feucht, Germany), 2 nm L-glutamine (Biochrom, Berlin, Germany), and 1% Pen/Strep/Fungi Mix (10,000 U Penicilin; 10 mg Streptomycin; 25 μg Amphotericin B/mL, Bio and Sell), or the complete osteoblast growth medium (OGM BulletKit; Szabo Scandic, Vienna, Austria). Cells were incubated at 37 °C and 5% CO$_2$. The first medium change was done after 24 h; after that, medium was changed in two day intervals. When cells started to grow out from the tissue pieces and attached to the plastic surface of the cell culture dish, the tissue pieces were detached mechanically from the plastic surface with a pipette tip to generate new spawning points within the well. At near-confluency, cells were trypsinized (Trypsin/EDTA solution, Merck, Darmstadt, Germany) and transferred to six-well plates (Sarstedt, Nümbrecht, Germany). After reaching near-confluency in the six-well plate, cells were transferred to 25 cm^2 cell culture flasks (Sarstedt) and expanded in 25 cm^2 and 75 cm^2 cell culture flasks (Sarstedt). Cells were frozen as soon as two 25-cm^2 cell culture flasks reached 80% confluency each, by resuspending trypsinized cells in a 1.5 M DMSO supplemented medium and using a CoolCell (Biozym, Vienna, Austria) to bring samples to -80 °C at a controlled cooling rate before storing them in liquid nitrogen.

For histological purposes, cells were scraped off a 25 cm^2 flask, at about 80% confluency and fixed in 4% buffered formaldehyde overnight. The cells were then pelleted by centrifugation (5000 g for 2 min) and the cell pellets pre-embedded in Histogel™ (Thermo Fischer Scientific, Vienna, Austria) and, subsequently, paraffin embedded.

2.3. Histology

FFPE samples from original tumor tissue and pellets of cell cultures were used for histological analysis. Sections measuring 3 μm were mounted on glutaraldehyde-activated 3-aminopropyl-triethoxysilane (APES)-coated glass slides.

2.4. Immunohistochemistry

A summary of the techniques and antibodies used in immunohistochemistry can be found in Table 2. For tissue unspecific alkaline phosphatase endogenous peroxidases were blocked using 0.6% H$_2$O$_2$ in 80% methanol. Epitope retrieval for tissue and cell pellets was done by steaming or microwaving as indicated in Table 2. 1.5% normal goat serum (Dako) was used for protein blocking. Sections/coverslip cultures were incubated with the respective primary antibody over night at 4 °C. For osteonectin, osteocalcin, vimentin, and cytokeratin, Alexa Fluor 488 goat-anti-mouse IgG (H + L) highly cross-adsorbed (Life Technologies; dilution 1:100 in PBS) was used as the secondary antibody. DAPI (Sigma Aldrich) was used for nuclear staining. The BrightVision Poly-HRP-anti-rabbit (ImmunoLogic, Duiven, Netherlands) was used as the secondary antibody for alkaline phosphatase and p53 staining, and slides were counterstained with haematoxylin. Sections prepared without primary antibody served as negative controls. For tissue unspecific alkaline phosphatase, osteocalcin canine phalanx and joint sections and feline femur sections were used as controls. Canine uterus was used as a control for vimentin and cytokeratin.

To determine a potential calcification of cultured osteosarcoma cells, slides of cell culture pellets and tumor were stained for 1 h in alizarin red (Morphisto, Frankfurt, Germany) pH 9.0 and 5 min alizarin red pH 7.0 (Morphisto).

Table 2. Details of procedures used for IHC staining.

Primary Antibody	Clone	Dilution	Antigen Retrieval		Source
Osteopontin	polyclonal	1:75	Tissue	30 min steamed in citric acid buffer pH 6.0	Biogenesis, Poole, UK
	rabbit		Cell pellet	2x 5 min microwaved in citric acid buffer pH 6.0	
Osteocalcin	polyclonal	1:400	Tissue	30 min steamed in citric acid buffer pH 6.0	Biogenesis
	rabbit		Cell pellet	2x 5 min microwaved in citric acid buffer pH 6.0	
Cytokeratin	monoclonal	1:250	Tissue	30 min steamed in Tris-EDTA buffer pH 9.0	Cell Marque, Rocklin, CA, USA
	mouse		Cell pellet	2x 5 min microwaved in Tris-EDTA buffer pH 9.0	
Vimentin	monoclonal	1:200	Tissue	20 min steamed in citric acid buffer pH 6.0	Dako, Glostrup, Denmark
	mouse		Cell pellet	2x 5 min microwaved in citric acid buffer pH 6.0	
Alkaline Phosphatase	polyclonal	Dog: 1:100	Tissue	30 min steamed in citric acid buffer pH 6.0	Genetex, Irvine, CA, USA
	rabbit	Cat: 1:250	Cell pellet	2x 5 min microwaved in citric acid buffer pH 6.0	
Osteonectin	polyclonal	1:1500	Tissue	none	Millipore, Billerica, MA, USA
	rabbit		Cell pellet	none	
p53	monoclonal	1:90	Tissue	3x 5 min microwaved in Tris-EDTA buffer pH 9.0	Enzo Life Sciences, Lausen, Switzerland
	mouse		Cell pellet	2x 5 min microwaved in Tris-EDTA buffer pH 9.0	

2.5. PCR

To verify the presence of ostecalcin (*BGLAP*), osteonectin (*SPARC*), and tissue unspecific alkaline phosphatase (*ALPL*), an mRNA amplicon dissociation assay was used. RNA was isolated from cells and corresponding tumours using the miRNeasy Mini kit (Qiagen, Hilden, Germany) and the RNeasy Fibrous Tissue Mini kit (Qiagen) according to the manufacturer's protocol, respectively. The amount of 500 ng RNA was transcribed into cDNA using the High-Capacity cDNA Reverse Transcription Kit (Applied Biosystems, Foster City, CA, USA). The reaction volume of 20 μl contained 2 μL 10 × RT Buffer, 0.8 μL 25 × dNTP Mix (100 mM of each dNTP), 2 μL 10 × RT random primers, 50 U multiscribe reverse transcriptase and 14.2 μL of RNase-free H_2O containing the 500 ng of RNA. The reaction was incubated for 10 min at 25 °C to initiate primer binding and was followed by 2 h at 37 °C for transcription. The reaction was stopped by heating to 85 °C for 5 s.

For PCR 5 ng of cDNA was mixed with 1 μL buffer BD (Solis Biodyne, Tartu, Estonia) 3.5 mM $MgCl_2$, 0.2 mM of each dNTP (Solis Biodyne) 0.4 × EvaGreen (Biotium, Hayward, CA, USA), 200 nM of each primer (Sigma-Aldrich) 0.5 unit hot-start Taq DNA polymerase (HOT FIREPol® DNA polymerase; Solis Biodyne) in a 10 μL reaction volume. Cycling conditions consisted of a hot start at 95 °C for 15 min followed by 40 cycles of denaturation for 15 s at 95 °C, annealing for 20 s at 60 °C and elongation for 20 s at 72 °C. For analysis a melting curve analysis was performed after the PCR, were the reaction mixture was heated from 60 °C to 95 °C at a ramp rate of 0.03 °C/s acquiring 20 data points per °C (primer sequences are given in Table 3).

Table 3. PCR-primer and assay details.

Gene / Symbol	Species	NCBI Ref Nr (Dog/Cat)	Foward Primer	Reverse Primer	Length (bp)
Osteocalcin /	Dog	XM_547536.4	GCTGGTCCAGCAGATGCAA	CCCAGCCCAGAGTCCAGGTA	125
BGLAP	Cat	XM_003999711.3	GCCCGGCAGATGCAAAG	CCCTCCTGCTTGGACACGA	70
Osteopontin/	Dog	XM_003434023.2	ACTGACATTCCAGCAACCCAA	CACAAGTGATGTGAAGTCCTCCTCT	168
SPP1	Cat	XM_006930977.2	CAATTTTTCACCCCAGCTGTC	CACAAGTGATGTGAAGTCCTCCTCT	150
Osteonectin /	Dog	XM_005619272.1	CACCCTGGAAGGCACCAA	CGCAGAGGGAATTCAGTCAGC	108
SPARC	Cat	XM_003981374.3	CCAAGAAGGGCCACAAACTC	GGAATTCGGTCAGCTCGGA	87
Alkaline phosphatase /	Dog	XM_005617214.1	GGCCTGAACCTCATCGACAT	GCGGTTCCAGACGTAGTGAGA	72
ALPL	Cat	NM_001042563.1	GGACGGCCTGAACCTCG	GAGTTCGGT GCGGTTCCA	85

All reactions were performed as technical duplicates with the inclusion of combined RT-controls and negative controls also performed in duplicate on a Light Cycler 480 (Roche Diagnostics, Vienna, Austria).

2.6. DNA-Fingerprint Assay

DNA of original fresh frozen tumor aliquots and primary cell cultures (passages used were: COS_1033: P5, FOS_1077: P12, COS_1140: P15, COS_1186h: P4, COS_1186w: P7, COS_1189: P23, COS_1220: P6) were isolated using the Nucleo Spin Tissue Kit (Macherey-Nagel, Düren, Germany). In brief, ~20 ng of tissue or a pellet of 10^5 to 10^6 cells was used as starting material. Tumor tissue samples were homogenized in T1 buffer (Macherey-Nagel) using zirconium beads (PEQLAB Biotechnologie, Erlangen, Germany) in the MagNA Lyser (Roche Diagnostics) for 2 times 20 s at 6500 rpm and were cooled on ice in between. Cultured tumour cells were homogenized by vortexing vigorously in T1 buffer (Macherey-Nagel). Homogenates were than lysed with proteinase K (Macherey-Nagel) for 15 min and DNA isolated as described in the manufacturers protocol.

DNA was sent to Laboklin (Bad Kissingen, Germany) for DNA fingerprinting determining 18/16 marker regions for dogs or cats, respectively [35].

3. Results

The canine osteosarcoma cells COS_1033, COS_1189 and COS_1220 were successfully grown to the passages 8, 25, and 6, respectively. The canine tumor 1186 macroscopically showed a distinct separation in a hard, bone- or cartilage-like area and a soft tissue-like area. Separate tissue cultures were established from both tumor parts and labelled as COS_1186h for the hard part and COS_1186w for the soft part, respectively. COS_1186h was grown to passage 4 and COS_1186w was grown to passage 7. The feline osteosarcoma cell lines were grown up to passage 21 for FOS_1077 and 19 for FOS_1140. Cells did not change their growth characteristics or proliferation within the stated number of passages. Most canine cell lines, namely COS_1033, COS_1186w, COS_1189, and COS_1220, showed a fibroblast-like morphology when grown as monolayers on plastic cell culture dishes or glass surfaces irrespective from the tumor subtype (Figure 1). In contrast, the "sister cell line" of COS_1186w (obtained from the same tumor), COS_1186h, showed a cobblestone epithelial-like morphology (Figure 1). Feline osteosarcoma cell lines (FOS_1077 and FOS_1140) had a mixed morphology of fibroblast-like cells and osteoblast like cells (Figure 1).

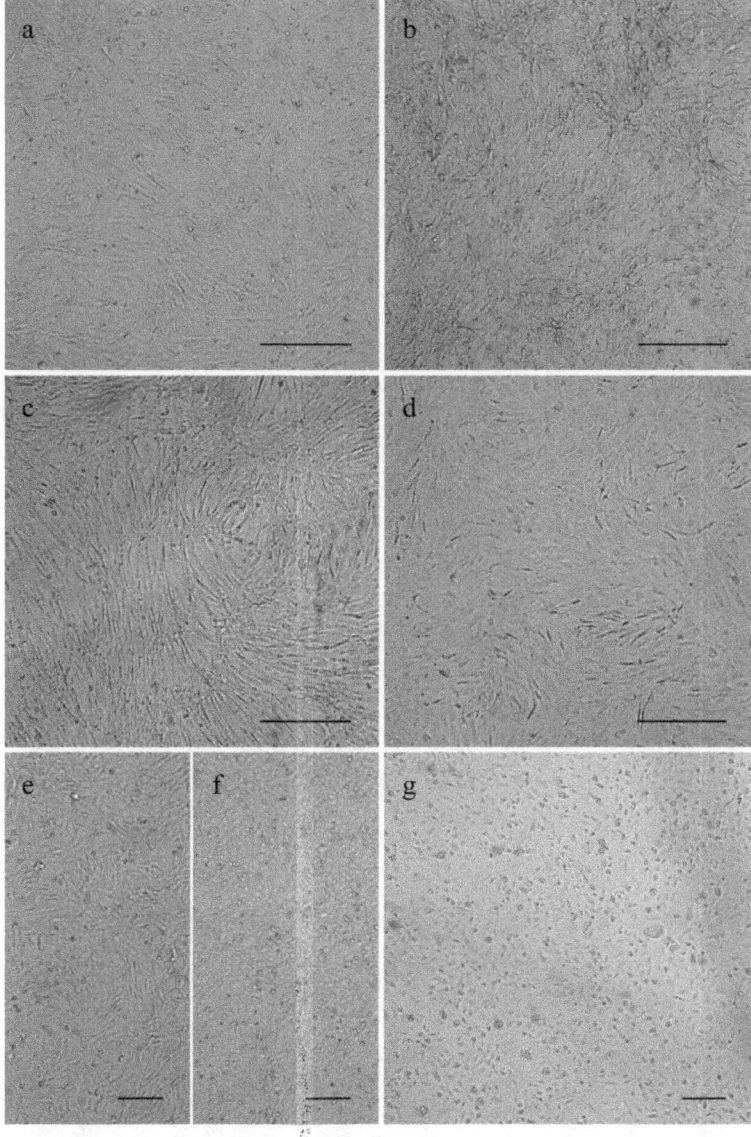

Figure 1. Phase contrast images showing growth morphology of (**a**) COS_1033 at P4; (**b**) COS_1189 at P7; (**c**) COS_1220 at P4; (**d**) FOS_1140 at P4; (**e**) COS_1186w at P3; (**f**) COS_1186h at P4; and (**g**) FOS_1077 at P4. Scale bars represent 100 μm for (**a**–**d**) and 200 μm for (**e**–**g**).

COS_1189 showed a weak attachment to plastic surfaces and once a continuous layer of cells was formed (~70%–80% confluency), even light agitation of the cell culture dish led to the detachment of sheets of cells which formed spheroids spontaneously.

Calcification of the tumors and tumor cell cultures was determined by alizarin red staining. Feline tumor 1077 and canine tumor 1186 showed large areas of calcification; in the latter both in the macroscopically hard and soft areas. The three other canine osteosarcomas showed only few calcified spots and no signs of calcification were found in feline osteosarcoma 1140. It has to be noted that the amount of calcification was observed to be very heterogeneous within the tumors. All canine and feline cell cultures were alizarin red negative after two (COS_1033), three (COS_1186w and COS_1220), four (COS_1186h), five (FOS_1077), seven (FOS_1140), or 11 (COS_1189) days of culture. The spontaneously-developing spheroids, as observed in COS_1189 cultures, showed strong calcification after three days in culture, as demonstrated by alizarin red staining (Figure 2), but the center of the spheroids also showed signs of necrosis.

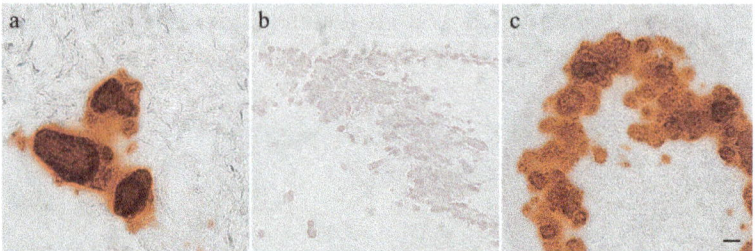

Figure 2. Alizarin red staining of (**a**) a tumor section of 1189; (**b**) a monolayer cell culture sample of COS_1189; and (**c**) a spheroid of COS_1189. Scale bar represents 20 μm.

3.1. Immunohistochemistry

The intermediate filament cytoskeleton of the cultivated cells, irrespective of their morphology, was composed of vimentin as expected for mesenchymal cells and as also seen in the corresponding histological tumor sections (Figure 3). Cytokeratin positive tumor cells were never observed, neither in the original tumors nor in the cultivated tumor cells (Figure 3). Immunohistochemistry demonstrated osteonectin and osteocalcin in every examined tumor, albeit in different intensity levels (Figure 4). Osteonectin was less abundant in cat tumors compared to their canine counterparts. The expression of these proteins was also detectable in the respective corresponding cell cultures of feline and canine osteosarcomas (Figure 4). All feline and canine osteosarcomas were positive for tissue unspecific alkaline phosphatase. This marker remained unchanged in the corresponding primary cell cultures with the exception of one canine cell line (COS_1220) where the original tumor was positive, but no expression was observed in the cell culture. The distribution of the signal was cytoplasmic, membrane bound or nuclear (Figure 4). p53 showed no staining in cats, whether the tumor itself or the corresponding cell culture, but was present in nuclei of all canine cell lines (Figure 5). It has to be noted that the tumor 1189 showed only very few stained cells, while the resulting cell line COS_1189 was clearly positive.

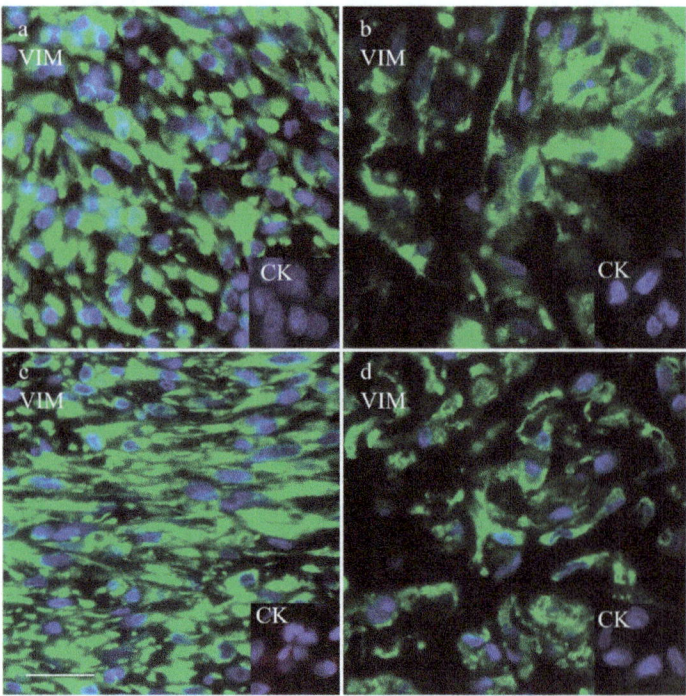

Figure 3. Immunofluorescence staining with anti-vimentin and anti-cytokeratin (inserts) of the canine tumor 1033 (**a**) and the resulting cell culture (**b**) as well as the feline tumor 1077 (**c**) and its resulting cell culture (**d**). Scale bar represents 25 μm.

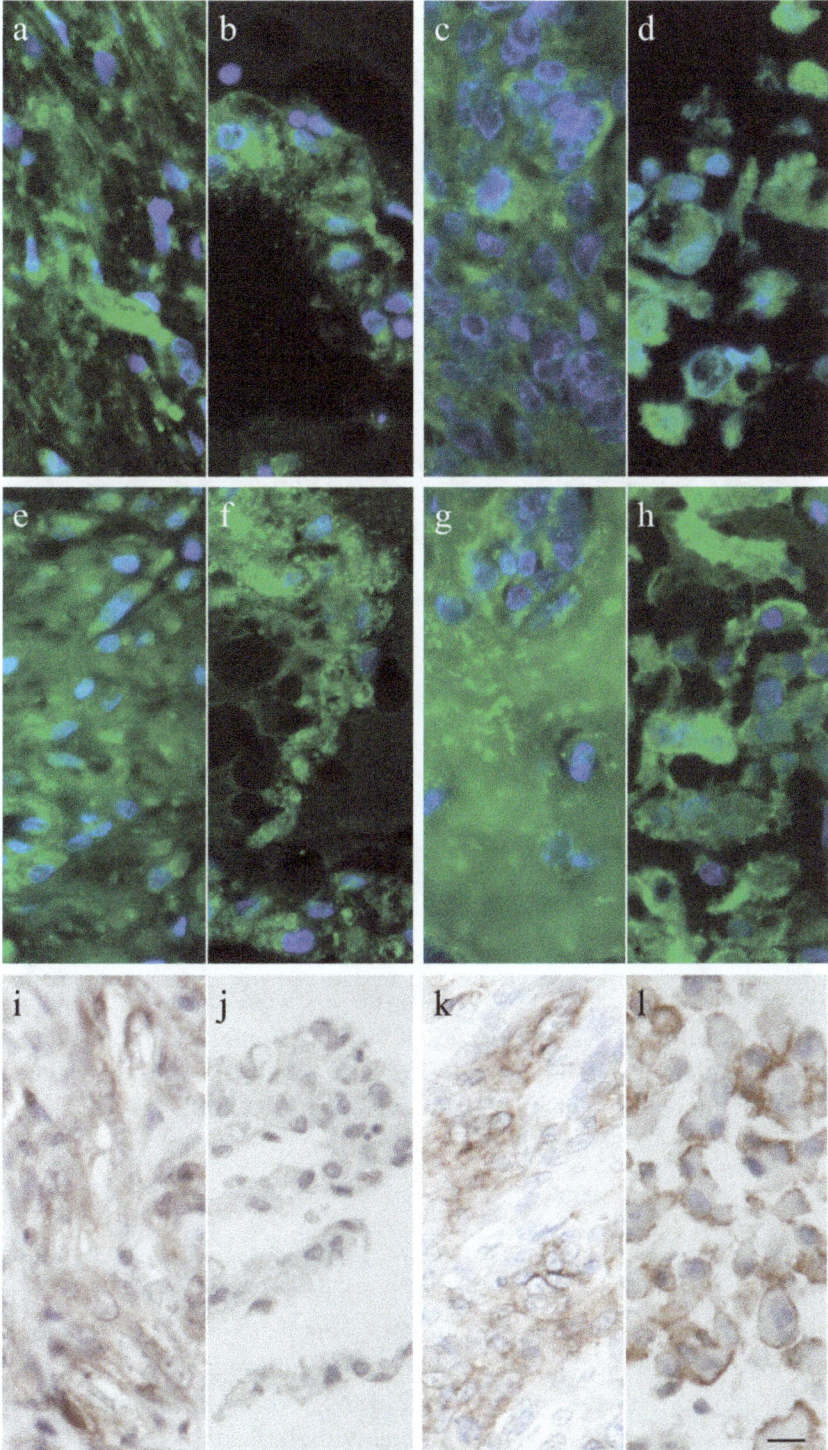

Figure 4. Immunhistochemistry and immunofluorescence of canine tumor 1220 (**a,e,i**) and its cell line (**b,f,j**), and the feline tumor 1077 (**c,g,k**) and its cell line (**d,h,l**) showing osteonectin (**a–d**), osteocalcin (**e–h**), and tissue unspecific alkaline phosphatase (**i–l**). Scale bar represents 10 μm.

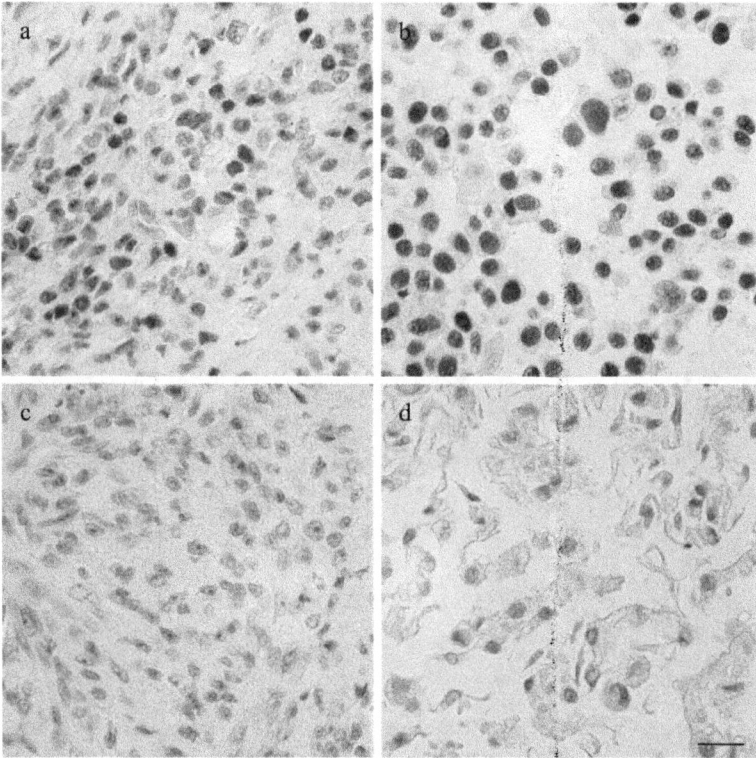

Figure 5. Imunhistological staining of p53 in the canine tumor 1189 (**a**) and feline osteosarcoma 1140 (**c**), and the cell lines COS_1189h (**b**) and FOS_1140 (**d**) derived from these tumors. Scale bar represents 20 μm.

3.2. PCR

By means of PCR, the presence of mRNA of tissue unspecific alkaline phosphatase (*ALPL*) and osteonectin (*SPARC*) was detected positively in all tested feline and canine tissue and cell culture samples, except for the cell culture samples of COS_1220 which lost ALPL expression, mirroring the results obtained by immunohistochemistry. However, we failed to amplify osteocalcin (*BGLAP*) mRNA in feline and canine samples (A list of the results is supplied in Supplementary Table S1).

3.3. DNA Fingerprint Assay

Microsatellite analysis of the established primary cell lines confirmed their origin from the corresponding tumor. In feline samples 16 markers were tested. All markers were identical between tumor tissue and cells in culture. In dogs, 18 markers were tested. COS_1033 and COS_1186h cells and tumor were completely identical in their marker setup, although one marker failed to amplify in the latter, both in tumor and in the cell line. COS_1220 showed one allele changed in a single marker, COS_1189 had alterations in two alleles. Three markers differed between COS_1186w and the tumor, although one marker failed to amplify in the tumor sample, but not in the cell line. A complete list of the obtained microsatellite data as first published in [35] is supplied in Supplementary Tables S2 and S3. These lists can be helpful in future experiments to exclude cross contaminations.

4. Discussion

Osteosarcomas are the most common bone neoplasms in humans [12], dogs [36], and cats [37]. Osteosarcomas in dogs are considered a valuable model for human osteosarcomas, because of the similar behavior of these two diseases concerning tumor progression and metastasis development in the lung [9,10,38]. In contrast, little research has been done on feline osteosarcomas, but current data points to a much less severe progress with less likelihood of metastasis in this species, although the histological properties of the primary tumor are very similar to its human and canine counterpart [26,27]. Osteosarcoma cell lines have been applied in many fields of research such as drug development [39,40], drug resistance development [41], and basic tumor research [42,43]. Mostly, these studies have been focused on human osteosarcoma cell lines [39,41–44], but also osteosarcomas of rat [45], mouse [46], and dog [40,43,46] were used for investigations. The use of canine and feline osteosarcoma cell cultures would be of particular interest allowing scientists to investigate the biological differences of these two species as reflected by the diverse metastatic behavior of these otherwise very similar tumors. Today, no feline osteosarcoma cell line is available or described in the literature to investigate their specificities and to use them in experimental applications.

We, therefore, developed five canine, and two feline, primary cell lines out of three canine osteosarcomas, one canine osteosarcoma-derived lung metastasis, and two feline osteosarcomas. Tumor cells attached to the plastic surface in a standard cell culture environment and were readily grown in provided media supplemented with fetal calf serum. Initially, two standard media (DMEM and Q286) and a medium specialized for the rearing of osteoblast cells (OGM), were chosen to initiate cell culture, however no preference to a single medium by a certain cell line was apparent. The applied method of establishment of the primary cell lines was robust and repeatable. There are two different main approaches for bringing osteosarcoma cells into culture, either by digesting the tumor matrix by collagenases [20,21] or by directly bringing minced pieces of osteosarcoma into cell culture [22,32]. While the digesting approach leads to a higher number of cells more quickly, and might be beneficial if cells need a high density for survival, it might damage the cells [47]. We have chosen the mincing approach because we are convinced that, preferably, tumor cells will grow out of the minced pieces, reducing contamination from non-tumor cells in the early passages.

Canine cell lines had a strong tendency to produce a fibroblast like morphology in cell cultures COS_1033, COS_1186w, COS_1189, and COS_1220, irrespective of the subtype. Only COS_1186h kept the osteoblastic morphology of the originally osteoblastic osteosarcoma in cell culture. Both feline cell lines showed a mixed phenotype of osteoblastic and fibroblastic cells. The differences in the morphology of the two sister cell lines COS_1186w and COS_1186h confirms the well-known inter-tumoral heterogeneity of the osteosarcoma [48,49]. Two tumor cell lines with basically the same genetic layout, but different morphological features, offers interesting prospects to further the understanding of tumor development, progression and drug response.

COS_1189 cells showed a strong tendency to adhere more strongly to each other than to the plastic surface of the dishes they were grown in. Depending on the confluency of cells and size of the dish, spheroids could be produced by simply shaking the dish. If done cautiously all cells tended to aggregate to one spheroid, but more likely two to four spheroids developed. Due to these large assembled spheroids, nutritional supply for cells in the middle was limited and these cells showed signs of degradation at the time of collection. In contrast to the cells grown as monolayers, cells within the spheroid deposited calcified osteoid-like areas, resembling the *in vivo* situation in osteosarcomas. We assume that a three-dimensional culture model would be preferable to better mimic the *in vivo* situation.

The established cell lines retained most of the characteristics of the tumors they derived from. We used the bone markers osteonectin [20,32,46], osteocalcin [31], and tissue unspecific alkaline phosphatase [29,30] at the protein and mRNA levels, confirming the origin of the cells that were obtained in cultures. These findings are in accordance with previously-established osteosarcoma cell lines that were positive for osteonectin, osteocalcin, and tissue unspecific alkaline phosphatase [30].

Alkaline phosphatase activities were found in other canine osteosarcoma cell lines [18,20,30] but also described as low [21]. Legare *et al.* [30] reported that most tested canine cell lines lost alkaline phosphatase immunoreactivity during culture time, however, only the very aggressive "Abrams" cell line consistently stained positive. In human osteosarcoma cells, tissue unspecific alkaline phosphatase activity was dependent on cell density [19], therefore, this condition has to be considered when comparing data about alkaline phosphatase. No data about alkaline phosphatase in feline osteosarcoma tumors or cell lines exist until now. Although higher serum levels of alkaline phosphatase have been correlated with shorter survival time [38], our results do not support tissue unspecific alkaline phosphatase as a distinguishing marker for the aggressive canine osteosarcoma from the low metastasizing feline osteosarcoma, as samples of both species were positive for tissue unspecific alkaline phosphatase, albeit the sampled tumor section of osteosarcoma 1189 showed only weak staining.

Osteocalcin, a small peptide hormone produced by osteoblasts, was used to verify the bony origin of our new cell lines. Immunhistochemistry was positive for osteocalcin in all tested samples, however, RT-PCR failed in all tested cases. Bioinformatically, osteocalcin is highly conserved and only one splice variant and one polycistronic mRNA containing BGLAP (PMF1-BGLAP) is known in the best-studied species, humans, and forms of these two transcripts are also predicted in cats and dogs. We are unsure why primers for this gene failed. Additionally, while all positive controls failed for this gene we do not consider it as evidence against the osteocalcin-antibody specificity.

Osteonectin is one of the most abundant proteins in the bone. It was present in all tested tumors and cell cultures, but its staining was notably weaker in feline tumors than it was canine osteosarcomas. Osteonectin is known to have tumor-progressing or -suppressing properties, depending on the surrounding cellular environment, and seems to be a negative prognostic marker in human osteosarcoma patients [50], indicating a valuable candidate gene that might influence the progression of osteosarcoma.

All established canine and feline cell cultures expressed vimentin irrespective of growth behavior but were negative for cytokeratin. This result is in contrast with the data from Nagamine et al. [51] who found canine osteosarcomas of various subtypes positive for cytokeratin and vimentin.

We tested calcification of tumor tissue and cell lines by alizarin red staining. All tumor samples showed calcified areas, except one feline tumor (1140), but no cell monolayer showed an alizarin positive staining. However, the spontaneous spheroids developed by COS_1189 showed alizarin red staining. While Mohseny et al. [33] showed that monolayers of HOS cells showed strong calcification, Martins-Neves et al. [34] showed only alizarin-positive spheroids, although both were grown in the media RPMI 1640. Prolonged sustaining the cells as a monolayer or differences in cell culture maintenances might influence calcification and explain these differences.

p53 is a transcription factor that is involved in cell cycle control [52] and it is known that disruption of p53 function strongly correlates with tumorigenesis [53]. In all our established canine cell lines p53 was present, as in their corresponding tumors. This is in accordance with the results of Bongiovanni et al. [54] who found p53 in canine appendicular osteosarcoma by means of immunohistochemistry. Moreover, p53 was correlated with the histological grade, as grade III tumors were 100% positive in canine osteosarcoma, and found to be a negative prognostic marker [54]. Interestingly, p53 was negative in both investigated feline tumors and the corresponding cell lines. It has been reported before that only about 50% of feline osteosarcomas express p53 [55] and that feline tumors tend to delete p53 [56]. Positivity might also be correlated to a certain subtype of osteosarcoma, however, tumor type was not stated in the report of Nasir et al. [55] and the number of cases investigated was low. Therefore, this hypothesis has to be verified on a statistically significant number of feline osteosarcomas. Further studies are needed to determine if p53 is involved in the characteristically lower tumor grades and enhanced survival of osteosarcoma affected cats.

The ability of tumor cell lines to produce tumors in immunodeficient laboratory animals is considered important for the characterization of neoplastic cell lines [18,20,21]. However, we consider the screened markers sufficient to confirm the origin of the newly produced cell lines as shown by other groups before [21,29,32]. However, comparative in vivo testing of the feline and canine osteosarcoma cell lines would, of course, add valuable data to their further experimental application. Therefore, their tumor formation capacity should be tested in future studies.

5. Conclusions

We have confirmed the osteosarcoma origin of the newly developed cell lines. They broaden the available species for *in vitro* osteosarcoma research to a species that is known to have a much better survival prognosis than humans or dogs. Species-specific differences, like the distinct expression of the oncogene p53, could be helpful to elucidate the biological reasons for the differences in feline and canine osteosarcoma progression. This research might also open interesting experimental tools to test potential therapeutic applications *in vitro*.

Acknowledgments: This study was funded by the Austrian Science Fund (FWF), grant number P 23336-B11. We would like to express our gratitude to Anne Fleming, Claudia Höchsmann, Hans Homola and Brigitte Machac for their technical support.

Author Contributions: Ingrid Walter conceived the study. Florian R.L. Meyer produced the cell lines. Florian R.L. Meyer and Ingrid Walter analyzed the samples, data, interpreted the results and wrote the manuscript.

References

1. World Cancer Research Fund International. Available online: https://www.wcrf.org/int/cancer-facts-figures/data-cancer-frequency-country (accessed on 31 May 2016).
2. Dorn, C.R.; Taylor, D.O.; Schneider, R.; Hibbard, H.H.; Klauber, M.R. Survey of animal neoplasms in Alameda and Contra Costa Counties, California. II. Cancer morbidity in dogs and cats from Alameda County. *J. Natl. Cancer Inst.* **1968**, *40*, 307–318. [PubMed]
3. Boerma, M.; Burton, G.R.; Wang, J.; Fink, L.M.; McGehee, R.E.; Hauer-Jensen, M. Comparative expression profiling in primary and immortalized endothelial cells: Changes in gene expression in response to hydroxy methylglutaryl-coenzyme A reductase inhibition. *Blood Coagul. Fibrinolysis* **2006**, *17*, 173–180. [CrossRef] [PubMed]
4. Lidington, E.; Moyes, D.; McCormack, A.; Rose, M. A comparison of primary endothelial cells and endothelial cell lines for studies of immune interactions. *Transpl. Immunol.* **1999**, *7*, 239–246. [CrossRef]
5. Rockwell, S. *In vivo-in vitro* tumour cell lines: Characteristics and limitations as models for human cancer. *Br. J. Cancer. Suppl.* **1980**, *4*, 118–122. [PubMed]
6. Wilson, H.; Huelsmeyer, M.; Chun, R.; Young, K.M.; Friedrichs, K.; Argyle, D.J. Isolation and characterisation of cancer stem cells from canine osteosarcoma. *Vet. J.* **2008**, *175*, 69–75. [CrossRef] [PubMed]
7. Levings, P.P.; McGarry, S.V.; Currie, T.P.; Nickerson, D.M.; McClellan, S.; Ghivizzani, S.C.; Steindler, D.A.; Gibbs, C.P. Expression of an exogenous human Oct-4 promoter identifies tumor-initiating cells in osteosarcoma. *Cancer Res.* **2009**, *69*, 5648–5655. [CrossRef] [PubMed]
8. Di Fiore, R.; Santulli, A.; Drago Ferrante, R.; Giuliano, M.; de Blasio, A.; Messina, C.; Pirozzi, G.; Tirino, V.; Tesoriere, G.; Vento, R. Identification and expansion of human osteosarcoma-cancer-stem cells by long-term 3-aminobenzamide treatment. *J. Cell. Physiol.* **2009**, *219*, 301–313. [CrossRef] [PubMed]
9. Vail, D.M.; Macewen, E.G. Spontaneously occurring tumors of companion animals as models for human cancer. *Cancer Investig.* **2000**, *18*, 781–792. [CrossRef]
10. Withrow, S.J.; Powers, B.E.; Straw, R.C.; Wilkins, R.M. Comparative aspects of osteosarcoma. Dog *versus* man. *Clin. Orthop.* **1991**, 159–168.
11. Bruland, O.S. Hematogenous micrometastases in osteosarcoma patients. *Clin. Cancer Res.* **2005**, *11*, 4666–4673. [CrossRef] [PubMed]
12. Mirabello, L.; Troisi, R.J.; Savage, S.A. Osteosarcoma incidence and survival rates from 1973 to 2004: Data from the surveillance, epidemiology, and end results program. *Cancer* **2009**, *115*, 1531–1543. [CrossRef] [PubMed]
13. Misdorp, W.; Hart, A.A. Some prognostic and epidemiologic factors in canine osteosarcoma. *J. Natl. Cancer Inst.* **1979**, *62*, 537–545. [PubMed]

14. Gelberg, K.H.; Fitzgerald, E.F.; Hwang, S.; Dubrow, R. Growth and development and other risk factors for osteosarcoma in children and young adults. *Int. J. Epidemiol.* **1997**, *26*, 272–278. [CrossRef] [PubMed]

15. Longhi, A.; Pasini, A.; Cicognani, A.; Baronio, F.; Pellacani, A.; Baldini, N.; Bacci, G. Height as a risk factor for osteosarcoma. *J. Pediatr. Hematol. Oncol.* **2005**, *27*, 314–318. [CrossRef] [PubMed]

16. Kelsey, J.L.; Moore, A.S.; Glickman, L.T. Epidemiologic studies of risk factors for cancer in pet dogs. *Epidemiol. Rev.* **1998**, *20*, 204–217. [CrossRef] [PubMed]

17. Fodstad, O.; Brøgger, A.; Bruland, O.; Solheim, O.P.; Nesland, J.M.; Pihl, A. Characteristics of a cell line established from a patient with multiple osteosarcoma, appearing 13 years after treatment for bilateral retinoblastoma. *Int. J. Cancer* **1986**, *38*, 33–40. [CrossRef] [PubMed]

18. Kadosawa, T.; Nozaki, K.; Sasaki, N.; Takeuchi, A. Establishment and characterization of a new cell line from a canine osteosarcoma. *J. Vet. Med. Sci.* **1994**, *56*, 1167–1169. [CrossRef] [PubMed]

19. Pautke, C.; Schieker, M.; Tischer, T.; Kolk, A.; Neth, P.; Mutschler, W.; Milz, S. Characterization of osteosarcoma cell lines MG-63, Saos-2 and U-2 OS in comparison to human osteoblasts. *Anticancer Res.* **2004**, *24*, 3743–3748. [PubMed]

20. Séguin, B.; Zwerdling, T.; McCallan, J.L.; DeCock, H.E.V.; Dewe, L.L.; Naydan, D.K.; Young, A.E.; Bannasch, D.L.; Foreman, O.; Kent, M.S. Development of a new canine osteosarcoma cell line. *Vet. Comp. Oncol.* **2006**, *4*, 232–240. [CrossRef] [PubMed]

21. Hong, S.H.; Kadosawa, T.; Mochizuki, M.; Matsunaga, S.; Nishimura, R.; Sasaki, N. Establishment and characterization of two cell lines derived from canine spontaneous osteosarcoma. *J. Vet. Med.* **1998**, *60*, 757–760. [CrossRef]

22. McAllister, R.M.; Gardner, M.B.; Greene, A.E.; Bradt, C.; Nichols, W.W.; Landing, B.H. Cultivation *in vitro* of cells derived from a human osteosarcoma. *Cancer* **1971**, *27*, 397–402. [CrossRef]

23. Ponten, J.; Saksela, E. Two established *in vitro* cell lines from human mesenchymal tumours. *Int. J. Cancer* **1967**, *2*, 434–447. [CrossRef] [PubMed]

24. Fogh, J.; Trempe, G. New human tumor cell lines. In *Human Tumor Cells in Vitro*; Fogh, J., Ed.; Springer U.S.: New York, NY, USA, 1975; pp. 115–159.

25. Billiau, A.; Edy, V.G.; Heremans, H.; Van Damme, J.; Desmyter, J.; Georgiades, J.A.; de Somer, P. Human interferon: Mass production in a newly established cell line, MG-63. *Antimicrob. Agents Chemother.* **1977**, *12*, 11–15. [CrossRef] [PubMed]

26. Riggs, J.L.; McAllister, R.M.; Lennette, E.H. Immunofluorescent studies of RD-114 virus replication in cell culture. *J. Gen. Virol.* **1974**, *25*, 21–29. [CrossRef] [PubMed]

27. Dimopoulou, M.; Kirpensteijn, J.; Moens, H.; Kik, M. Histologic prognosticators in feline osteosarcoma: A comparison with phenotypically similar canine osteosarcoma. *Vet. Surg.* **2008**, *37*, 466–471. [CrossRef] [PubMed]

28. Heldmann, E.; Anderson, M.A.; Wagner-Mann, C. Feline osteosarcoma: 145 Cases (1990–1995). *J. Am. Anim. Hosp. Assoc.* **2000**, *36*, 518–521. [CrossRef] [PubMed]

29. Holmes, K.E.; Thompson, V.; Piskun, C.M.; Kohnken, R.A.; Huelsmeyer, M.K.; Fan, T.M.; Stein, T.J. Canine osteosarcoma cell lines from patients with differing serum alkaline phosphatase concentrations display no behavioural differences *in vitro*: OSA cell lines differing in serum ALP. *Vet. Comp. Oncol.* **2015**, *13*, 166–175. [CrossRef] [PubMed]

30. Legare, M.E.; Bush, J.; Ashley, A.K.; Kato, T.; Hanneman, W.H. Cellular and phenotypic characterization of canine osteosarcoma cell lines. *J. Cancer* **2011**, *2*, 262. [CrossRef] [PubMed]

31. Fanburgsmith, J.; Bratthauer, G.; Miettinen, M. Osteocalcin and osteonectin immunoreactivity in extraskeletal osteosarcoma: A study of 28 cases. *Hum. Pathol.* **1999**, *30*, 32–38. [CrossRef]

32. Loukopoulos, P.; O'Brien, T.; Ghoddusi, M.; Mungall, B.; Robinson, W. Characterisation of three novel canine osteosarcoma cell lines producing high levels of matrix metalloproteinases. *Res. Vet. Sci.* **2004**, *77*, 131–141. [CrossRef] [PubMed]

33. Mohseny, A.B.; Machado, I.; Cai, Y.; Schaefer, K.-L.; Serra, M.; Hogendoorn, P.C.W.; Llombart-Bosch, A.; Cleton-Jansen, A.-M. Functional characterization of osteosarcoma cell lines provides representative models to study the human disease. *Lab. Investig.* **2011**, *91*, 1195–1205. [CrossRef] [PubMed]

34. Martins-Neves, S.R.; Lopes, Á.O.; do Carmo, A.; Paiva, A.A.; Simões, P.C.; Abrunhosa, A.J.; Gomes, C.M. Therapeutic implications of an enriched cancer stem-like cell population in a human osteosarcoma cell line. *BMC Cancer* **2012**, *12*, 139. [CrossRef] [PubMed]

35. Meyer, F.R.L.; Steinborn, R.; Grausgruber, H.; Wolfesberger, B.; Walter, I. Expression of platelet-derived growth factor BB, erythropoietin and erythropoietin receptor in canine and feline osteosarcoma. *Vet. J.* **2015**, *206*, 67–74. [CrossRef] [PubMed]

36. Morello, E.; Martano, M.; Buracco, P. Biology, diagnosis and treatment of canine appendicular osteosarcoma: Similarities and differences with human osteosarcoma. *Vet. J.* **2011**, *189*, 268–277. [CrossRef] [PubMed]

37. Pool, R.R.; Thompson, K.G. *Tumors of joints*. In *Tumors in Domestic Animals*; Meuten, D.J., Ed.; Iowa State Press: Ames, IA, USA, 2002; pp. 199–243.

38. Mueller, F.; Fuchs, B.; Kaser-Hotz, B. Comparative biology of human and canine osteosarcoma. *Anticancer Res.* **2007**, *27*, 155–164. [PubMed]

39. Chang, Y.S.; Graves, B.; Guerlavais, V.; Tovar, C.; Packman, K.; To, K.-H.; Olson, K.A.; Kesavan, K.; Gangurde, P.; Mukherjee, A.; Baker, T.; *et al.* Stapled α-helical peptide drug development: A potent dual inhibitor of MDM2 and MDMX for p53-dependent cancer therapy. *Proc. Natl. Acad. Sci. USA* **2013**, *110*, 3445–3454. [CrossRef] [PubMed]

40. Couto, J.I.; Bear, M.D.; Lin, J.; Pennel, M.; Kulp, S.K.; Kisseberth, W.C.; London, C.A. Biologic activity of the novel small molecule STAT3 inhibitor LLL12 against canine osteosarcoma cell lines. *BMC Vet. Res.* **2012**, *8*, 244. [CrossRef] [PubMed]

41. Lourda, M.; Trougakos, I.P.; Gonos, E.S. Development of resistance to chemotherapeutic drugs in human osteosarcoma cell lines largely depends on up-regulation of Clusterin/Apolipoprotein J. *Int. J. Cancer* **2007**, *120*, 611–622. [CrossRef] [PubMed]

42. Montanini, L.; Lasagna, L.; Barili, V.; Jonstrup, S.P.; Murgia, A.; Pazzaglia, L.; Conti, A.; Novello, C.; Kjems, J.; Perris, R.; *et al.* MicroRNA cloning and sequencing in osteosarcoma cell lines: Differential role of miR-93. *Cell. Oncol. Dordr.* **2012**, *35*, 29–41. [CrossRef] [PubMed]

43. Sharili, A.-S.; Allen, S.; Smith, K.; Price, J.; McGonnell, I.M. Snail2 promotes osteosarcoma cell motility through remodelling of the actin cytoskeleton and regulates tumor development. *Cancer Lett.* **2013**, *333*, 170–179. [CrossRef] [PubMed]

44. Rimann, M.; Laternser, S.; Gvozdenovic, A.; Muff, R.; Fuchs, B.; Kelm, J.M.; Graf-Hausner, U. An *in vitro* osteosarcoma 3D microtissue model for drug development. *J. Biotechnol.* **2014**, *189*, 129–135. [CrossRef] [PubMed]

45. Majeska, R.J.; Rodan, S.B.; Rodan, G.A. Parathyroid hormone-responsive clonal cell lines from rat osteosarcoma. *Endocrinology* **1980**, *107*, 1494–1503. [CrossRef] [PubMed]

46. Mohseny, A.B.; Hogendoorn, P.C.W.; Cleton-Jansen, A.-M. Osteosarcoma Models: From cell lines to Zebrafish. *Sarcoma* **2012**. [CrossRef] [PubMed]

47. Mather, J.P.; Roberts, P.E. *Introduction to Cell and Tissue Culture: Theory and Technique*; Springer Science & Business Media: Berlin, Germany, 2007.

48. Hiddemann, W.; Roessner, A.; Wörmann, B.; Mellin, W.; Klockenkemper, B.; Bösing, T.; Büchner, T.; Grundmann, E. Tumor heterogeneity in osteosarcoma as identified by flow cytometry. *Cancer* **1987**, *59*, 324–328. [CrossRef]

49. Kunz, P.; Fellenberg, J.; Moskovszky, L.; Sápi, Z.; Krenacs, T.; Poeschl, J.; Lehner, B.; Szendrõi, M.; Ewerbeck, V.; Kinscherf, R.; *et al.* Osteosarcoma microenvironment: Whole-slide imaging and optimized antigen detection overcome major limitations in immunohistochemical quantification. *PLoS ONE* **2014**, *9*, e90727. [CrossRef] [PubMed]

50. Dalla-Torre, C.A.; Yoshimoto, M.; Lee, C.-H.; Joshua, A.M.; de Toledo, S.R.; Petrilli, A.S.; Andrade, J.A.; Chilton-MacNeill, S.; Zielenska, M.; Squire, J.A. Effects of THBS3, SPARC and SPP1 expression on biological behavior and survival in patients with osteosarcoma. *BMC Cancer* **2006**, *6*, 237. [CrossRef] [PubMed]

51. Nagamine, E.; Hirayama, K.; Matsuda, K.; Okamoto, M.; Ohmachi, T.; Kadosawa, T.; Taniyama, H. Diversity of histologic patterns and expression of cytoskeletal proteins in canine skeletal osteosarcoma. *Vet. Pathol.* **2015**. [CrossRef] [PubMed]

52. Kastan, M.B.; Canman, C.E.; Leonard, C.J. P53, cell cycle control and apoptosis: Implications for cancer. *Cancer Metastasis Rev.* **1995**, *14*, 3–15. [CrossRef] [PubMed]

53. Donehower, L.A.; Harvey, M.; Slagle, B.L.; McArthur, M.J.; Montgomery, C.A.; Butel, J.S.; Bradley, A. Mice deficient for p53 are developmentally normal but susceptible to spontaneous tumours. *Nature* **1992**, *356*, 215–221. [CrossRef] [PubMed]

54. Bongiovanni, L.; Mazzocchetti, F.; Malatesta, D.; Romanucci, M.; Ciccarelli, A.; Buracco, P.; de Maria, R.; Palmieri, C.; Martano, M.; Morello, E.; *et al.* Immunohistochemical investigation of cell cycle and apoptosis regulators (survivin, β-catenin, p53, caspase 3) in canine appendicular osteosarcoma. *BMC Vet. Res.* **2012**, *8*, 78. [CrossRef] [PubMed]

55. Nasir, L.; Rutteman, G.R.; Reid, S.W.; Schulze, C.; Argyle, D.J. Analysis of p53 mutational events and MDM2 amplification in canine soft-tissue sarcomas. *Cancer Lett.* **2001**, *174*, 83–89. [CrossRef]

56. Mayr, B.; Reifinger, M.; Loupal, G. Polymorphisms in feline tumour suppressor gene p53. Mutations in an osteosarcoma and a mammary carcinoma. *Vet. J.* **1998**, *155*, 103–106. [CrossRef]

12

Sentinel Animals in a One Health Approach to Harmful Cyanobacterial and Algal Blooms

Lorraine C. Backer [1,*] and Melissa Miller [2,3]

1   National Center for Environmental Health, Centers for Disease Control and Prevention,
    4770 Buford Highway NE, MS F-60, Chamblee, GA 30341, USA
2   Office of Spill Prevention and Response, Department of Fish and Wildlife,
    Marine Wildlife Veterinary Care and Research Center, 1451 Shaffer Rd, Santa Cruz, CA 95060, USA;
    melissa.miller@wildlife.ca.gov
3   School of Veterinary Medicine, University of California at Davis, Davis, CA 95616, USA
*   Correspondence: lfb9@cdc.gov

Academic Editors: Peter M. Rabinowitz and Lisa A. Conti

Abstract: People, domestic animals, and wildlife are all exposed to numerous environmental threats, including harmful algal blooms (HABs). However, because animals exhibit wide variations in diet, land use and biology, they are often more frequently or heavily exposed to HAB toxins than are people occupying the same habitat, making them sentinels for human exposures. Historically, we have taken advantage of unique physiological characteristics of animals, such as the sensitivity of canaries to carbon monoxide, to more quickly recognize threats and help protect human health. As HAB events become more severe and widespread worldwide, exposure and health outcome data for animals can be extremely helpful to predict, prevent, and evaluate human exposures and health outcomes. Applying a One Health approach to investigation of HABs means that lessons learned from animal sentinels can be applied to protect people, animals and our shared environment.

Keywords: algae; biotoxin; cyanobacteria; cyanotoxin; domoic acid; freshwater; harmful algal bloom; marine water; one health; saxitoxin; sentinel

---

1. Introduction

Like humans, domestic animals and wildlife can experience acute and chronic health impacts following exposure to environmental threats, such as air or water pollution. Because of their unique habitat use, behavior, and biology, animals may be exposed to environmental pollutants more rapidly and at higher concentrations than humans residing in the same areas, making them potential sentinels for emerging threats to human health. Animal-based sentinel systems can expedite recognition of dangerous environmental conditions, illustrate pollutant bioavailability, and clarify health hazards associated with known contaminants, providing an approximation of what people might experience [1]. Historically, animal sentinels have been used *in situ* to monitor potentially dangerous environments. One well-known example is the use of canaries and mice in coal mines to warn miners when carbon monoxide was present at dangerous levels [2]. Animals live alongside humans in diverse environments, including homes, workplaces and natural aquatic or terrestrial ecosystems, and study of their pollutant exposure trends can provide early warnings of potential human health hazards [1].

As one important example, investigation of deaths of domestic animals and wildlife has expedited recognition of human health threats associated with exposure to harmful cyanobacterial and algal blooms (herein referred to as HABs) in water and food worldwide. The first published description of animals as sentinels for a dangerous HAB event was a short report by Francis [3] describing poisonings of domestic animals that drank from lakes of the Murray River estuary system in Australia. A severe cyanobacterial bloom was tentatively identified as *Nodularia spumigera*, and horses, sheep, dogs, and pigs died within hours of drinking from bloom-contaminated waters. Schwimmer and Schwimmer [4] reviewed historical reports of domestic and wild animal poisonings during freshwater HAB events, and Stewart *et al.* [5] published an updated review as part of a compendium on the current state of knowledge about cyanobacteria and future research needs.

Synergizing efforts to monitor sentinel animal events and sentinel animal systems with human disease surveillance activities is a critical component of the "One Health" approach for identifying and addressing environmental threats. One Health is a global initiative to link human, animal, and environmental health [6]. One Health principles encompass data integration, collaboration, and cooperation across all health disciplines, synergizing the study of human and animal health and disease in shared habitats. One of the greatest challenges is facilitating and expediting communication across human and animal health disciplines. HABs affect every aspect of global aquatic environments and thus represent a unique opportunity and an obvious need for interdisciplinary collaboration to identify, mitigate, and prevent adverse health outcomes. In this paper we review examples of sentinel animal events that have contributed to our collective understanding of potential public health threats from HABs, and discuss opportunities whereby investigation of HAB events using the One Health approach can expedite, optimize and guide current and future public health protections.

2. Example Animal Sentinel Systems and Events

2.1. Aquatic Species

Aquatic animals, including invertebrates, fish and marine animals, provide some of the earliest alerts regarding potential adverse effects from HABs, and face numerous health and survival threats from toxin exposure.

2.1.1. Invertebrates

Marine and freshwater invertebrates, including mussels, clams and crabs, comprise an important food resource for animals and people living in both coastal and inland communities. Invertebrate population health reflects the quality of local marine waters and adverse changes may signal subsequent health risks for the people and animals that consume them or otherwise share the local environment. Invertebrates have served as sentinels for coastal and freshwater environmental contamination for at least 30 years. One example is the Mussel Watch program, the longest-running chemical contaminant monitoring program in U.S. coastal and Great Lakes Waters [7]. This program has monitored over 150 organic and inorganic contaminant concentrations in water and bivalves since 1986, including trends for polyaromatic hydrocarbons and polychlorinated biphenyls in sediments and bivalve tissues [8].

In addition to these legacy contaminants, the program has evolved to measure emerging contaminants of concern, including polybrominated biphenyl ethers (flame retardants) and pharmaceuticals. Mussel Watch data can be used to assess how increased regulation of these chemicals affects their environmental distributions and concentrations, and can help assess human health risks from consuming invertebrates, fish, or drinking water, or via recreational water contact. Archived specimens allow retrospective assessment of contaminants of concern, including new compounds and existing chemicals with newly discovered environmental distributions.

Over the past 20 years environmental monitoring programs have been expanded to include freshwater and marine HABs and their associated toxins. Like Mussel Watch, the sentinel animal event for these programs is the detection of toxins at concentrations of concern in shellfish. These programs monitor blooms and shellfish quality along coastlines where toxin-producing blooms occur, and provide early warnings of shellfish contamination specifically to protect human health (e.g., [9]). For example, Florida prevents most cases of neurotoxic shellfish poisoning through monitoring shellfish for brevetoxin, and posting harvest bans when levels are high [10].

In the Northeast, new technologies detect *Alexandrium fundyense,* which can develop into HABs often called "red tides". During bloom events, dinoflagellates like *A. fundyense* can produce large concentrations of a potent neurotoxin (saxitoxin) that can bioaccumulate in shellfish and cause paralytic shellfish poisoning in animals and people. Models used data from ocean observing sensors to predict the concentrations of Alexandrium produce seasonal forecasts that support decisions to open or close commercial and sport shellfisheries for human consumption in the Gulf of Maine [11]. Data from these bivalve monitoring programs provide an evolving picture of coastal contaminants that can be used to assess risk for regional human exposure, to inform epidemiologic studies of exposures and health effects, and to optimize regional prevention, education, and outreach programs.

Dinoflagellate HAB events with abundant saxitoxin production are also an annual occurrence along the Pacific Coast of North America, and were the main catalyst for developing regional shellfish-based HAB monitoring programs. The Olympic Region Harmful Algal Bloom (ORHAB) partnership identified sampling sites along the coast and monitors for rapid increases in *Pseudo-nitzschia* cells and for the presence of toxin in seawater [12,13]. Using data from this monitoring program, resource managers can predict when domoic acid levels will be high in local shellfish and can target which recreational shellfish harvesting areas should be closed to prevent human poisonings. During the summer 2015, the largest and most extensive *Pseudo-nitzschia* bloom event ever recorded was documented off the Pacific Coast, extending from California to Alaska [14]. *Pseudo-nitzschia* produces domoic acid, and routine monitoring of ocean water and marine organisms detected elevated toxin levels beginning in May 2015. High domoic acid concentrations were documented in marine bivalves and crabs, resulting in extensive shellfish harvest closures [15]. High domoic acid levels in shellfish from these areas and could be an underlying cause of reported marine mammal deaths [16].

A common HAB event in Southeastern North America is Florida red tide, comprising seasonal blooms of the dinoflagellate *Karenia brevis* in the Gulf of Mexico. *Karenia brevis* produces the neurotoxin brevetoxin, which accumulates in the marine food web (e.g., [17]). Ongoing monitoring of shellfish and water by the Florida Fish and Wildlife Conservation Commission supports the management of commercial and recreational shellfish harvesting [18]. Shellfish beds are closed when *Karenia brevis* cells in water exceed 5000 per L, or when shellfish meat contains ≥20 mouse units of toxin [19]. Because of this diligence, very few cases of human intoxication from brevetoxins occur in Florida, and those typically involve visitors who may not understand or heed posted warnings. Florida provides public information on red tides, including when and where Florida red tide events occur and the status of shellfish harvesting beds, on the website of the Florida Fish and Wildlife Conservation Commission [20].

Finally, filter-feeding estuarine and marine invertebrates are a potential source of human and animal exposure to freshwater cyanotoxins originating in coastal rivers [21–25]. For example, filter-feeding invertebrates from regions of microcystin-contaminated coastal freshwater outflow are the most likely source of microcystin intoxication for threatened southern sea otters (*Enhydra lutris nereis*) in Monterey Bay, California [21]. As part of their investigation, Miller *et al.* (2010) [21] conducted laboratory studies showing that marine shellfish maintained under ambient conditions following exposure to cyanobacterial scum from a Pinto Lake bloom rapidly accumulate microcystins and only slowly depurate them, even when maintained in clean, uncontaminated seawater. Significant bioconcentration of microcystin by marine bivalves (clams, mussels and oysters) and snails, but not large marine crabs, was documented, with tissue concentrations of microcystin-LR up to 107 times higher in invertebrate hepatopancreas than in adjacent seawater. Findings from this investigation revealed a new environmental health threat for sea otters and people by tracing marine contamination by microcystins derived from fresh water, and demonstrating that marine shellfish consumed by both marine mammals and people can accumulate microcystins.

Microcystins have also been detected in wild and commercially-raised marine and estuarine mussels (*Mytilus trossulus*) from Puget Sound, Washington, D.C., U.S.; Nile tilpaia (*Oreochromis nitoticus*) from Chian Rai, Thailand; and other aquatic foods intended for human consumption [26–28]. Routine seawater and aquatic animal monitoring in areas where cyanotoxins have been found could provide early that warning that animal and human shellfish consumers could be at risk. However, the accuracy of detection requires further study, especially when attempting microcystin detection from biological samples [29]. Analytic detection of microcystins is complicated by the large diversity of microcystin congeners, challenges with congener extraction from biological samples, and a large range of abiotic and biotic processes that can alter the toxicity and structure of microcystin molecules [30]. When possible the most sensitive and specific sample extraction and detection methods should be used to screen biological samples, such as liquid chromatography-mass spectrometry (LC-MS), or liquid chromatography tandem mass spectrometry (LC-MS/MS).

The above summaries provide a snapshot of key HAB events that occur repeatedly along North American coastlines where invertebrates are exposed to HABs. Monitoring programs for these invertebrates can serve as sentinels for human and animal exposure, in addition to preventing foodborne exposures. Additional bloom events occur that are not captured in this overview. For example, the Florida coastline also experiences intermittent dinoflagellate blooms with saxitoxin production where invertebrate bioconcentration plays a key role in public health monitoring efforts [31]. In addition, commercial shellfish beds along the Gulf Coast have faced closures due to HAB-associated production of okadaic acid, a source of diarrheic shellfish poisoning (DSP) [32]. Large inland freshwater bodies, such as Lake Erie, are also exhibiting increased frequency and severity of HAB events [33].

2.1.2. Fish

Fish have been indicators of environmental contamination as part of the National Status and Trends Program (NS&T) in the U.S. since 1984 [1]. NS&T includes histopathologic assessments of fish tissues; and these assessments were used to link environmental exposures to the formation of lesions, which often resembled those identified in laboratory animals with similar chemical exposures [1]. Confirmation of similar adverse effects in fish and laboratory animals suggests that similar effects could occur in people sharing the same environments. The first record of a massive fish kill associated with harmful algal bloom formation occurred approximately 1000 years BC in Egypt, and was noted in the bible [34]. HAB-associated fish kills are now commonly recognized, and may serve as rapid indicators of HAB development. HAB-associated fish deaths may occur due to a variety of factors, including direct toxicity of the toxins [15] and hypoxia secondary to high respiration by the algae or increased bacterial respiration during bloom decay [34]. Algae and their products can also cause mechanical or hemolytic damage to gills, ultimately resulting in respiratory failure or fatal metabolic disturbances [34]. Given the complexity of methods by which these events can trigger fish deaths, and the rapid decomposition of fish involved in such events, the pathophysiology of massive, HAB-associated fish kills is often speculative or unknown.

In the late 1990s, investigation of massive fish kills in southeastern U.S. estuaries prompted discovery of an estuarine dinoflagellate, *Pfiesteria piscicida* [35]. Investigators reported human illness following occupational exposure to laboratory cultures of the organism, and fish collected from areas of *P. piscicida* blooms exhibited superficial ulcers [36,37]. Notably, even without evidence that local seafood was contaminated with either *P. piscicida* or any associated toxin, consumers chose not to eat seafood caught from the Chesapeake Bay, or served in restaurants along the shoreline [38]. There is conflicting evidence regarding whether *Pfiesteria piscicida* kills fish by a combination of toxic and physical means or whether the fish kills were due to anoxia or hypoxia with superficial ulcers attributed to *Aphanomyces invadans* infections [39–42]. Ultimately, no statistical associations were found between exposure to *P. piscicida* cultures or their derivatives and human illness [43,44]. Although the initial concerns about health risks due to *P. piscicida* exposure were not supported by later scientific studies, the attention given to the organism raised public and political awareness about algal bloom events, HABs and their potential ecologic, economic, and health effects.

Recent research demonstrated that microcystins can accumulate in freshwater fish. For example, microcystins were detected in both fresh water samples and fish in aquaculture ponds in Thailand [26].

In the mid-2000s, the Nature Conservancy began restoring the Williamson River Delta Preserve in Oregon, USA with the goal of regenerating habitats essential for the survival of the endangered Lost River sucker (*Deltistes luxatus*), and short-nose sucker (*Chasmistes brevirostris*) [45]. However, lack of recruitment into spawning populations in Upper Klamath Lake is preventing recovery of these typically long-lived species [46]. This disappearance of juvenile suckers coincides with a decrease in water quality, which supported massive cyanobacteria blooms. Bloom decay resulted in high concentrations of cyanotoxins and hypoxic conditions in the Upper Klamath. Short-term microcystin feeding trials, using concentrations approximating those in Upper Klamath Lake, revealed microscopic lesions in exposed suckers similar to those described from other fish species following sub-lethal microcystin exposure [46].

The detrimental impacts of impaired water quality leading to dense cyanobacteria blooms extend well beyond Upper Klamath Lake. Suckerfish are highly valued by the indigenous Klamath Tribe for food and ceremonial purposes [47]. Local cyanobacteria blooms and associated toxins threaten the local ecology, a traditional food source, and ceremonial heritage. Ongoing water and fish monitoring programs can help protect Klamath Tribe members by notifying them when cyanobacteria toxins are accumulating in water and/or fish tissue.

One fish species that has served as a unique local indicator of algal proliferation in freshwater is the pike (*Esox lucius*) [48]. These fish can modify their coloration somewhat to reflect their local environment. During summer 2015, fishermen reported catching "glowing neon fish." Local fish and wildlife authorities explained that the edges of the pike's fins, tails, and mouths turn bright neon green as an adaptation for hunting among reeds with admixed algae. While these algae may not produce toxins, the annual appearance of bright green fish signals adaptation to algal proliferation.

Fish are highly susceptible to the toxins produced by another microalga, *Prymnesium parvum* (also known as "golden algae". *Prymnesium parvum* was first confirmed in west Texas in 1985, and blooms have killed millions of fish; however, it is also likely that the organism was killing fish in the 1950s [49]. Golden algae produce a toxin that asphyxiates gilled animals, including fish, freshwater mollusks, and juvenile frogs. Extended *P. parvum* blooms can drastically affect local ecology with long-term adverse effects on fisheries and economic hardship for those serving recreational anglers [50]. *Prymnesium parvum* was first noticed in Arizona in 2005, possibly carried into the state by migrating water-birds, fishing equipment, water transport, or wind dispersal of dust contaminated with cysts [51]. Although not considered a threat to birds or mammals, golden algae blooms can persist under environmental conditions less favorable to other microalgae, such as cold weather, suggesting that these blooms may be indicators for local or regional ecologic changes.

Because of their high numbers and fixed location, with inability to escape bloom events, farmed fish are especially vulnerable to bloom events and may serve as sensitive bioindicators of HAB formation. In addition, negative economic impacts of HAB events on coastal mariculture can be substantial. . Net-pen liver disease (NLD), is a common disease of farmed Atlantic salmon (*Salmo salar*) from British Columbia and Washington State [52]. Development of severe liver disease appears to be associated with ingestion of microcystin-LR when feeding on natural biota that can proliferate in the nutrient-rich environment of net-pens [53].

Other events associated with toxic algae exposure of fish can be harder to detect, because these events can be small, focal, and ephemeral. Additionally, HAB-exposed fish may be relatively resistant to the toxin's effects. One example is ciguatera fish poisoning (or ciguatera), a human illness caused by consuming fish that appear to be healthy, but that contain toxins or metabolites produced by the microalga *Gambierdiscus toxicus* [54]. Associated clinical signs in humans include nausea, vomiting, and neurologic symptoms such as tingling fingers or toes. Ciguatera fish poisoning is most commonly associated with ingestion of predatory reef fish harvested from tropical and subtropical waters, such as the Caribbean Sea and the Pacific and Indian Oceans.

2.1.3. Marine Mammals

Marine mammals are long-lived species that tend to live in coastal waters shared by people and feed at the same trophic level as humans. They are susceptible to many recognized human pathogens, including emerging and resurging pathogens such as methicillin-resistant *Staphylococcus aureus*, and *Toxoplasma gondii* [55–57]. The health of marine mammals reflects the health of coastal marine waters, including environmental changes triggered by climate change, and presence of chemical contaminants and pathogens. In turn, these animals can serve as "early warning systems" for toxin exposures and potential HAB-associated health effects for people who share the same coastal environments and consume similar foods. HABs are common coastal events, and fossil evidence suggests that repeated mass-strandings of Miocene-era marine mammals in the Atacama Region of Chili may have been HAB-associated [58].

Because many toxins are capable of concentrating and spreading through food webs, one of the most common sources for HAB exposure of marine mammals is their food, including both fish and invertebrates. In this capacity marine mammals often alert resource managers to potential human health risks from consumption of aquatic foods harvested during, or following HAB events. One excellent example is the potent excitatory neurotoxin, domoic acid, which was associated with human amnesic shellfish poisoning Canada in 1987 [59]. In 1998, hundreds of California sea lions (*Zalophus californianus*) died after consuming anchovies (*Engraulis mordax*) that had accumulated high levels of domoic acid after feeding on toxin-producing *Pseudo-nitzschia* spp. [60]. Clinical signs exhibited by domoic acid-exposed sea lions included seizures, head weaving, obtundation, and pruritis. Because no specific antidote exists to treat domoic acid intoxication, affected animals received supportive and symptomatic care, including fluids, diazepam, lorazepam, and phenobarbitone. Despite treatment, over half of the clinically affected animals died, and many animals that were rehabilitated and released re-stranded within four months [61]. Many of the sea lions that survived acute domoic acid intoxication displayed clinical and physical signs of chronic, irreversible brain damage, which was especially apparent in the hippocampus [61].

Many additional California sea lions died from domoic acid poisoning along the California coast during subsequent years [61,62]. In addition to acute death due to neurotoxicity, domoic acid exposure has also been shown to cause cardiac disease [63], abortion, premature parturition, and death of pregnant sea lions [64], thus raising the possibility that similar, non-acute health impacts could also be occurring in humans but are currently under-recognized. Interestingly, the symptomatology and epidemiology of domoic acid toxicosis in California sea lions has evolved over time in response to an apparent increase in toxin-producing blooms [65]. Two distinct clinical syndromes can now be identified; acute domoic acid toxicosis, and chronic epilepsy, reflecting neurologic damage induced by sub-lethal doses of domoic acid. The importance of sub-lethal domoic acid exposure as a cause of epilepsy in humans is unknown.

In addition to consumption of biotoxin-contaminated food and water, both marine mammals and humans can be poisoned via inhalation of aerosolized toxins. In 1996, unprecedented mortality of nearly 150 endangered West Indian manatees (*Trichechus manatus latirostris*) occurred along the southwest Florida coast in association with a bloom of brevetoxin-producing *Gymnodinium breve* (now called *Karenia brevis*) [66]. Affected animals exhibited multi-organ congestion, nasopharyngeal and pulmonary edema and hemorrhage suggestive of brevetoxin poisoning [66], and lymphocytes and macrophages in multiple tissues were immunopositive for brevetoxin. The manatees were thought to have been exposed to brevetoxin through both ingestion and inhalation. Interestingly, weak positive brevetoxin staining was also observed in tissues from control animals, suggesting that manatees are likely repeatedly exposed to brevetoxins [66].

Historically, it was presumed that organisms other than filter-feeding shellfish would not accumulate brevetoxins via the food web. For example, during previous manatee mortality events, brevetoxin exposure was presumed to be via inhalation, as evidenced by pulmonary pathology. However, in 2005, Flewelling *et al.* [17] described two mortality events in which marine mammals were fatally poisoned by brevetoxins during a period when no *K. brevis* bloom was apparent. In 2002, 34 West Indian manatees died in southwest Florida, and in 2004, 107 bottlenose dolphins (*Tursiops truncatus*) died in waters off the Florida panhandle. Although *K. brevis* cell counts were low in seawater samples, brevetoxins were detected in locally-collected fish and seagrass. Exposure was confirmed through biochemical analysis of stomach contents collected during necropsy.

In addition to serving as indicator species for toxic marine HAB events, marine mammals have also been implicated as sentinels for coastal outflows of freshwater HAB toxins. During 2007, 11 dead or dying southern sea otters were recovered from Monterey Bay, California with mild to severe icterus and enlarged, friable livers [21]. Microscopic examination revealed liver lesions consistent with a hepatotoxin, such as mushroom or cyanobacterial poisoning, and biochemical tests confirmed the presence of the potent hepatotoxins, microcystins [21]. Microcystins are typically associated with cyanobacteria found in fresh or estuarine waters, and the findings prompted a search for potential freshwater sources. Pinto Lake, located about 8.5 km inland from where some affected otters were recovered in Monterey Bay, historically had severe *Microcystis* spp. blooms that produced high concentrations of microcystins, and health warnings had been posted near the lake during fall 2007. Miller *et al.* (2010) [21] sampled water and surface algae scum from Pinto Lake through its tributaries to the Pajaro River, which drains directly into Monterey Bay. Microcystin concentrations in Pinto Lake surface scum were extremely high (2.1 million ppb microcystin LA, and 2.9 million ppb total microcystins), and decreased progressively to about 1 ppb in the lower reaches of the Pajaro River. Importantly, both microcystins and the parent cyanobacterium (*Microcystis* spp.) were detected throughout this water system, from Pinto Lake, to within sight of the ocean. Nearly every year since 2007, large and intense *Microcystis* blooms have occurred in Pinto Lake. Although ocean waters and the marine interfaces of coastal rivers flowing into Monterey Bay were biochemically negative for microcystins, samples from the marine outfalls of the Pajaro and Salinas Rivers tested positive for microcystins during the rainy season, when coastal freshwater runoff was highest. A subsequent study has identified microcystin contamination in 15 of 21 freshwater outflows draining into the Monterey Bay National Marine Sanctuary [22]. Nutrient loading was a significant predictor of microcystin concentrations in affected watersheds. In a related study, 100% of assessed coastal fresh water bodies in Southern California tested positive for at least one cyanotoxin, including microcystin, and three sites exceeded California action levels [67].

2.2. Birds

In part due to their unique biology, habits and physiology, birds are highly sensitive indicators of local environmental quality. Raptors at the top of the food web, and aquatic birds residing at the land-sea interface often succumb to environmental hazards posed by HABs and their associated toxins. Because birds are numerous and highly visible, avian mass-mortality events often serve as early warning systems for the presence of pesticides and toxins, highlighting local and regional environmental health risks for other animals and people.

For example, the first scientific report of animal mass-mortality due to domoic acid poisoning occurred in brown pelicans (*Pelecanus occidentalis*) and Brandt's cormorants (*Phalacrocorax penicillatus*) along the central California coast in 1991 [68]. This discovery, along with subsequent mass-mortality of California sea lions due to domoic acid intoxication in 1998, prompted scientists to revisit an avian mass-mortality event in the same region that resulted in deaths of numerous sooty shearwaters (*Puffinus griseus*) in 1961. Large numbers of affected birds acted abnormally, crashed into buildings and regurgitated anchovies throughout the central coast community of Capitola, California. Alfred Hitchcock was a local resident at the time, and researched this event, providing inspiration for his 1963 movie, "The Birds". Fifty one years later, Bargu *et al.* [69] identified frustules (silica-based exoskeletons) of potentially toxic *Pseudo-nitzschia* spp. in the gastrointestinal tracts of preserved zooplankton collected in 1961 during the same time period and from the same region, strongly supporting the possibility of large-scale avian mortality due to domoic acid intoxication. Numerous additional bird deaths have been associated with domoic acid intoxication in recent years [70,71].

Aquatic birds can also serve as sensitive sentinels for *K. brevis* blooms with brevetoxin production. Kreuder *et al.* [72] investigated sporadic appearance of neurological disease in double-crested cormorants (*P. auritus*) in Florida that may have extended back as much as 30 years. Clinical signs consisted of severe cerebellar ataxia, characterized by a broad-based stance, truncal incoordination, hypermetric gait, and intention tremors. Histopathologic findings were mild and nonspecific, but immunohistochemical staining was positive for brevetoxin. Admittance of cormorants to the Clinic for the Rehabilitation of Wildlife (Sanibel Island, FL, U.S.) with outbreak-specific clinical signs was positively correlated ($p < 0.05$) with concurrent concentrations of *K. brevis* in local water. This cross-correlation coefficient was also significant when increased *K. brevis* levels preceded cormorant admittances by 2, 4, 6, and 8 weeks, suggesting associations between *K. brevis* blooms and local cormorant morbidity.

Interestingly, freshwater and marine-associated toxins can cause avian mortality even when bloom events are not apparent. Avian vacuolar myelinopathy (AVM) is a neurologic disease of birds associated with consumption of submerged vegetation colonized with a toxin-producing cyanobacteria [73,74]. The cyanobacterium *Aetokthonos hydrillicola* has been tentatively identified as the source of this toxin [75]. While the toxin(s) produced have not been fully characterized, these organisms are known to grow abundantly on both introduced *Hydrilla* spp. and on native aquatic plants [76]. Another fascinating aspect of AVM is the ability of these uncharacterized toxins to kill both direct consumers (e.g., American coots, *Fulica americana*), and predatory birds such as bald eagles (*Haliaeetus leucocephalus*) [77]. Coots are exposed through grazing on cyanobacterium-contaminated aquatic vegetation, and affected eagles were shown to develop AVM after consuming affected coots. To date, disease has not been documented in mammals and people, including hunters and others who consume waterfowl [77]. Although there is no direct evidence that humans could be affected, out of an abundance of caution, federal and state agencies have created outreach materials that outline precautions to take when handling and consuming waterfowl that could have vacuolar myelinopathy.

In November–December 2007, a widespread seabird mortality event occurred in Monterey Bay, California (USA) in conjunction with a massive bloom of the dinoflagellate *Akashiwo sanguinea* that deposited piles of a foamy substance onshore [78]. Affected birds had water-soaked feathers covered with yellow-green slimy material, and were severely hypothermic. Investigators determined that foam produced by the bloom contained proteins with surfactant properties, which coated the birds' feathers and neutralized their natural water repellency and insulation [78]. In September 2009, a similar bloom developed off the coast of Washington state, and there was concern about surfers' exposure to the foam and surfactants generated by *A. sanguinea*. A small study (n = 20) of surfers found that, of 10 respondents who reported no symptoms before surfing, 8 reported nasal congestion or burning post-exposure (Personal communication, Myduc Ta, 19 July 2010). Although this pilot study did not definitively demonstrate that exposure to the chemicals produced by *A. sanguinea* caused specific symptoms in people, the effects observed in birds suggest that humans should avoid exposure to the foams that are the hallmark of this type of bloom.

2.3. Domestic Animals

The death of a domestic animal, particularly a pet dog, may be the first indication that a local waterbody has an ongoing toxin-producing HAB event. Dogs are particularly vulnerable because they may swim in waters that smell bad or are visually unappealing to people. They are also likely to lick algae from their fur after they leave the water. Backer *et al.* [79] published a review of canine cyanobacteria poisonings from three different data sources—the Harmful Bloom Related Illness Surveillance System supported by the National Center for Environmental Health, Centers for Disease Control and Prevention; retrospective case files from the Veterinary Medical Teaching Hospital (VMTH), University of California, Davis; and an extensive review of written media reports, scientific and medical manuscripts, and web-based reports of canine cyanobacteria intoxications. Between the 1920s and 2012,

231 unique events and 368 poisonings were reported [79]. Between 2007 and 2011, Departments of Health/Environment from 13 states (California, Florida, Iowa, Kansas, Maryland, Minnesota, Montana, New York, North Carolina, Oregon, Texas, Virginia, and Wisconsin) reported 67 confirmed or suspected cases of HAB-related canine poisonings [79]. Thirty-eight (58%) of the poisonings were fatal. Of the 67 cases, 63 were possibly or confirmed to be associated with exposure to freshwater cyanobacteria HABs. The retrospective review of suspected and confirmed canine cyanobacteria toxin poisoning accessions between 1984 and 2012 from the VMTH necropsy and biopsy cases identified 71 cases that met selection criteria as possible or confirmed cyanotoxin poisoning cases. Of these, 43 dogs (61%) had a moderate to high possibility of microcystin poisoning based on clinical presentation, lesion descriptions, listed differential diagnoses, pathologist comments, and diagnostic test results. Between the late 1920s and mid-2012, historical reports, including media reports, state and federal agency reports, and published literature identified 115 cyanobacteria HAB-related events involving 260 dogs [79]. Two hundred and fifteen (83%) dogs died from the exposures, and 45 (17%) became ill and then recovered.

Stewart *et al.* [5] reviewed reports of cyanobacteria-related poisonings in livestock, wild mammals, and birds. Poisonings have occurred on every continent, and pre-historic mass mortalities of unrelated fauna have been attributed to cyanotoxin poisoning. The early reports of cyanobacteria poisonings included in this review tended to be anecdotal, but included detailed descriptions of bloom events that were temporally and geographically linked with animal deaths. The later reports are less subjective and include clinical and postmortem findings, as well as results from analytic tests developed to detect toxins in clinical specimens. Livestock poisonings are sentinel events indicating contamination of ponds and other water resources that are not routinely monitored. They signal a poisoning risk for other animals using the pond for drinking water and for people using the pond for recreation, including swimming and fishing.

2.4. A One Health Approach to HABs

We live in a complex and rapidly changing environment where protection of human health is a growing challenge. Because HAB-associated illness occurs with higher frequency and severity in animals [80], careful investigation and monitoring of animal illnesses and deaths due to biotoxin exposure can expedite recognition and mitigation of potential human health risks. A One Health approach that incorporates animals as key HAB sentinels is needed. The overarching concept of One Health approach includes using exposure and health outcome information learned from animal exposures and outbreaks as components in human risk assessment; applying what we know about human illnesses to animals that might experience similar exposures; developing new public health activities that integrate animal and human data, such as cross-species disease surveillance [80,81]; and creating an environment that facilitates cross-disciplinary collaboration among scientists, veterinarians, medical professionals, and many others [82].

HAB-related animal monitoring coupled with animal and human health event response can be used iteratively to enhance our knowledge of, response to, and prevention of HAB-related exposures and associated illnesses. For example, Amnesic shellfish poisoning from exposure to domoic acid produced by the diatom *Pseudo-nitzschia multiseries* was first documented along the Northeast coast of North America in 1987, when three people died and 100 became ill after eating mussels collected offshore of Prince Edward Island, Canada [59,83]. The first scientific report of domoic acid intoxication of animals or people along the Pacific Coastal North America occurred at about the same time, in 1991 in Monterey Bay, California [70]; although it is possible that earlier west coast events had simply been missed [84]. Additionally associated with blooms of *Pseudo-nitzschia* spp., studies have confirmed bioaccumulation of domoic acid in diverse marine and estuarine invertebrates, characterized by high bioconcentration and slow depuration in some species, notably razor clams [12] mole crabs (*Emerita analoga*) and fat innkeeper worms (*Urechis caupo*) [85]. This was confirmed in work done by Cook *et al.* [86], who reported impaired memory and impaired hippocampal activity in California sea lions (*Alophus califonianus*) exposed to domoic acid. Because these animals rely on spatial memory for foraging and navigation, impaired memory may affect survival in the wild [86]. *Pseudo-nitzschia* blooms of varying intensity with variable domoic acid production are now recognized as an annual event along the Pacific Coast [9], and bloom frequency and severity may be increasing over time [12]. Communication between the human medical community and veterinarians during bloom events could result in both a more proactive response for poisoned marine mammals (e.g., conducting surveillance for strandings) and earlier shellfish bed closings to protect human consumers.

Manatees have also served as sentinels for adverse health outcomes in people. Studies by Bossart *et al.* [66] describing the effects of brevetoxins on wild manatees provided a hypothesis of what human health effects might be expected following brevetoxin exposures. This research indicated that manatees are exposed to brevetoxins by drinking seawater, eating contaminated seagrass, and by breathing contaminated air at the ocean/air interface. These results highlighted the need for a closer look at the effects of both chronic low-level and periodic high-level brevetoxin exposures in people, including lifeguards who are occupationally exposed, and people with underlying respiratory conditions such as asthma. A study by Backer *et al.* [87] assessed Florida lifeguards over time and found that, while the lifeguards reported respiratory symptoms associated with exposure to brevetoxins during Florida red tide events, they did not appear to have adverse effects on respiratory function, as measured by pulmonary function testing [87]. In contrast, Fleming *et al.* [88] reported subtle changes in pulmonary function and increased self-reported respiratory symptoms in people with asthma following exposure to aerosolized brevetoxins. Studies with the same group of asthmatics revealed increases in self-reported symptoms unaccompanied by changes in pulmonary function, even when brevetoxin exposures were low [89]. Linking the manatee epizootic with exposure to brevetoxins revealed a potential gap in information about human exposures. Prior to investigation of the manatee mass-mortality, scientists and beach managers were aware that beach visitors coughed during periods when there was a *K. brevis* bloom event, but potential health consequences were under-recognized. This gap was addressed with scientific studies that revealed not only potential human health effects from these exposures, but also useful clinical information about how asthmatics understand and communicate the severity of their illness [88,89].

Animals may also serve as sentinels for adverse human health effects from freshwater or estuarine cyanobacteria blooms. As noted above, southern sea otters were poisoned by microcystins produced by a freshwater bloom that drained into Monterey Bay [21]. This event, coupled with studies demonstrating microcystin bioaccumulation by *Microcystis*-exposed marine invertebrates could indicate that seafood harvested by people may be unfit to eat due to elevated microcystin concentrations. Also, medical advances in treating microcystin-poisoned animals could help improve medical care for poisoned people. A recent case report documenting successful treatment of confirmed, severe microcystin poisoning in a dog by Rankin *et al.* [90] provided details of the clinical presentation, successful therapy, and subsequent recovery. The dog was exposed to a *Microcystis* spp.-dominated cyanobacterial bloom in a Montana lake. Within hours, the dog was lethargic and anorexic, and clinical signs rapidly progressed to severe depression and vomiting. A complete blood count and serum chemistry panel were indicative of acute hepatic damage, and feces were positive for microcystin-LA on liquid chromatography/mass spectrometry (LCMS). The dog was hospitalized for eight days and treated supportively. Its clinical condition and hematological parameters continued to decline over the first few days of hospitalization. On day 5 of hospitalization, oral treatment with the bile acid sequestrant cholestyramine was inititated, and marked clinical improvement was noted within 48 h. After seventeen days post-exposure, the dog was clinically normal and remained clinically normal at one year post-exposure. Selection of cholestyramine as an inexpensive, easily administered oral medication with the potential to bind microcystin in the digestive tracts of exposed dogs was based on its efficacy in microcystin-exposed rats [91].

Another medication with potential although unproven benefits for treatment of microcystin poisoning in dogs is silibinin. When administered intravenously as Legalon® SIL, this plant derivative has demonstrated efficacy for treatment of Amanita phalloides hepatoxicity [92–94]. This flavonolignan appears to interact with specific hepatic transport proteins, blocking cellular amatoxin re-uptake and thus interrupting enterohepatic recirculation [94]. Because microcystin causes hepatic damage through a similar mechanism as amatoxin, administering intravenous silibinin may also limit the effects of microcystin intoxication in exposed animals and people. This possibility appears to be supported by experimental data in microcystin-exposed mice and rats; although livers from rats and mice exposed to microcystin-LR revealed severe hepatocellular necrosis, pre-treatment with silymarin abolished the negative effects of microcystin exposure [92] The successful use of cholestyramine and intravenous silibinin to treat microcystin poisoning in animals provides information to support research on similar medical treatments for people.

Surveillance for HAB-related illnesses in people and animals would enhance our knowledge about the occurrence and distribution of these events. For example, the Centers for Disease Control and Prevention (CDC) supported the Harmful Algal Bloom-related Illness Surveillance System (HABISS) from 2009 until 2013. For the period of 2007–2011, Departments of Health and/or Environment from 11 states funded by the National Center for Environmental Health (NCEH), CDC contributed reports for 4534 HAB events, including environmental data and information on animal and human illnesses [80]. More detailed information describing HAB-related canine poisonings from HABISS and other sources were described by Backer *et al.* [79]. The information recorded in HABISS and efforts to apply these data to support a wide range of state-based public health prevention and response activities indicate that HABs are an environmental One Health issue that needs continuing attention (e.g., [95–97]). A new system for surveillance of HAB-related events, disease outbreaks, and cases of illness in people and animals is under development by an internal CDC collaboration between the NCEH and The National Center for Zoonotic, Enteric, and Infectious Diseases. States and other partners will be able to report HAB events, as well as outbreaks and individual cases of HAB-related diseases in people and animals [98].

The number of HAB-related adverse health events affecting animals and people continues to grow. In a one-health approach, information learned about the biological effects from and treatments for exposure to HAB toxins in animals can help determine how to protect and treat humans. Similarly, knowledge gained from the study of human HAB exposures can be used to help protect and treat wild and domestic animals. Table 1 has a summary of the events described in this paper.

Table 1. Summary of animal sentinel systems and events described in this paper.

Animal Sentinel	Event	References
Aquatic invertebrates and fish		
Marine food web organisms	Brevetoxin bioaccumulation associated with *Karenia brevis* blooms in the Gulf of Mexico and subsequent human poisonings.	Flewelling *et al.* (2005) [17]
Invertebrates	Okadaic acid bioaccumulation in Gulf coast oysters associated with algal blooms.	Gulf Coast oyster reefs may be home to emerging infection threat [32]
Mussels, bivalves, other invertebrates	Environmental contaminant bioaccumulation.	Kimbrough *et al.* (2008) [7]
Marine bivalves, crabs	Domoic acid bioaccumulation in marine bivalves and crabs associated with *Pseudonitzschia* spp. blooms in along western coast of US, from southern California to Alaska, subsequent human and animal (e.g., marine mammals, seabirds) poisonings.	Large bloom of toxic algae underway in Monterey Bay and beyond (2015) Massive domoic acid event in Monterey Bay (2015) [14]
Mussels and clams	Saxitoxin bioaccumulation in mussels and clams, subsequent human paralytic shellfish poisonings.	Lewitis *et al.* (2012) [9]
Mussels	Domoic acid bioaccumulation in mussels, subsequent human amnesic shellfish poisonings.	Perl *et al.* (1960); Bates *et al.* (1998) [59,83]
Invertebrates	Saxitoxin bioaccumulation during dinoflagellate blooms, subsequent poisonings.	Shellfish poisonings [31]

Table 1. *Cont.*

Animal Sentinel	Event	References
Aquatic invertebrates and fish		
Diverse species, including razor clams (*Siliqua patula*), mole crabs (*Emerita analoga*), fat innkeeper worms (*Urechis caupo*)	Domoic acid bioconcentration and slow depuration during *Pseudonitzschia* spp. blooms.	Trainer and Suddleson (2005) Goldberg (2003) [12,85]
Pike (*Esox Lucius*)	Algal chemical bioaccumulation make the edges of the pike's fins, tails, and mouths turn bright neon green	The strange case of Yellowknife's neon green pike [48]
Fish, freshwater mollusks, juvenile frogs	Gill-damaging toxin exposure associated with blooms of *Prymnesium parvum*, subsequent asphyxiation.	Toxic golden alga in Texas [49]
Lost River sucker (*Deltistes luxztus*) and shortnose sucker (*Chasmistes brevirostris*)	Cyanobacteria toxins accumulate in rivers and produce hypoxic conditions, subsequent interference with population recovery.	Burdick and Hewitt (2012); Martin *et al.* (2015); Suckerfish and the Klamath Tribe [45–47]
Fish	Cyanobacteria blooms (respiration and bloom decay) produce hypoxic conditions and/or mechanical or hemolytic gill damage and respiratory failure, subsequent fish kills.	Hallegraef (1993) [34]
Commercially-raised marine and estuarine mussels, fish, and other aquatic foods intended for human consumption	Microcystins bioaccumulation associated with cyanobacteria blooms in aquaculture ponds, subsequent poisonings, including net-pen liver disease.	Whangchai *et al.* (2013); Kent *et al.* (1996); Anderson *et al.* (1993) [26,52,53]
Commercially-raised marine and estuarine mussels, fish, and other aquatic foods intended for human consumption	Microcystins bioaccumulation associated with coastal river cyanobacteria blooms contaminating freshwater-to-marine outflows, subsequent animal poisonings.	De Pace *et al.* (2014); Preece *et al.* (2015) [27,28]
Coastal mariculture, including caged yellowtail fish	Toxin bioaccumulation associated with algae blooms.	Hallegraef (1993) [43]
Menhaden and other estuarine fish	Unknown toxin exposure thought to be associated with the presence of *Pfiesteria piscicida*, subsequent fish morbidity and mortality.	Steidinger *et al.* (1996); Glasgow *et al.* (1995); Burkholder *et al.* (1992) [35–37]
Marine mammals		
Miocene-era marine mammals	Hypothesized marine HAB-associated toxins bioaccumulation, subsequent mass strandings.	Peyson *et al.* (2013) [58]
Southern sea otters	Microcystins bioaccumulation in oysters, mussels, clams, and snails associated with coastal river cyanobacteria blooms contaminating freshwater-to-marine outflows, subsequent Southern sea otter poisoning.	Miller *et al.* (2010); Lehman *et al.* (2005); Tanner (2005); Gibble *et al.* (2014); Takahashi *et al.* (2014); Wall (2012) [21–25,29]
California sea lions (*Zalophus californianus*)	Domoic acid bioaccumulation associated with a *Pseudo-nitzschia* spp. bloom, subsequent morbidity and mortality of hundreds of sea lions.	Scholin *et al.* (2000); Gulland *et al.* (2002); Bargu *et al.* (2010); Zabka *et al.* (2009); Brodie *et al.* (2006); Goldstein *et al.* (2007) [60–65]
West Indian (Florida) manatees (*Trichechus manatus latirostris*)	Brevetoxin bioaccumulation associated with *Karenia brevis* bloom, subsequent morbidity and mortality.	Flewelling *et al.* (2005); Bossart *et al.* (1998) [17,66]
Bottlenose dolphins (*Tursiops truncatus*)	Brevetoxin bioaccumulation associated with *Karenia brevis* bloom, subsequent morbidity and mortality.	Flewelling *et al.* (2005) [17]
Birds		
Brown Pelicans (*Pelecanus occidentalis*) and Brandt's Cormorants (*Phalacrocorax penicillatus*) in California	Domoic acid bioaccumulation in anchovies during a large *Pseudonitzchia australis* bloom off the California coast, subsequent seabird poisonings.	Work *et al.* (1993); Algae bloom kills sea birds, other sea life in Southern California in record numbers [68,71]
Sooty shearwaters (*Puffinus griseus*)	Domoic acid accumulation in food web, particularly anchovies.	Bargu *et al.* (2012) [69]
Double crested cormorants (*Phalacrocorax auritus*)	Brevetoxin bioaccumulation associated with *Karenia brevis* bloom, subsequent morbidity and mortality.	Kreuder *et al.* (2002) [72]
Bald eagles (*Haliaeetus leucocephalus*), American coots (*Fulica americana*), and other water birds	Cyanobacteria toxin bioaccumulation in association with eating cyanobacterium-contaminated vegetation.	Fischer *et al.* (2006) [77]
Seabirds	Domoic acid bioaccumulation in association with *Pseudonitzchia* spp. blooms, subsequent mortalities.	Fritz *et al.* (1992) [70]

Table 1. *Cont.*

Animal Sentinel	Event	References
Birds		
Seabirds	Accumulation of surfactant in coastal waters in association with *Akashiwo sanguinea* bloom, subsequent morbidities and mortalities.	Jessup *et al.* (2009) [78]
Terrestrial animals		
Domestic animals	Cyanobacteria toxins accumulation during cyanobacteria bloom in the Murray River water and subsequent animal poisonings.	Francis (1878) [3]
Domestic and wild animals	Cyanobacteria toxins accumulation in drinking water associated with cyanobacteria blooms, subsequent animal poisonings.	Schwimmer and Schwimmer (1968) [4]
Domestic and wild animals	Cyanobacteria toxins accumulation in river water, subsequent poisonings in animals drinking the water.	Stewart *et al.* (2008) [5]
Dogs	Cyanobacteria toxins accumulation in waterbodies, subsequent poisonings from drinking water, swimming, or licking algae from fur.	Backer *et al.* (2013) [79]
Dog	Microcysin exposure associated with swimming in a blooming lake, subsequent poisoning.	Rankin *et al.* (2013) [90]

3. Summary and Conclusions

In the U.S. current state-supported monitoring efforts have prevented many acute foodborne HAB toxin poisonings (*i.e.*, the shellfish poisonings). However, fewer sustainable programs are available to prevent human exposures from HABs in drinking and recreational waters. There are many animals that can serve as sentinels for HAB events, and these sentinels can provide information for public health decision-making. A One Health approach may provide a more complete characterization of HAB events and their consequences, thus limiting both human and animal exposures. Synergized datasets that include simultaneous monitoring of water, algae, people, and animals can more effectively identify high risk areas for HAB events, expedite recognition of potential public health risks, and help catalyze and optimize mitigation and management efforts. Communication and data-sharing across disciplines is critical to our understanding the many nuances of HAB ecology and HAB effects on animals and people.

Author Contributions: Lorraine Backer contributed substantially to the manuscript. Melissa Miller contributed substantially to the manuscript.

References

1. National Research Council. *Animals as Sentinels of Environmental Health Hazards*; National Research Council: Washington, DC, USA, 1991; p. 160.
2. Burrell, G.A.; Siebert, F.M. *Gases Found in Coal Mines*; Miner's Circular 14; Bureau of Mines, Department of the Interior: Washington, DC, USA, 1916.
3. Francis, G. Poisonous Australian Lake. *Nature* **1878**, *18*, 11–12. [CrossRef]
4. Schwimmer, M.; Schwimmer, D. Medical aspects of phycology. In *Algae, Man, and the Environment*; Jackson, A.F., Ed.; Syracuse University Press: Syracuse, NY, USA, 1968; pp. 279–358.
5. Stewart, I.; Seawright, A.A.; Shaw, G.R. Cyanobacterial poisoning in livestock, wild mammals, and birds—An overview. In *Cyanobacterial Harmful Algal Blooms, State of the Science and Research Needs*; Hudnell, H.K., Ed.; Springer: New York, NY, USA, 2008; pp. 613–636.
6. One Health Initiative. Available online: http://onehealthinitiative.com/ (accessed on 1 February 2016).

7.   Kimbrough, K.L.; Johnson, W.E.; Lauenstein, G.G.; Christensen, J.D.; Apeti, D.A. *An Assessment of Two Decades of Contaminant Monitoring in the Nation's Coastal Zone*; NOAA Technical Memorandum NOS NCCOS 74; Silver Spring, MD, USA, 2008; p. 105. Available online: http://ccma.nos.noaa.gov/publications/MWTwoDecades.pdf (accessed on 9 September 2015).

8.   National Status and Trends Mussel Watch Program. Available online: http://www.coris.noaa.gov/metadata/records/html/mw_project.html (accessed on 7 October 2015).

9.   Lewitus, A.J.; Horner, R.A.; Caron, D.A.; Garcia-Mendoza, E.; Hickey, B.M.; Hunter, M.; Huppert, D.D.; Kudela, R.M.; Langlois, G.W.; Largier, J.L.; *et al.* Harmful algal blooms along the North American west coast region: History, trends, causes, and impacts. *Harmful Algae* **2012**, *19*, 133–159. [CrossRef]

10.   Rapid Toxin Testing for Shellfish in FLORIDA. Available online: http://m.myfwc.com/research/redtide/research/current/toxin-testing/ (accessed on 8 September 2015).

11.   New Sensor Array to Monitor Impacts of Changing Gulf of Maine Conditions on New England Red Tide. Available online: http://www.whoi.edu/news-release/redtide (accessed on 8 September 2015).

12.   Trainer, V.L.; Suddleson, M. Monitoring approaches for early warning of domoic acid events in Washington State. *Oceanography* **2005**, *18*, 228–237. [CrossRef]

13.   Trainer, V.L.; Cochlan, W.P.; Erickson, A.; Bill, B.D.; Cox, F.H.; Borchert, J.A.; Lefebvre, K.A. Recent domoic acid closures of shellfish harvest areas in Washington State inland waterways. *Harmful Algae* **2007**, *6*, 449–459. [CrossRef]

14.   Large Bloom of Toxic Algae Underway in Monterey Bay and Beyond. Available online: http://news.ucsc.edu/2015/05/algal-bloom.html (accessed on 8 September 2015).

15.   Massive Domoic Acid Event in Monterey Bay. Available online: http://sanctuarysimon.org/news/2015/05/massive-domoic-acid-event-in-monterey-bay/ (accessed on 5 October 2015).

16.   West Coast Harmful Algal Bloom NOAA Responds to Unprecedented Bloom that Stretches from Central California to the Alaska Peninsula. Available online: http://oceanservice.noaa.gov/news/sep15/westcoast-habs.html (accessed on 4 December 2015).

17.   Flewelling, L.J.; Naar, J.P.; Abbot, J.P.; Baden, D.G.; Barros, N.B.; Bossart, G.D.; Bottein, M.-Y.D.; Hammond, D.G.; Haubold, E.M.; Heil, C.A.; *et al.* Red tides and marine mammal mortalities: Unexpected brevetoxin vectors may account for deaths long after or remote from an algal bloom. *Nature* **2005**, *435*, 755–756. [CrossRef] [PubMed]

18.   Florida Fish and Wildlife Conservation Commission, Fish and Wildlife Research Institute. Available online: http://myfwc.com/research/redtide/ (accessed on 2 October 2015).

19.   Open/Closed Status of Shellfish Areas for Harvesting. Available online: http://shellfish.floridaaquaculture.com/seas/seas_centralgulf.htm (accessed on 5 October 2015).

20.   Florida Fish and Wildlife Conservation Commission, Red Tide Current Status. Available online: http://myfwc.com/research/redtide/statewide/ (accessed on 2 October 2015).

21.   Miller, M.A.; Kudela, R.M.; Mekebri, A.; Crane, D.; Oates, S.C.; Tinker, T.M.; Staedlers, M.; Millere, W.A.; Toy-Choutka, S.; Dominik, C.; *et al.* Evidence for a Novel Marine Harmful Algal Bloom: Cyanotoxin (Microcystin) Transfer from Land to Sea Otters. *PLoS ONE* **2010**, *5*. [CrossRef] [PubMed]

22.   Lehman, P.W.; Boyer, G.; Hall, C.; Waller, S.; Gehrts, K. Distribution and toxicity of a new colonial *Microcystis aeruginosa* bloom in San Francisco Bay Estuary, California. *Hydrogiologia* **2005**, *541*, 87–90. [CrossRef]

23.   Tanner, R.; Kangur, K.; Spoof, L.; Meriluoto, J. Hepatotoxic cyanobacterial peptides in Estonian freshwater bodies and inshore marine water. *Proc. Estonian Acad. Sci. Biol. Ecol.* **2005**, *54*, 40–52.

24.   Gibble, C.M.; Kudela, R.M. Detection of persistent microcystin toxins at the land-sea interface in Monterey Bay, California. *Harmful Algae* **2014**, *39*, 146–153. [CrossRef]

25.   Takahashi, T.; Umehara, A.; Tsutsumi, H. Diffusion of microcystins (cyanobacteria hepatotoxins) from the reservoir of Isahaya Bay, Japan, into the marine and surrounding ecosystems as a result of large-scale drainage. *Mar. Pollut. Bull.* **2014**, *89*, 250–258. [CrossRef] [PubMed]

26.   Whangchai, N.; Wannom, S.; Gutierrez, R.; Kannikia, K.; Promna, R.; Iwami, N.; Itayama, T. Accumulation of microcystins in water and economic fish in Phayap Lake, and fish ponds along the Ing River tributary in Chiang Rai, Thailand. *J. Agric. Sci.* **2013**, *4*, 52–56.

27. De Pace, R.; Valeria, V.; Bucci, M.S.; Gallo, P.; Milena, B. Microcystin contamination in sea mussel farms from the Italian southern Adriatic coast following cyanobacterial blooms in an artificial reservoir. *J. Ecosyst.* **2014**. Available online: http://www.hindawi.com/journals/jeco/2014/374027/ (accessed on 6 October 2015).

28. Preece, E.P.; Moorea, B.C.; Hardy, F.J.; Deobald, L.A. First Detection of Microcystin in Puget Sound, Washington, Mussels (Mytilus trossulus). *Lake Reserv. Manag.* **2015**, *31*, 50–54. [CrossRef]

29. Wall, J.M. Identification and Detection of Cyanobacteria and Their Toxins in Pacific Oysters. Master's Thesis, Master of Science, University of Otago, New Zealand, 2012. Available online: http://hdl.handle.net/10523/2621 (accessed on 28 October 2015).

30. Schmidt, J.R.; Wilhelm, S.W.; Boyer, G.L. The Fate of Microcystins in the Environment and Challenges for Monitoring. *Toxins* **2014**, 3354–3387. [CrossRef] [PubMed]

31. Shellfish Poisonings. Available online: http://www.floridahealth.gov/environmental-health/aquatic-toxins/shellfish-poisoning.html (accessed on 5 October 2015).

32. Gulf Coast Oyster Reefs may be Home to Emerging Infection Threat. Available online: http://blog.al.com/live/2010/04/gulf-coast-oyster-reefs-may-be.html (accessed on 5 October 2015).

33. Great Lakes Environmental Research Laboratory. Available online: http://www.glerl.noaa.gov/res/waterQuality/?targetTab=habs (accessed on 5 October 2015).

34. Hallegraeff, G.M. A review of harmful algal blooms and their apparent global increase. *Phycologia* **1993**, *32*, 79–99. [CrossRef]

35. Steidinger, K.A.; Burkholder, J.M.; Glasgow, H.B.; Hobbs, C.W.; Garrett, J.K.; Truby, E.W.; Noga, E.J.; Smith, S.A. *Pfiesteria piscicida* gen. et sp. nov. (Pfiesteriaceae fam. nov.), a new toxic dinoflagellate with a complex life cycle and behavior. *J. Phycol.* **1996**, *32*, 157–164. [CrossRef]

36. Glasgow, H.B., Jr.; Burkholder, J.M.; Schmechel, D.E.; Tester, P.A.; Rublee, P.A. Insidious effects of a toxic estuarine dinoflagellate on fish survival and human health. *J. Toxicol. Environ. Health* **1995**, *46*, 501–522. [CrossRef] [PubMed]

37. Burkholder, J.M.; Noga, E.J.; Hobbs, C.W.; Glasgow, H.B., Jr. New "phantom" dinoflagellate is the causative agent of major estuarine fish kills. *Nature* **1992**, *358*, 407–410. [CrossRef] [PubMed]

38. Parsons, G.R.; Morgan, A.; Whitehead, J.C.; Haab, T.C. The welfare effects of Pfiesteria-Related fish kills: A contingent behavior analysis of seafood consumers. *Agric. Res. Econ. Rev.* **2006**, *35*, 348–356.

39. Vogelbein, W.K.; Lovko, V.J.; Reece, K.S. Pfiesteria. In *Oceans and Human Health*; Walsh, P.J., Smith, S.L., Fleming, L.E., Solo-Gabriel, H.M., Gerwick, W.H., Eds.; Academic Press: Burlington, MA, USA, 2006; pp. 297–325.

40. Brownie, C.; Glasgow, H.B.; Burkholder, J.M.; Reed, R.; Tang, Y. Re-evaluation of the relationship between *Pfiesteria* and estuarine fish kills. *Ecosystems* **2003**, *6*, 1–10. [CrossRef]

41. Burkholder, J.M.; Marshall, H.G. Toxigenic *Pfiseteria* species—Updates on biology, ecology, toxins, and impacts. *Harmful Algae* **2012**, *14*, 196–230. [CrossRef]

42. Moestrup, O.; Hansen, G.; Daugbjerg, N.; Lundholm, N.; Overton, J.; Vestergard, M.; Steenfeldt, S.J.; Calado, A J.; Hansen, P.J. The dinoflgaellates *Pfiesteria shumwayae* and *Luciella masanensis* cause fish kills in recirculation fish farms in Denmark. *Harmful Algae* **2014**, *32*, 33–39. [CrossRef]

43. Swinker, M.; Koltai, D.; Wilkins, J.; Stopford, W. Is there an estuary associated syndrome in North Carolina? *NCMJ* **2001**, *62*, 126–132. [PubMed]

44. Morris, J.G.; Grattan, L.M.; Wilson, L.A.; Meyer, W.A.; McCarter, R.; Bowers, H.A.; Hebel, J.R.; Matuszak, D.L.; Oldach, D.W. Occupational exposure to *Pfiesteria* species in estuarine waters is not a risk factor for illness. *Environ. Health Perspect.* **2006**, *114*, 1038–1043. [CrossRef] [PubMed]

45. Burdick, S.M.; Hewitt, D.A. *Distribution and Condition of Young-of-Year Lost River and Shortnose Suckers in the Williamson River Delta Restoration Project and Upper Klamath Lake, Oregon, 2008–10—Final Report*; Open-File Report 2012-1098; U.S. Geological Survey: Seattle, WA, USA, 2012; p. 52.

46. Martin, B.; Echols, K.; Feltz, K.; Elliot, D.; Conway, C.M. Effects of microcystin on juvenile Lost River Suckers. In Proceeding of the 145th Annual Meeting, Portland, Oregon, 16–20 August 2015; American Fisheries Society: Bethesda, MD, USA, 2015.

47. Suckerfish and the Klamath Tribe. Available online: http://indiancountrytodaymedianetwork.com/print/2011/02/14/suckerfish-and-klamath-tribe-16763 (accessed on 4 September 2015).

48. The Strange Case of Yellowknife's Neon Green Pike. Available online: http://www.fieldandstream.com/blogs/the-lateral-line/the-strange-case-of-yellowknifes-neon-green-pike (accessed on 17 September 2015).

49. Toxic Golden Alga in Texas. Available online: https://tpwd.texas.gov/landwater/water/environconcerns/hab/media/report.pdf (accessed on 6 October 2015).

50. Golden Alga, What is It? Available online: http://tpwd.texas.gov/landwater/water/environconcerns/hab/ga/ (accessed on 6 October 2015).

51. Golden Alga Frequently Asked Questions. Available online: http://www.azgfd.gov/temp/golden_alga_faqs.shtml (accessed on 6 October 2015).

52. Kent, M.L.; Dawe, S.C.; St. Hilaire, S.; Andersen, R.J. Effects of feeding rate, seawater entry, and exposure to natural biota on the severity of net-Pen liver disease among pen-Reared Atlantic salmon. *Prog. Fish Cult.* **1996**, *58*, 43–46. [CrossRef]

53. Andersen, R.J.; Lu, H.A.; Chen, D.Z.; Holmes, C.F.; Kent, M.L.; Le Blanc, M.; Taylor, F.J.; Williams, D.E. Chemical and biological evidence links microcystins to salmon "netpen liver disease". *Toxicon* **1993**, *10*, 1315–1323. [CrossRef]

54. Friedman, M.A.; Fleming, L.E.; Fernandez, M.; Bienfang, P.; Schrank, K.; Dickey, R.; Bottein, M.-Y.; Backer, L.; Ayyar, R.; Weisman, R.; *et al.* Giguatera fish poisoning: Treatment, prevention, and management. *Mar. Drugs* **2008**, *6*, 456–479. [CrossRef] [PubMed]

55. Bossart, G.D. Marine mammals as sentinel species of oceans and human health. *Vet. Pathol.* **2010**. [CrossRef] [PubMed]

56. Fravel, V.; Van Bonn, W.; Rios, C.; Gulland, F. Meticillin-resistant *Staphylococcus aureus* in a harbor seal (*Phoca vitulina*). *Vet. Rec.* **2011**. [CrossRef] [PubMed]

57. Mazzillo, F.F.M.; Shapiro, K.; Silver, M.W. A new pathogen transmission mechanism in the ocean: The case of sea otter exposure to the land—parasite *Toxoplasma gondii*. *PLoS ONE* **2013**, *8*, e82477. [CrossRef] [PubMed]

58. Peynson, N.D.; Gutstein, C.S.; Parham, J.F.; Le Roux, J.P.; Chavarria, C.C.; Little, H.; Metallo, A.; Rossi, V; Valenzuela-Toro, A.M.; Velez-Juarbe, J.; *et al.* Repeated mass strandings of Miocene marine mammals from Atacama Region of Chile point to sudden death at sea. *Proc. R. Soc. B* **2014**, *281*, 1–9. Available online: http://www.ncbi.nlm.nih.gov/pubmed/24573855 (accessed on 17 September 2015).

59. Perl, T.M.; Bedard, L.; Kosatsky, T.; Hockin, J.C.; Todd, E.C.D.; Remis, R.S. An outbreak of toxic encephalopathy caused by eating mussels contaminated with domoic acid. *N. Engl. J. Med.* **1990**, *322*, 1775–1780. [CrossRef] [PubMed]

60. Scholin, C.A.; Gulland, F.; Doucette, G.J.; Benson, S.; Busman, M.; Chavez, F.P.; Cordaro, J.; DeLong, R.; De Voeglaera, A.; Harvey, J.; *et al.* Mortality of sea lions along the central California coast linked to a toxic diatom bloom. *Nature* **2000**, *403*, 80–84. [CrossRef] [PubMed]

61. Gulland, F.M.D.; Haulena, M.; Fauquier, D.; Langlois, G.; Lander, M.E.; Zabka, T.; Duerr, R. Domoic acid toxicity in California sea lions (*Zalophus californianius*): Clinical signs, treatment and survival. *Vet. Rec.* **2002**, *150*, 475–480. [CrossRef] [PubMed]

62. Bargu, S.; Silver, M.; Goldstein, T.; Roberts, K.; Gulland, F. Complexity of domoic acid-related sea lion strandings in Monterey Bay, California: Foraging patterns, climate events, and toxic blooms. *Mar. Ecol. Prog. Ser.* **2010**, *418*, 213–222. [CrossRef]

63. Zabka, T.S.; Goldstein, T.; Cross, C.; Mueller, R.W.; Kreuder-Johnson, C.; Gill, S.; Gulland, F.M.D. Characterization of a degenerative cardiomyopathy associated with domoic acid toxicity in California sea lions (*Zalophus californianus*). *Vet. Pathol.* **2009**, *46*, 105–119. [CrossRef] [PubMed]

64. Brodie, E.C.; Gulland, F.M.D.; Greig, D.J.; Hunter, M.; Jaakola, J.; St. Leger, J.; Leighfield, T.A.; Van Dolah, F.M. Domoic acid causes reproductive failure in California sea lions (*Zalophus califonianus*). *Mar. Mammal Sci.* **2006**, *22*, 700–707. [CrossRef]

65. Goldstein, T.; Mazet, J.A.K.; Zabka, T.S.; Langlois, G.; Colegrove, K.M.; Silver, M.; Bargu, S.; Van Dolah, F.; Leighfield, T.; Conrad, P.A.; *et al.* Novel symptomatology and changing epidemiology of domoic acid toxicosis in California sea lions (*Zalophus californianus*): An increasing risk to marine mammal health. *Proc. R. Soc. B* **2008**, *275*, 267–276. [CrossRef] [PubMed]

66. Bossart, G.D.; Baden, D.G.; Ewing, R.Y.; Roberts, B.; Wright, S.C. Brevetoxicosis in manatees (*Trichechus manatus latirostris*) from the 1996 epizootic: Gross, histologic, and immunohistochemical features. *J. Environ. Toxicol. Pathol.* **1998**, *26*, 276–282. [CrossRef]

67. The Prevalence of Cyanotoxins in Southern California Waterbodies. Available online: http://www.mywaterquality.ca.gov/monitoring_council/bioaccumulation_oversight_group/docs/2012/nov/150pm_howard_fetscher.pdf (accessed on 6 October 2015).

68. Work, T.M.; Barr, B.; Beale, A.M.; Fritz, L.; Quilliam, M.A.; Wright, J.L.C. Epidemiology of domoic acid poisoning in brown pelicans (*Pelecanus occidentalis*) and Brandt's cormorants (*Phalacrocorax penicillatus*) in California. *J. Zoo Wildl. Med.* **1993**, *24*, 54–62.

69. Bargu, S.; Silver, M.W.; Ohman, M.D.; Benitez-Nelson, C.R.; Garrison, D.L. Mystery behind Hitchcock's birds. *Nat. Geosci.* **2012**, *5*, 2–3. [CrossRef]

70. Fritz, L.; Quilliam, M.A.; Wright, J.L.C.; Beale, A.M.; Work, T.M. An outbreak of domoic acid poisoning attributed to the pennate diatom *Pseudo-nitzschia australis*. *J. Phycol.* **1992**, *28*, 439–442. [CrossRef]

71. Algae Bloom Kills Sea Birds, Other Sea Life in Southern California in Record Numbers. Available online: http://www.sciencedaily.com/releases/2007/04/070427084149.htm (accessed on 6 October 2015).

72. Kreuder, C.; Mazet, J.A.; Bossart, G.D.; Carpenter, T.E.; Holyoak, M.; Elie, M.S.; Wright, S.D. Clinicopathologic features of suspected brevetoxicosis in double-crested cormorants (*Phalacrocorax auritus*) along the Florida Gulf Coast. *J. Zoo Wildl. Med.* **2002**, *33*, 8–15. [PubMed]

73. Thomas, N.J.; Meteyer, C.U.; Sileo, L. Epizootic vacuolar myelinopathy of the central nervous system of bald eagles (*Haliaeetus leucocephalus*) and American coots (*Fulica americana*). *Vet. Pathol.* **1998**, *35*, 479–487. [CrossRef] [PubMed]

74. Rocke, T.E.; Miller, K.; Augspurger, T.; Thomas, N.J. Epizootiologic studies of avaian vacularo melinopathy in water birds. *J. Wildl. Dis.* **2002**, *38*, 678–684. [CrossRef] [PubMed]

75. Wilde, S.B.; Murphy, T.M.; Hope, C.P.; Habrun, S.K.; Kempton, J.; Birrenkott, A.; Wiley, F.; Bowerman, W.W.; Lewitus, A.J. Avian vacuolar myelinopathy linked to exotic aquatic plants and a novel cyanobacteria species. *Environ. Toxicol.* **2005**, *20*, 348–353. [CrossRef] [PubMed]

76. Wilde, S.B.; Johansen, J.R.; Wilde, H.D.; Jiang, P.; Bartelme, B.A.; Haynie, R.S. Aetokthonos hydrillicola gen. et sp. nov: Epiphytic cyanobacteria on invasive aquatic plants implicated in avian vacuolar myelinopathy. *Phytotaxa* **2014**, *181*, 243–260. [CrossRef]

77. Fischer, J.R.; Lewis-Weis, L.A.; Tate, C.M.; Gaydos, J.K.; Gerhold, R.W.; Poppenga, R.H. Avian vacuolar myelinopathy outbreaks at a southeaster reservoir. *J. Wildl. Dis.* **2006**, *42*, 501–510. [CrossRef] [PubMed]

78. Jessup, D.A.; Miller, M.A.; Ryan, J.P.; Nevins, H.M.; Kerkering, H.A.; Mekebri, A.; Crane, D.B.; Johnson, T.A.; Kudela, R.M. Mass stranding of marine birds caused by a surfactant-producing red tide. *PLoS ONE* **2009**, *4*. [CrossRef] [PubMed]

79. Backer, L.C.; Landsberg, J.H.; Miller, M.; Keel, K.; Taylor, T.K. Canine Cyanotoxin Poisonings in the United States (1920s–2012): Review of Suspected and Confirmed Cases from Three Data Sources. *Toxins* **2013**, *5*, 1597–1628. [CrossRef] [PubMed]

80. Backer, L.C.; Manasaram-Baptiste, D.; LePrell, R.; Bolton, B. Cyanobacteria and algae blooms: Review of health and environmental data from the harmful algal bloom-related illness surveillance system (HABIS) 2007–2011. *Toxins* **2015**, *7*, 1048–1064. [CrossRef] [PubMed]

81. CDC. One Health. Available online: http://www.cdc.gov/onehealth/ (accessed on 1 February 2016).

82. Fleming, L.E.; Kirpatrick, B.; Backer, L.C.; Walsh, C.J.; Nierenberg, K.; Clark, J.; Reich, A.; Hollenbeck, J.; Benson, J.; Cheng, Y.S.; *et al.* Review of Florida red tide and human health effects. *Harmful Algae* **2011**, *10*, 224–233. [CrossRef] [PubMed]

83. Bates, S.S.; Bird, C.J.; de Freitas, A.S.W.; Foxall, R.; Gilgan, M.; Hanic, L.A.; Johnson, G.R.; McCulloch, A.W.; Odense, P.; Pocklington, R.; *et al.* Pennate Diatom *Nitzschia pungens* as the Primary Source of Domoic Acid, a Toxin in Shellfish from Eastern Prince Edward Island, Canada. *Can. J. Fish Aquat. Sci.* **1989**, *46*, 1203–1215. [CrossRef]

84. Mos, L. Domoic acid: A fascinating marine toxin. *Environ. Toxicol. Pharmcol.* **2001**, *9*, 79–85. [CrossRef]

85. Goldberg, J.D. Domoic Acid in the Benthic Food Web of Monterey Bay, California. Master's Thesis, University Monterey Bay, Moss Landing Marine Laboratories, Moss Landing, CA, USA, 2003.

86. Cook, P.F.; Reichmuth, C.; Rouse, A.A.; Libby, L.A.; Dennison, S.E.; Carmichael, O.T.; Kruse-Elliot, K.T.; Bloom, J.; Singh, B.; Fravel, V.A.; *et al.* Algal toxin impairs sea lion memory and hippocampal connectivity, with implications for strandings. *Sciencexpress* **2015**. [CrossRef] [PubMed]

87. Backer, L.C.; Kirkpatrick, B.; Fleming, L.E.; Cheng, Y.S.; Pierce, R.; Bean, J.A.; Clark, R.; Johnson, D.; Wanner, A.; Tamer, R.; *et al.* Occupational Exposure to Aerosolized Brevetoxins during Florida Red Tide Events: Impacts on a Healthy Worker Population. *Environ. Health Perspect.* **2005**, *113*, 644–649. [CrossRef] [PubMed]

88. Fleming, L.E.; Kirkpatrick, B.; Backer, L.C.; Bean, J.A.; Wanner, A.; Dalpra, D.; Tamer, R.; Zaias, J.; Cheng, Y.S.; Pierce, R.; *et al.* Initial Evaluation of the Effects of Aerosolized Florida Red Tide Toxins (Brevetoxins) in Persons with Asthma. *Environ. Health Perspect.* **2005**, *113*, 650–657. [CrossRef] [PubMed]

89. Fleming, L.E.; Kirkpatrick, B.; Backer, L.C.; Bean, J.A.; Wanner, A.; Reich, A.; Zaias, J; Cheng, Y.S.; Pierce, R.; Naar, J.; *et al.* Aerosolized Red Tide Toxins (Brevetoxins) and Asthma. *Chest* **2006**, *13*, 187–194. [CrossRef] [PubMed]

90. Rankin, K.A.; Alroy, K.A.; Kudela, R.M.; Oates, S.C.; Murray, M.J.; Miller, M.A. Treatment of cyanobacteria (microcystin) toxicosis using oral cholestyramine: Case report of a dog from Montana. *Toxins* **2013**, *5*, 1051–1063. [CrossRef] [PubMed]

91. Dahlem, A.M.; Hassan, A.S.; Swanson, S.P.; Carmichael, W.W.; Beasley, V.R. A model system for studying the bioavailablity of intestinally administered microcystin-LR, a hepatotoxic peptide from the cyanobacterium *Microcystis Aeruginosa. Pharm. Toxicol.* **1989**, *64*, 177–181. [CrossRef]

92. Mereish, K.A.; Bunner, D.L.; Ragland, D.R.; Creasia, D.A. Protection against microcytsin-LR-induced hepatotoxicity by silymarin: Biochemistry, histopathology, and lethality. *Pharm. Res.* **1991**, *8*, 273–277. [CrossRef] [PubMed]

93. Saller, R.; Meier, R.; Brignoli, R. The use of silymarin in the treatment of liver diseases. *Drugs* **2001**, *61*, 2035–2063. [CrossRef] [PubMed]

94. Mengs, U.; Pohl, R.-T.; Mitchell, T. Legalon® SIL: The antidote of choice in patients with acute hepatotoxicity from amatoxin poisoning. *Curr. Pharm. Biotechnol.* **2012**, *13*, 1964–1970. [CrossRef] [PubMed]

95. Florida Department of Environmental Protection. Information on Freshwater Algal Blooms. Available online: http://dep.state.fl.us/labs/biology/hab/index.htm (accessed on 1 February 2016).

96. Virginia Department of Health. Harmful Algal Blooms (HABS). Available online: https://www.vdh.virginia.gov/epidemiology/DEE/HABS/index.htm (accessed on 1 February 2016).

97. Anderson-Abbs, B.A.; Howard, M.; Taberski, K.M.; Worcester, K.R. California Freshwater Harmful Algal Blooms Assessment and Support Strategy. Available online: http://www.waterboards.ca.gov/sanfranciscobay/water_issues/programs/SWAMP/HABstrategy_phase%201.pdf (accessed on 1 February 2016).

98. Centers for Disease Control and Prevention. National Outbreak Reporting System. Available online: http://www.cdc.gov/nors/ (accessed on 2 September 2015).

13

An Alternative Vaccination Approach for The Prevention of Highly Pathogenic Avian Influenza Subtype H5N1 in The Red River Delta, Vietnam — A Geospatial-Based Cost-Effectiveness Analysis

Chinh C. Tran [1,2,*], John F. Yanagida [1], Sumeet Saksena [2] and Jefferson Fox [2]

[1] Department of Natural Resources and Environmental Management, University of Hawaii at Manoa, 1910 East-West Road, Honolulu, HI 96822, USA; jyanagid@hawaii.edu

[2] East-West Center, 1601 East-West Road, Honolulu, HI 96848, USA; saksenas@eastwestcenter.org (S.S.); foxj@eastwestcenter.org (J.F.)

* Correspondence: chinh.tran@hawaii.edu

Academic Editors: Duncan C. Ferguson and Margarethe Hoenig

Abstract: This study addresses the tradeoff between Vietnam's national poultry vaccination program, which implemented an annual two-round HPAI H5N1 vaccination program for the entire geographical area of the Red River Delta during the period from 2005–2010, and an alternative vaccination program which would involve vaccination for every production cycle at the recommended poultry age in high risk areas within the Delta. The *ex ante* analysis framework was applied to identify the location of areas with high probability of HPAI H5N1 occurrence for the alternative vaccination program by using boosted regression trees (BRT) models, followed by weighted overlay operations. Cost-effectiveness of the vaccination programs was then estimated to measure the tradeoff between the past national poultry vaccination program and the alternative vaccination program. *Ex ante* analysis showed that the focus areas for the alternative vaccination program included 1137 communes, corresponding to 50.6% of total communes in the Delta, and located primarily in the coastal areas to the east and south of Hanoi. The cost-effectiveness analysis suggested that the alternative vaccination program would have been more successful in reducing the rate of disease occurrence and the total cost of vaccinations, as compared to the national poultry vaccination program.

Keywords: HPAI H5N1; alternative vaccination program; national poultry vaccination program; Red River Delta

---

1. Introduction

The Highly Pathogenic Avian Influenza (HPAI) subtype H5N1 has had serious, detrimental effects on the economy and human health in Vietnam since the first reported outbreak on 27 December 2003 [1]. Millions of poultry were culled due to disease occurrences, causing an estimated economic loss of 3 trillion VND (approximately U.S. $187.15 million) [2,3]. The average growth rate of poultry population was reduced from 7.6% for the period 2000–2003 (before HPAI H5N1 occurrence) to 3.8% for the period 2003–2006 (during HPAI H5N1 disease occurrence) [4]. Market demand and price decreases caused further economic losses to poultry producers [5,6]. The disease also seriously affected human health. By 19 November 2010, a total of 119 human cases of HPAI H5N1 were reported, with 59 deaths [7].

Financial support from many international organizations, including the Food and Agriculture Organization (FAO) of the United Nations, the World Bank, the World Health Organization, and others, helped to contain the disease as designed in the Integrated National Operational Program for

Avian and Human Influenza (OPI) which is also known as the *Green Book* [8]. The overall objective of the OPI was to reduce the health risk to humans by controlling the HPAI H5N1 disease at the source in domestic poultry. The national poultry vaccination campaign was a key strategic plan in the OPI [8] (we hereby use the term "national poultry vaccination program" throughout the study). After the pilot vaccinations implemented in Nam Dinh and Tien Giang provinces in August 2005, a mass vaccination campaign was conducted nationally from late September to the beginning of November, 2005 and continued until the end of 2010. The vaccination was applied nationally in two rounds per year with the first round from April–May and the second round from October–November. The vaccination program continued in later years, but on a smaller scale, and was primarily determined and implemented by provincial authorities.

Vaccination has been shown to be a viable means of protection against the HPAI H5N1 virus [9]. While the campaign was carried out only twice a year in April–May and October–November, poultry production, however, occurs all year round. A previous study confirmed that November to January and April to June were the periods that are most vulnerable for disease occurrence [5]. A sizeable proportion of poultry population remained unvaccinated at different times of the year. Therefore, unvaccinated poultry between the two rounds of vaccinations will be at risk of infection. As a result, the disease has been repeatedly reported over the years. Circulation of the HPAI H5N1 virus was found mostly in unvaccinated waterfowl, especially ducks [10,11]. Additionally, the cost of the vaccination program was estimated to be approximately U.S. $10 million per round [7,12,13].

Therefore, it is critical to explore implications of an alternative vaccination program, which is likely to be more successful in containing and preventing the disease from recurrence in the Red River Delta, Vietnam, and reducing total vaccination costs as compared to the national poultry vaccination program implemented in the period 2005–2010. This study focuses on the Red River Delta of Vietnam. This area has been identified as a high-risk area for the disease [10,14]. Vaccination was implemented across all geographical areas for all provinces in the Delta under the national poultry vaccination program.

A number of studies have identified factors affecting the occurrence and spread of the HPAI H5N1 virus in Vietnam, in general, and in the Red River Delta, in particular. It was suggested that higher average monthly temperatures and poultry density in combination with lower average monthly precipitation, humidity, and elevation significantly affected the occurrence of HPAI H5N1 in the Delta [5]. Other factors linked with the disease at the national level were a higher proportion of land used for rice paddy fields and aquaculture, increases in production, trade and movement of live poultry, and the expansion of free-grazing ducks [14–17].

Given these findings, it is not likely that all areas within the Red River Delta are equally susceptible to the disease. We propose an alternative vaccination program which involves shifting from a less frequent blanket vaccination for the entire Delta to more frequent vaccination in high probability areas for disease occurrence within the Delta. This modification would involve vaccination for every production cycle at the recommended poultry age in high risk areas. Two key questions emerge with this proposal: (i) Where are the higher probability areas (focus areas) for the alternative vaccination program? (ii) Is it beneficial for the Government to switch to the alternative vaccination program in terms of the cost-effectiveness of vaccination programs? To answer questions and fulfill the objective, this study (i) identifies the focus areas for the alternative vaccination program to be implemented in the Red River Delta, and (ii) estimates the tradeoff between the national poultry vaccination program and the alternative vaccination program based on the cost-effectiveness analysis of vaccination programs.

2. Methods

2.1. Study Area and Data Sources

This study focuses on the Red River Delta of Vietnam (Figure 1), which represents one of the two largest flood plains in Vietnam. The Delta includes two large river systems—the Red river and Thai Binh river systems—that support agricultural and livestock activities. The Red River Delta includes eight provinces and two municipalities, the capital city of Hanoi and the main port of Hai Phong. The Delta plays an important role and interacts with a wide range of environmental and socioeconomic sectors, including industry, commerce, services, agriculture, tourism, *etc.* Livestock production is among the main activities in the Delta, including poultry, pig, and cow husbandry. Poultry production has faced serious problems caused by the HPAI H5N1 disease.

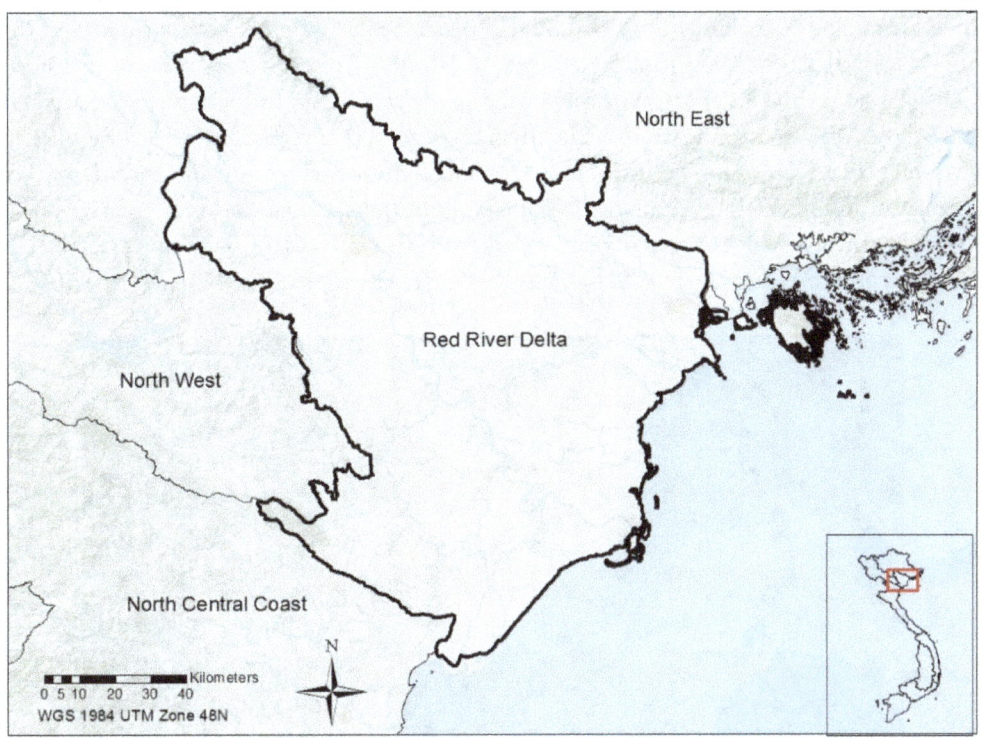

Figure 1. The study area—the Red River Delta, Vietnam.

The HPAI H5N1 outbreak data are routinely collected and reported by the Vietnam Department of Animal Health. The Red River Delta has been identified as a high-risk area for the disease [10,14]. The Delta has been severely affected by three out of the five large epidemic waves of HPAI H5N1 outbreaks reported in Vietnam. These three waves included the first wave, which occurred from December 2003–February 2004, the third wave was recorded from October–December 2005, and the fifth wave reported from May–September 2007 [14,18]. A number of outbreaks in the second epidemic wave which was from November 2004 to March 2005 were also reported in the Red River Delta despite the primary effects occurring in the Mekong Delta. Other sporadic outbreaks occurred over the period from December 2003 to the present, with recent reported outbreaks in Bac Ninh and Nam Dinh provinces in January and February 2014 [1]. Although the disease occurred in the Delta with the first epidemic wave reported from the end of 2003, the dates and locations of occurrences were not formally reported until the end of March 2004 [14]. Therefore, this study analyzed reported disease data for the period starting from the end of March, 2004, to the end of December, 2007, which included four large epidemic waves of HPAI H5N1 outbreaks with 267 confirmed HPAI H5N1 outbreaks in the Red River Delta. The data were reported at the commune level and coded as 1 if the disease was found or 0 if there was no disease reported.

Other risk factors used for the analysis were identified based on earlier studies of HPAI H5N1 in Vietnam. These included the percentage of land used for rice paddy fields and aquaculture [14,19], chicken and water bird density [4,14,15] and elevation [5,14,17]. Land use diversity was found to be significantly associated with disease occurrence [19]. Land use/land cover is dominated by forests and permanent vegetation in high elevation areas, and characterized by agriculture and a mixed uses of land in low elevation areas [17]. Disease occurrence was also found around heavily-populated cities in different regions in Vietnam such as Ho Chi Minh city in the South, Da Nang city in the central part, and Hanoi and Hai Phong cities in the north [14]. Therefore, two other land use factors, characterizing built-up and forest/perennial trees features, were also included.

These variables, percentage of land use for rice paddy fields, aquaculture, built-up and forest/perennial trees, and chicken and water bird density, were measured at the commune level and obtained from The 2006 Vietnam Rural, Agricultural and Fishery Census provided by the East West Center–National Science Foundation project, "Coupled Natural-Human Systems and Emerging Infectious Diseases: Anthropogenic environmental change and avian influenza in Vietnam". Elevation data were obtained from the Shuttle Radar Topography Mission (SRTM) 90-m resolution Digital Elevation Model (DEM) [20]. These data were then retrieved for each commune and merged with other data using commune codes for the statistical analysis. Remotely sensed Landsat TM/ETM+ Bands 1–5, 7 data that cover the study area were downloaded from the USGS EROS Data Center [21]. The Red River Delta is covered by four Landsat tiles: P126R045, P126R046, P127R045, and P127R046 (Figure 2).

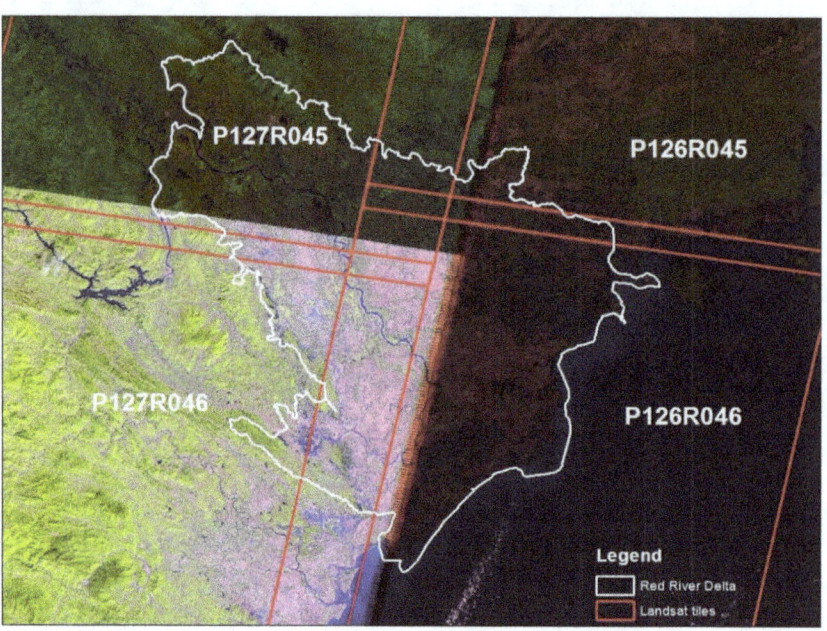

Figure 2. Landsat tiles covering the Red River Delta of Vietnam.

2.2. Statistical Analysis

For the first objective involving identification of focus areas for the alternative vaccination program in the Red River Delta, this study adopted the *ex ante* analysis framework. Outbreak data were divided into two datasets. The first dataset contained the data before the launch of the national poultry vaccination program in 2005, which included the second and the third epidemic waves, with a total of 193 outbreaks. The second dataset consisted of outbreak data that occurred after 2005 which comprised the fifth epidemic wave with 74 outbreaks. The use of the first dataset was to identify focus locations for the alternative vaccination program. The second dataset would be used to evaluate the cost and effectiveness of the vaccination program in analyzing the tradeoff between the national poultry vaccination program and alternative vaccination program.

2.2.1. *Ex Ante* Analysis

For *ex ante* analysis, weighted overlay analysis was applied to identify the focus locations for the alternative vaccination program. This method has been considered as one of the most suitable techniques and is frequently used for site selection and suitability models in spatial analysis [22].

It has been widely applied in several fields, e.g., disease management, climate change, habitat conservation, sustainable ecosystems, and land-use planning, *etc.* [23–27]. This technique requires that all input factors are classified into different groups and weighted to determine their weight accordingly. The analytical procedure for weighted overlay analysis in this study involved a two-stage process: (1) boosted regression trees (BRT), followed by (2) weighted overlay operations.

The first step is to run BRT to determine the appropriate weighting for the main factors that were previously found to have significant effects on disease occurrence, including water bird density, chicken density, elevation, and land use/land cover (Table 1). BRT utilizes a combination of decision trees and boosting algorithms to improve prediction accuracy through an iterative process [28,29]. This method has been popularly applied for predicting the distribution of HPAI H5N1 disease [19,30–33]. Several combinations of the learning rate and tree complexity were tested to choose the best setting for evaluating model performance which was determined through cross-validation (CV). The final model setting was the combination of a tree complexity of 4 and a learning rate of 0.005, with a bag fraction of 0.75, which were also previously used in [30]. The results present which factors appear to have more influence on the disease occurrence in the Red River Delta.

Table 1. Critical factors affecting the disease occurrence.

Factors	Data Sources	Attribute Values of Factors
Water bird density (heads/km^2)	The 2006 Vietnam Rural, Agricultural and Fishery Census	0–892 893–2097 2098–4299 >4299
Chicken density (heads/km^2)	The 2006 Vietnam Rural, Agricultural and Fishery Census	0–1738 1739–3992 3993–9472 >9472
Elevation (m)	SRTM 90-m resolution DEM: http://srtm.csi.cgiar.org/ [20]	$\leqslant$5 >5–15 >15–200 >200
Land use/land cover (%)	The 2006 Vietnam Rural, Agricultural and Fishery Census	Agriculture Aquaculture Built-up Forest/perennial trees

Each factor has its own characteristics that also have impacts on the disease. The next step is to measure the weights of attribute values of each factor. The land use/land cover included land for agriculture, aquaculture, built-up purposes, and forest/perennial tree areas. The Red River Delta topography was reclassified into four groups of elevation (above 200 m, from 15 m to 200 m, from 5 m to 15 m, and less than 5 m) and coded from 1 to 4, respectively, to represent upland, midland, lowland, and coastal areas (see [5]). Other factors were categorized into four groups by using the commonly-used Jenks natural breaks classification method [34] in ArcGIS to group data into categories (Table 1).

The second step determined the potential focus area for the vaccination program by performing weighted overlay analysis in ArcGIS 10.1 (ESRI, Redlands, CA, USA). The analysis was operated in raster layers. Therefore, vector layers detailing water bird density and chicken density at the commune level were converted to corresponding raster layers. The elevation data were originally stored in raster format. For the spatial distribution of land use/land cover, a support vector machine (SVM) was applied to classify remotely-sensed imagery data in the Red River Delta into four categories that represent built-up, agriculture, forest/perennial trees, and water areas. The SVM method has been successfully applied in several studies on biophysical tasks, land cover/land use including vegetation, agriculture, and impervious surfaces, such as urban areas, *etc.* [35–37]. The classification process was performed using ENVI version 4.8 (Exelis Visual Information Solutions, Boulder, CO, USA) and ArcGIS version 10.1 (ESRI, Redlands, CA, USA). Outputs were the classification maps of land use/land cover for each subset and were mosaiced together to produce the final land use/land cover classification map for the Red River Delta.

All raster layers were then reclassified using the corresponding weight obtained from BRT results for the weighted overlay operations processed in ArcGIS version 10.1 to find the suitable areas for the alternative vaccination program. The analysis provides suitability maps with suitability scores in integer numbers scaled from 0 to 100. The higher suitability scores represent the higher probability of contracting the HPAI H5N1 disease. Areas with higher suitability scores are suggested as good candidates where the alternative vaccination program should be focused.

2.2.2. The Cost-Effectiveness Analysis

For the tradeoff between the past national poultry vaccination program and the alternative vaccination program, the cost and effectiveness of the vaccination program were estimated for each program. The second dataset which included data for the fifth epidemic wave with 74 affected communes was used in addition to the first dataset. To implement the vaccination program, the government is responsible for all the costs, including the costs of vaccine, labor, and other costs associated with vaccination. The costs for the vaccination program are the product of the number of birds vaccinated, the cost of vaccination per bird, and the number of vaccination rounds per year. When the disease occurs, the Vietnamese government implements the stamping out method, which culls all birds in affected communes and emergency vaccination is deployed to vaccinate all birds in surrounding communes in order to contain and prevent the disease from spreading. These are extra costs of the vaccination program. The total cost of the vaccination program is comprised of the cost of the government vaccination program, the cost of emergency vaccination, government compensation for birds culled, and farmer's losses because of the value difference between market price and the government's compensation when the disease occurs.

$$\text{Cost} = A \times C \times N + B \times C + I \times G + (P - G) \times I \tag{1}$$

where A is the number of birds vaccinated; C is the costs of vaccination per bird; N is the number of vaccination rounds per year; B is the number of birds vaccinated because of emergency vaccination; I is the number of birds culled due to the disease occurrence; G is the government compensation per bird culled; and P is the market price per bird.

The effectiveness of the vaccination program is the measure of proportionate reduction in the rate of disease occurrence as the result of the vaccination program. This can be achieved through the calculation based on the relative risk of the disease [38].

$$\text{Effectiveness} = \frac{\text{ARU-ARV}}{\text{ARU}} \times 100 \tag{2}$$

where ARU and ARV are, respectively, the infection rates before and after the launch of the vaccination program. The infection rate is the number of affected communes divided by the total communes in the Red River Delta.

3. Results and Discussion

3.1. Results

3.1.1. *Ex Ante* Analysis

The BRT results (see Table 2) suggest that water bird density had the largest effect on disease occurrence with the weight estimated at 19%. Ducks, as a reservoir host for the HPAI H5N1 virus, have been discussed in earlier studies [10,16,17,39–42]. The number of recorded duck-related disease occurrences steadily increased from 11% in 2003/2004 to its peak of 78% in 2006/2007 [10]. The next highest weight factors were land used for rice paddy field, elevation, land used for aquaculture, land used for built-up purposes, chicken density, and land used for forest/perennial trees. Land used for forest/perennial trees had the smallest effect with 2% weight.

Table 2. Estimated weight of each factor to the HPAI H5N1 occurrences.

Variable	Weight (%)
Water bird density	19
Land used for rice paddy field	18
Elevation	18
Land used for aquaculture	17
Land used for built-up purposes	14
Chicken density	12
Land used for forest/perennial trees	2

Table 3 reveals the weight of attribute values of each factor; lower water bird density and chicken density were found to have higher weight as compared to other groups within each factor. Specifically, water bird density ranging from 893–2097 heads/km^2 had the highest weight of 76% for the water bird density factor. Chicken density attributes ranging from 0–1738 heads/km^2 showed the highest weight of 37%. Elevation less than 5 m was estimated to have a 73% weight. These were flat plain areas where rice production was the predominant agricultural activity in the Red River Delta. Lowlands with elevation ranging from 5–15 m, and midland areas with elevation ranging from 15–200 m, were ranked the second and third with 26% and 11% weights, respectively. These areas were located to the west of the Delta, including the capital city of Hanoi. Land used for rice production also had the highest contribution to disease occurrence with a 46% weight and followed by land used for built-up purposes at 35%.

Table 3. Attribute weight of each group within a factor.

Factors	Attribute Values of Factors	Attribute Weight (%)
Water bird density (heads/km^2)	0–892	11
	893–2097	76
	2098–4299	7
	>4299	6
Chicken density (heads/km^2)	0–1738	37
	1739–3992	27
	3993–9472	25
	>9472	11
Elevation (m)	⩽5	73
	>5–15	16
	>15–200	11
	>200	0
Land use/land cover (%)	Agriculture	46
	Built-up	35
	Aquaculture	17
	Forest/perennial trees	2

The BRT estimation results provided essential information for weighted overlay analysis. The weight of each attribute in Table 3 was assigned to corresponding groups in each raster layer through raster reclassification processes. For instance, in the land-use raster, agriculture, built-up, water, and forest/perennial trees groups were, respectively, assigned their corresponding weight values of 46,

35, 17, and 2 (Table 3). The same procedure was applied to other raster layers detailing water bird density, chicken density, and elevation. Each of the input rasters was then weighed using the weighted values from Table 2. In this weighted overlay analysis, water bird density had a 19% weight, land used for rice paddy field an 18% weight, elevation an 18% weight, land used for aquaculture a 17% weight, land used for built-up purposes a 14% weight, chicken density a 12% weight, and land used for forest/perennial trees a 2% weight. The output suitability map is shown in Figure 3.

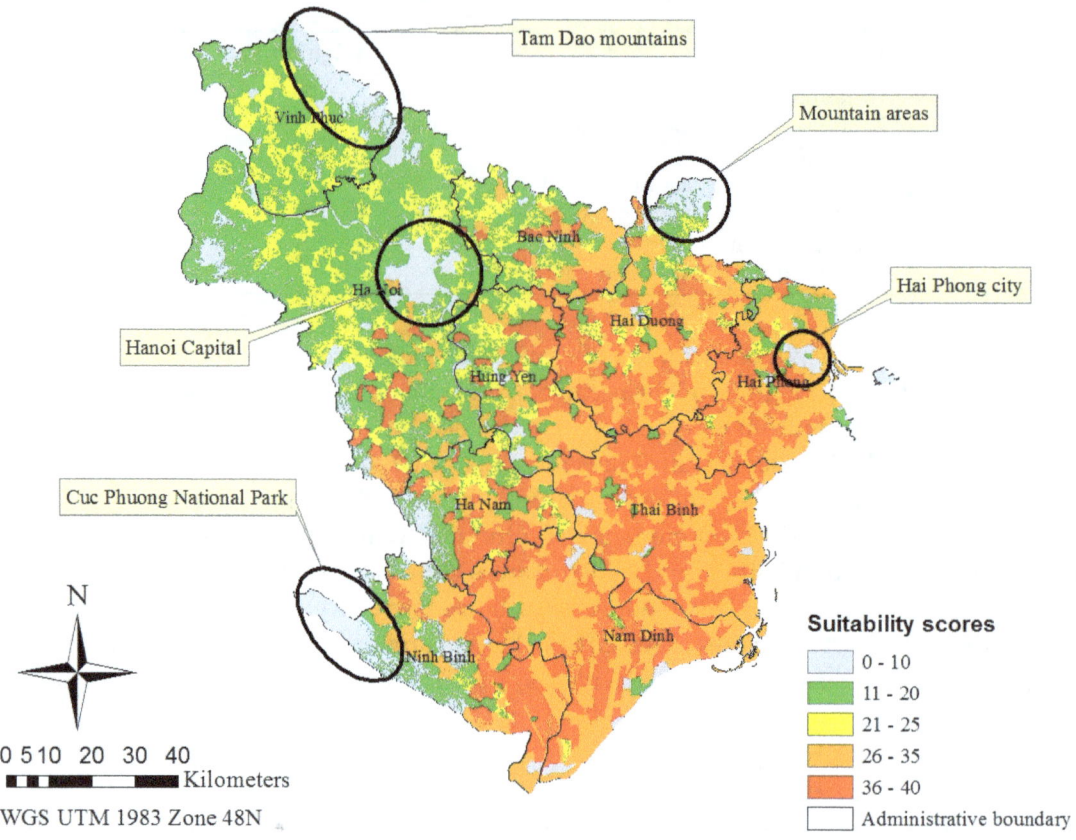

Figure 3. Weighted overlay analysis results for the HPAI H5N1 occurrence in the Red River Delta.

The highest suitability score areas were shown in red, followed by orange. Yellow, green, and blue areas have lower suitability scores. These areas (suitability scores ranging from 0–10, 11–20, and 21–25, respectively) were mostly located to the west and northwest of the Red River Delta. The areas with high suitability scores (ranging from 26–40), as shown in red and orange, were chosen as the focus areas for the alternative vaccination program against HPAI H5N1.

3.1.2. Cost-Effectiveness Analysis of Vaccination Programs and Policy Implications

The focus areas for the alternative vaccination program were extracted and overlaid with the spatial distribution of the fifth HPAI H5N1 (Figure 4a) for the cost-effectiveness analysis. The fifth wave of outbreak, with 74 affected communes, was the result of the national poultry vaccination program. Based on the Vietnam follow-up disease report No. 45 released by OIE (The World Organisation for Animal Health) for the period from December 2006 to December 2010 [43], we found that the disease was mostly reported in unvaccinated poultry. Vaccines mainly used in Vietnam contain a killed antigen combined with an oil-based adjuvant: (1) A/TK/England/N-28/73, subtype H5N2 (referred to as N28); and (2) a genetically modified reassortant H5N1 low-pathogenic virus, A/Harbin/Re-1/2003 (referred to as Re-1) [44]. Vaccines were found to provide protection against the disease and reduction of viral shedding on both chickens and ducks [44]. The vaccination program proved to be a viable means of protection against the HPAI H5N1 virus [9]. Given this information, this study assumed 100%

vaccine efficacy in order to evaluate the tradeoff in cost-effectiveness between the two vaccination programs. As a result, it is expected that the focus areas are protected from the HPAI H5N1 disease as the result of frequent vaccinations under the alternative vaccination program. Figure 4b showed that a total of 61 out of 74 infected communes in the fifth epidemic was correctly predicted in the focus areas for the alternative vaccination program. As a result, the alternative vaccination program would protect these 61 communes from the disease. However, the other 13 communes which were not covered by this program could be affected by the disease.

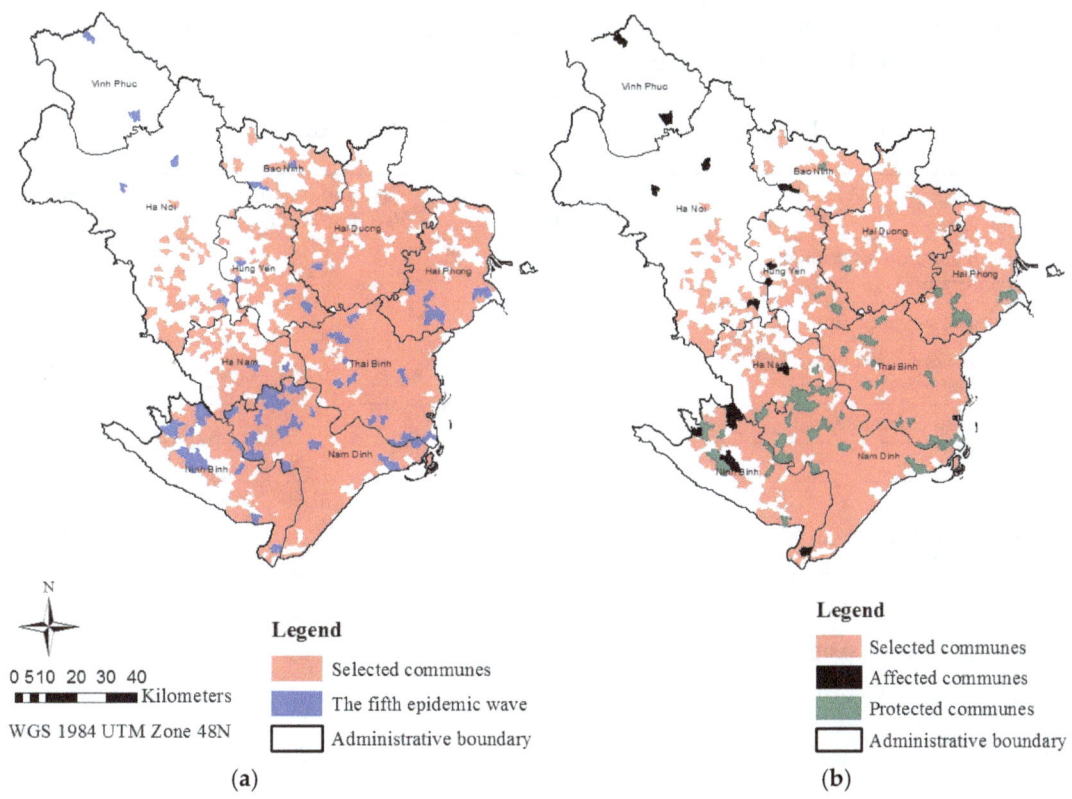

Figure 4. (a) Spatial distribution of the fifth epidemic wave in the Red River Delta and the focus areas for the alternative vaccination program; and (b) spatial distribution of the estimated affected communes and protected communes under the alternative vaccination program.

The cost-effectiveness analysis of the vaccination programs was conducted by using Equations (1) and (2) to investigate which program would be more successful in preventing the disease occurrence. The results of the analysis are shown in Table 4.

Of the total number of 2248 communes in the River Delta, there were 193 communes affected by the disease before the implementation of the national poultry vaccination program. This resulted in the infection rate ARV = 8.59. The national poultry vaccination program contributed to the reduction of the affected communes to 74 as reported in the fifth epidemic waves, resulting in the infection rate ARU = 3.29. The alternative vaccination program was expected to further reduce the number of communes affected to 13 communes which yields the infection rate ARU = 0.58. The effectiveness results suggested that the alternative vaccination program would be more successfully in reducing the rate of disease occurrence measured at 93.26%, compared to the national poultry vaccination program at 61.66%.

It was previously estimated that the optimal length of both chicken and duck production cycles were 10 weeks, including a two-week cleaning period [45,46]. Assuming that producers are continuously engaged in production, there would be five duck production cycles per year. Therefore, the alternative vaccination program would involve five vaccination campaigns throughout the year.

It was noted that the national poultry vaccination program covered the entire poultry population in the Red River Delta and was conducted twice a year. The cost of a HPAI H5N1 vaccination in Viet Nam was estimated to be U.S. $0.038/head, including the vaccine cost of U.S. $0.016 per dose, labor cost of U.S. $0.013, and other costs associated with vaccination of U.S. $0.009 [47]. As a result, the cost of the national poultry vaccination program was estimated at U.S. $4.50 million per year. The alternative vaccination program consists of about half of the total communes in the Delta, covering 1137 communes with poultry population of 31,171 thousand birds. Having vaccinated poultry five times per year would cost U.S. $5.92 million per year. By examining the costs of vaccination only, the cost of the alternative vaccination program appears to be higher than the national poultry vaccination program (U.S. $5.92 million *vs.* U.S. $4.50 million).

Table 4. Cost-effectiveness analysis of the two programs.

Content	Before Vaccination Program	National Poultry Vaccination Program	Alternative Vaccination Program
Total number of communes involved in vaccination program	0	2248	1137
Number of rounds of vaccination per year	0	2	5
Number of birds vaccinated per round (Thousand heads)	0	59,241	31,171
Number of affected communes	193	74	13
Infection rate (%)	8.59	3.29	0.58
Effectiveness (%)		61.66	93.26
Vaccination cost (Million U.S. $)	0	4.50	5.92
Number of birds culled (Thousand heads)	6375	2165	395
Cost of culling birds (Million U.S. $)	1.59	0.54	0.10
Government compensation (Million U.S. $)	7.95	2.68	0.49
Number of communes included in emergency vaccination	543	304	92
Number of birds vaccinated in emergency vaccination (Thousand heads)	0	8625	2898
Cost of emergency vaccination (Million U.S. $)	0	0.33	0.11
Farmers loss (Million U.S. $)	4.95	1.65	0.30
Total loss (Million U.S. $)	14.49	9.70	6.92

When the disease occurs, all birds in affected communes are culled due to the stamping out program and all birds in surrounding communes are vaccinated. Before the official vaccination campaign was launched at the end of 2005, the only emergency response to the disease occurrence was the stamping out program. This resulted in 6.375 million. birds in 193 affected communes culled in the second and third epidemic waves. After the implementation of the national poultry vaccination program, a total of 2.165 million birds were affected and culled, and 8.625 million birds were vaccinated, as the result of the emergency response to the disease occurrence. Under the alternative vaccination program, it was estimated that 395,000 birds in 13 communes were affected and culled by the disease. Another 2.898 million birds in 92 surrounding communes were vaccinated due to the emergency vaccination.

The government incurred more losses from the stamping out and emergency vaccination. The cost of culling birds in the stamping out process was estimated at U.S. $0.25/head [47]. Total culling cost was estimated at U.S. $1.59 million before the implementation of the national poultry vaccination program. This cost was much smaller as a result of either the national poultry vaccination program (U.S. $0.54 million) or the proposed alternative vaccination program (U.S. $0.10 million). The average amount of compensation per bird culled due to the disease occurrence was regulated at U.S. $1.24/head

(23,000 VND/head) (exchange rate at 1 USD = 18,500 VND), in Decision No 719/QD-TTg, dated 5 June 2008. In addition, the average market value of a bird was estimated at U.S. $2 [12]. The farmers also suffered losses of U.S. $0.76/head from production because of the value difference between the market price and the government compensation. This resulted in the Government's additional losses from compensation and farmers' losses of U.S. $7.95 million and U.S. $4.95 million, respectively, in the second and third epidemic waves. Under the national poultry vaccination program, emergency vaccination was implemented which caused the government an estimated U.S. $0.33 million in losses in addition to the government compensation and farmers losses measured at, respectively, U.S. $2.68 million and U.S. $1.65 million. These losses were also estimated at U.S. $0.49 million, U.S. $0.11 million, and U.S. $0.30 million for the government and farmers under the alternative vaccination program. Except for the costs of vaccination (U.S. $4.50 million *vs.* U.S. $5.92 million), and other costs, the alternative vaccination program costs were lower than the national poultry vaccination program.

Total losses imposed on the government and farmers were highest without vaccination and estimated at U.S. $14.49 million, as compared to U.S. $9.70 million for the national poultry vaccination program, and U.S. $6.92 million for the alternative vaccination program.

3.2. Discussion

A vaccination program was identified as a key strategic plan in preventing the HPAI H5N1 disease in Vietnam in the period 2006–2010 [8]. Although the implementation of the national poultry vaccination program resulted in the reduction in disease outbreaks and number of infected birds [44], the disease was repeatedly reported during this period. The third epidemic wave of outbreaks occurred during the first vaccination campaign (September–December 2005). The fourth and fifth waves occurred in between two rounds of vaccination which were from December 2006–March 2007 and May–September 2007, respectively. Infection was reported in unvaccinated ducks based on routine surveillance [10,44]. During the time between the two rounds of vaccinations, the unvaccinated poultry are susceptible to the disease. Additionally, the best vaccination immunity occurs when poultry is vaccinated at the recommended ages suggested by vaccine manufacturers [12]. The national poultry vaccination program scheduled vaccinations at a certain time in each province. It is highly unlikely that the vaccination program exactly matches the optimal timing for vaccination recommended for poultry at various ages.

The alternative vaccination program seeks to fill this gap between the two vaccination rounds and focus more on high risk areas of disease occurrences. The alternative vaccination program was proposed to vaccinate poultry for every production cycle at the recommended poultry ages in high risk areas. Vaccinating poultry at early age provides high level of immunity [44]. A two-dose vaccine given to ducks at one day of age and a booster at four weeks of age produced effective protection [44,48]. It is critical to understand what factors potentially affect the disease occurrence in order to locate susceptible areas where the disease is likely to occur. These factors have been analyzed in previous studies. This study incorporated these factors to spatially identify the focus areas for the proposed alternative vaccination program.

Traditional production methods with free range water bird farming and backyard chicken farming have been considered to be typical Asian production methods which had the potential of contracting and spreading the HPAI H5N1 virus to other neighboring farms [49,50]. These methods were found popular in the poultry sectors 3 and 4 (as classified by [51]) which have small scale production with less than 2000 birds [4]. Poultry sectors 1 and 2, on the other end, are characterized by industrial and commercial poultry production which operate with standard procedures and keep poultry indoors continuously during production to maintain high biosecurity standards against diseasesh, including HPAI H5N1 [51,52]. The BRT results showed the same trend. Water bird density ranging from 893–2097 heads/km^2 and chicken density ranging from 0–1738 heads/km^2 were found to have higher impacts on the disease occurrence as their weights were estimated at 76% for water bird density factor and 37% in water bird and chicken density factors, respectively. Therefore, it was expected that poultry sectors 3 and 4 would fall more in the lower density group. This result also agreed with the study by [9], which suggested communes with medium water bird density to have an increased risk of contracting the disease. Communes with higher water bird and chicken density would be expected to fall in poultry sectors 1 and 2, which have more secure closed farming methods against the disease than the free range farming.

Lower elevation was previously identified to be correlated with the HPAI H5N1 disease in Vietnam, in general, and in the Red River Delta, Vietnam, in particular [5,17]. This finding was further confirmed by BRT estimation. It was suggested that topographic elevation features noticeably contributed differently to the disease occurrence. Coastal areas with elevation less than 5 m contributed to the likelihood of disease occurrence. In contrast to lower elevation areas, upland areas with elevation greater than 200 m were found not likely to affect the disease. Evergreen forests or forestry production dominates these areas [53]. This was also consistent with BRT estimation for land use/land cover which showed that the weight of land used for forest/perennial trees was small and measured at 2% (see Table 2).

The BRT results for land use/land cover were in agreement with studies by [14] and [17] which suggested the link between HPAI H5N1 occurrence and the higher proportion of land use for rice paddy fields and closer distance to higher-density human population areas. Water bird movement through rice paddy fields has been defined as a potential source for spreading the HPAI H5N1 virus [10,14,16,17,54]. The built-up areas characterizes urban and peri-urban areas. It was found that peri-urban areas were the hotspot for the occurrence of the disease. These are the places where land-use changes, interaction, and contact between human and poultry become more frequent and, therefore, they were found to be at significantly higher risk for HPAI H5N1 occurrence [19].

The suitable areas for the vaccination campaign are shown in Figure 3. These suggested areas are characterized by low and high suitability scores. The lowest suitability score areas were either in urban cores or mountainous areas. They included urban core areas of Hanoi, Hai Phong, Hai Duong, Bac Ninh, Hung Yen, Nam Dinh, and Thai Binh provinces and mountain areas of Ba Vi of Hanoi, Tam Dao of Vinh Phuc, Cuc Phuong national park of Ninh Binh, and mountain areas located to the north of the Chi Linh district of Hai Duong province. The highest suitability score areas were mostly located in the coastal areas to the east and south of Hanoi. These areas were chosen to have frequent vaccinations against the HPAI H5N1 disease in the Red River Delta. A total of 1137 communes, corresponding to 50.6% of total communes in the Delta, were selected for the alternative vaccination program, including provinces near the Gulf of Tonkin—Hai Phong, Thai Binh, Nam Dinh, Hai Duong, and the eastern parts of Hung Yen and Ha Nam provinces. These areas were also previously identified to have the highest probability of disease occurrence in the Delta [5]. Almost the entire areas of Hai Duong, Hai Phong, Thai Binh, and Nam Dinh provinces were identified as the focus areas for the alternative vaccination program except urban cores and mountains in the north of Hai Duong. Water bird production with free range farming was found to be the most intensive in the Red River Delta together with the Mekong Delta [55]. Thanh Oai, Thuong Tin, Ung Hoa, and Phu Xuyen districts of Hanoi were also identified as focus areas. These areas are famous for high-quality free-range duck meat provided to consumers in Hanoi.

The cost-effectiveness analysis indicated that the alternative vaccination program would better prevent the occurrence of the disease at lower costs associated with disease prevention than the national poultry vaccination program. Although the cost of the alternative vaccination program was estimated to be higher than that of the national poultry vaccination program (U.S. $5.92 million *vs.* U.S. $4.50 million), it resulted in reducing the rate of disease occurrence by 93.26% as compared to 61.66% of the national poultry vaccination program. As a result, this reduced the cost of immediate responses to the disease occurrence, including stamping out and emergency vaccination, government compensation, and farmers' losses. This contributed to lower total costs associated with the alternative vaccination program as compared to the national poultry vaccination program (U.S. $6.92 million *vs.*

U.S. $9.70). The results of the analysis suggested that Vietnam may face lower costs with the alternative vaccination program.

Poultry production is much more complicated in reality. Producers may have different production cycles. Therefore, for the implementation of the alternative vaccination program, it is recommended that vaccination occurs at the commune level where the commune veterinary officers are required to monitor and vaccinate all poultry at recommended ages for every production cycle.

4. Conclusions

The national poultry vaccination program in the period 2006–2010, which implemented an annual two round vaccination plan for the entire geographical area of the Red River Delta, did not successfully control the disease. This study explored implications of an alternative vaccination program. This alternative vaccination program involves vaccination for every production cycle at the recommended poultry age in high risk areas. This alternative plan would have to be enacted at the local level for all production cycles.

This study identified the focus areas for the alternative vaccination program which were located mostly in the coastal areas to the east and south of Hanoi. A total of 1137 communes, corresponding to 50.6% of total communes in the Delta, were selected for the alternative vaccination program. The alternative vaccination program would have been less costly as compared to the national poultry vaccination program. Effectiveness analysis found that the alternative vaccination program would have been more successful in reducing the rate of disease occurrence from 61.66% rate of reduction (the national poultry vaccination program) to 93.26% rate of reduction (the alternative vaccination program). The cost analysis indicated that the alternative vaccination program would have saved the government and farmer resources because of lower total costs associated with prevention. Total losses imposed on both the government and farmers were higher for the national poultry vaccination program (U.S. $9.70 million) than for the alternative vaccination program (U.S. $6.92 million).

Acknowledgments: This study is a contribution to the project "Coupled Natural-Human Systems and Emerging Infectious Diseases: Anthropogenic environmental change and avian influenza in Vietnam", funded by the U.S. National Science Foundation Grant # DEB-0909410. We would like to thank the East-West Center for providing computer laboratory facilities and support. Thanks to the Vietnam Department of Animal Health and the General Statistic Office of Vietnam for providing data for the study.

Author Contributions: All the authors contributed to this study are as follows: Chinh C. Tran designed, carried out the analysis, interpreted the results and wrote this manuscript. John F. Yanagida supervised the methods of statistical and geostatistical analysis and contributed to the design and revision of the article. Sumeet Saksena provided advice for the Boosted Regression Trees model and reviewed the manuscript for intellectual content. Jefferson Fox reviewed the manuscript for intellectual content and contributed to the revision of the article. All the authors read and approved the final manuscript.

References

1. OIE. Follow-Up Report No. 8. Available online: http://www.oie.int/wahis_2/temp/reports/en_fup_0000014834_20140225_152400.pdf (accessed on 5 September 2014).
2. Phan Dang, T.; Duquesne, B.; Lebailly, P.; Vu Dinh, T. Diversification and epidemic risks of poultry production systems in Hanoi suburban. *J. Sci. Dev.* **2010**, *8*, 203–215.
3. Peyre, M.; Desvaux, S.; Phan Dang, T.; Rossi, V.; Renard, J.F.; Vu Dinh, T.; Roger, F. Financial evaluation of vaccination strategies against HPAI. A modeling approach. In Proceedings of AI Research to Policy International Workshop, FAO, Hanoi, Vietnam, 16–18 June 2008.
4. Desvaux, S.; Ton, V.D.; Phan Dang, T.; Hoa, P.T.T. *A General Review and Description of the Poultry Production in Vietnam*; Agricultural Publishing House: Hanoi, Vietnam, 2008.
5. Tran, C.C.; Yost, R.S.; Yanagida, J.F.; Saksena, S.; Fox, J.; Sultana, N. Spatio-temporal occurrence modeling of highly Pathogenic Avian Influenza subtype H5N1: A case study in the Red River Delta, Vietnam. *ISPRS Int. J. Geo-Inf.* **2013**, *2*, 1106–1121. [CrossRef]

6.   World Bank. *The Avian Influenza Emergency Recovery Project: Implementation completion and Results Report*; World Bank: Washington, DC, USA, 2007.

7.   CAP. *Policy Analysis of HPAI Strategy Including Analysis of Collaboration and Partnership between Public and Private Sectors: Gathering Evidence for A Transitional Strategy (GETS) for HPAI H5N1 Vaccination in Vietnam*; Center for Agricultural Policy: Hanoi, Vietnam, 2011.

8.   MARD & MOH. *Vietnam: Integrated National Operational Program for Avian and Human Influenza (OPI) 2006–2010*; MARD & MOH: Hanoi, Vietnam, 2006.

9.   Henning, K.A.; Henning, J.; Morton, J.; Long, N.T.; Ha, N.T.; Meers, J. Farm-and flock-level risk factors associated with Highly Pathogenic Avian Influenza outbreaks on small holder duck and chicken farms in the Mekong Delta of Viet Nam. *Prev. Vet. Med.* **2009**, *91*, 179–188. [CrossRef] [PubMed]

10. Minh, P.Q.; Morris, R.S.; Schauer, B.; Stevenson, M.; Benschop, J.; Nam, H.V.; Jackson, R. Spatio-temporal epidemiology of highly Pathogenic Avian Influenza outbreaks in the two deltas of Vietnam during 2003–2007. *Prev. Vet. Med.* **2009**, *89*, 16–24. [CrossRef] [PubMed]

11. Taylor, N.; Dung, D.H. *An Analysis of Data Generated by Post-Vaccination Sero-Monitoring and Surveillance Activities, Following HPAI Vaccination in Viet Nam (2005–2006)*; FAO: Hanoi, Vietnam, 2007; p. 46.

12. Sims, L.; Do, H.D. *Vaccination of Poultry in Vietnam against H5N1 Highly Pathogenic Avian Influenza*; Australian Government Department of Agriculture, Fisheries and Forestry: Canberra, Australia, 2009.

13. MARD & MOH. Avian and pandemic influenza Vietnam's experience. In Proceedings of International Ministerial Conference on Animal and Pandemic Influenza, Hanoi, Vietnam, 19–21 April 2010.

14. Pfeiffer, D.U.; Minh, P.Q.; Martin, V.; Epprecht, M.; Otte, M.J. An analysis of the spatial and temporal patterns of highly Pathogenic Avian Influenza occurrence in Vietnam using national surveillance data. *Vet. J.* **2007**, *174*, 302–309. [CrossRef] [PubMed]

15. Desvaux, S.; Grosbois, V.; Pham, T.T.H.; Fenwick, S.; Tollis, S.; Pham, N.H.; Tran, A.; Roger, F. Risk factors of highly Pathogenic Avian Influenza H5N1 occurrence at the village and farm levels in the Red River Delta Region in Vietnam. *Transbound. Emerg. Dis.* **2011**, *58*, 492–502. [CrossRef] [PubMed]

16. Gilbert, M.; Chaitaweesup, P.; Parakamawongsa, T.; Premashthira, S.; Tiensin, T.; Kalpravidh, W.; Wagner, H.; Slingenbergh, J. Free-grazing ducks and highly Pathogenic Avian Influenza, Thailand. *Emerg. Infect. Dis.* **2006**, *12*, 227–234. [CrossRef] [PubMed]

17. Gilbert, M.; Xiao, X.; Pfeiffer, D.U.; Epprecht, M.; Boles, S.; Czarnecki, C.; Chaitaweesub, P.; Kalpravidh, W.; Minh, P.Q.; Otte, M.J.; *et al.* Mapping H5N1 highly Pathogenic Avian Influenza risk in southeast Asia. *Proc. Natl. Acad. Sci. USA* **2008**, *105*, 4769–4774. [CrossRef] [PubMed]

18. FAO Summary of Highly Pathogenic Avian Influenza (HPAI) Situation in Viet Nam 31 December 2008. Available online: http://www.un.org.vn/images/stories/press_centre/2008_hpai_update_31dec08.pdf (accessed on 21 October 2010).

19. Saksena, S.; Fox, J.; Epprecht, M.; Tran, C.; Nong, D.; Spencer, J.; Nguyen, L.; Finucane, M.; Tran, V.; Wilcox, B. Evidence for the convergence model: The emergence of highly Pathogenic Avian Influenza (H5N1) in Viet Nam. *PLoS ONE* **2015**, *10*, e0138138. [CrossRef] [PubMed]

20. CGIAR-CSI. Shuttle Radar Topography Mission (SRTM) 90-m Resolution Digital Elevation Model (DEM). Available online: http://srtm.csi.cgiar.org/ (accessed on 2 March 2015).

21. USGS. USGS EROS Data Center. Available online: http://glovis.usgs.gov/ (accessed on 28 October 2013).

22. ESRI. How Weighted Overlay Works. Available online: http://resources.arcgis.com/en/help/main/10.1/index.html#//009z000000s1000000 (accessed on 10 September 2014).

23. Gilbert, M.; Xiao, X.; Domenech, J.; Lubroth, J.; Martin, V.; Slingenbergh, J. Anatidae migration in the western Palearctic and spread of highly Pathogenic Avian Influenza H5N1 virus. *Emerg. Infect. Dis.* **2006**, *12*, 1650–1656. [CrossRef] [PubMed]

24. Shahid, S. Impact of climate change on irrigation water demand of dry season Boro rice in northwest Bangladesh. *Clim. Change* **2011**, *105*, 433–453. [CrossRef]

25. Jayakumar, S.; Arockiasamy, D.I.; Britto, S.J. Conserving forests in the eastern Ghats through remote sensing and GIS-A case study in Kolli hills. *Curr. Sci.* **2002**, *82*, 1259–1266.

26. Münch, Z.; Conrad, J. Remote sensing and GIS based determination of groundwater dependent ecosystems in the Western Cape, South Africa. *Hydrogeol. J.* **2007**, *15*, 19–28. [CrossRef]

27. Diamond, J.T.; Wright, J.R. Design of an integrated spatial information system for multiobjective land-use planning. *Environ. Plan. B-Plan. Design* **1988**, *15*, 205–214. [CrossRef]

28. Elith, J.; Leathwick, J.R.; Hastie, T. A working guide to boosted regression trees. *J. Anim. Ecol.* **2008**, *77*, 802–813. [CrossRef] [PubMed]

29. Elith, J.; Catherine, G.; Anderson, P.R.; Dudík, M.; Ferrier, S.; Guisan, A.; Hijmans, J.R.; Huettmann, F.; Leathwick, R.J.; Lehmann, A.; *et al.* Novel methods improve prediction of species' distributions from occurrence data. *Ecography* **2006**, *29*, 129–151. [CrossRef]

30. Martin, V.; Pfeiffer, D.U.; Zhou, X.; Xiao, X.; Prosser, D.J.; Guo, F.; Gilbert, M. Spatial distribution and risk factors of highly Pathogenic Avian Influenza (HPAI) H5N1 in China. *PLoS Pathog.* **2011**, *7*, e1001308. [CrossRef] [PubMed]

31. Gilbert, M.; Newman, S.H.; Takekawa, J.Y.; Loth, L.; Biradar, C.; Prosser, D.J.; Balachandran, S.; Rao, M.V.S.; Mundkur, T.; Yan, B.; *et al.* Flying over an infected landscape: Distribution of highly Pathogenic Avian Influenza H5N1 risk in south Asia and satellite tracking of wild waterfowl. *Ecohealth* **2010**, *7*, 448–458. [CrossRef] [PubMed]

32. Stevens, K.B.; Pfeiffer, D.U. Spatial modelling of disease using data-and knowledge-driven approaches. *Spat. Spatio-Temporal Epidemiol.* **2011**, *2*, 125–133. [CrossRef] [PubMed]

33. Van Boeckel, T.P.; Thanapongtharm, W.; Robinson, T.; Biradar, C.M.; Xiao, X.; Gilbert, M. Improving risk models for avian influenza: The role of intensive poultry farming and flooded land during the 2004 Thailand epidemic. *PLoS ONE* **2012**, *7*, e49528. [CrossRef] [PubMed]

34. Jenks, G.F. The data model concept in statistical mapping. *Int. Yearb. Cartogr.* **1967**, *7*, 186–190.

35. Castrence, M.; Nong, D.H.; Tran, C.C.; Young, L.; Fox, J. Mapping urban transitions using multi-temporal Landsat and DMSP-OLS night-time lights imagery of the Red River Delta in Vietnam. *Land* **2014**, *3*, 148–166. [CrossRef]

36. Schneider, A. Monitoring land cover change in urban and peri-urban areas using dense time stacks of Landsat satellite data and a data mining approach. *Remote Sens. Environ.* **2012**, *124*, 689–704. [CrossRef]

37. Mountrakis, G.; Im, J.; Ogole, C. Support vector machines in remote sensing: A review. *ISPRS J. Photogramm. Remote Sens.* **2011**, *66*, 247–259. [CrossRef]

38. Weinberg, G.A.; Szilagyi, P.G. Vaccine epidemiology: Efficacy, effectiveness, and the translational research roadmap. *J. Infect. Dis.* **2010**, *201*, 1607–1610. [CrossRef] [PubMed]

39. Pfeiffer, D.U. Assessment of H5N1 HPAI risk and the importance of wild birds. *J. Wildl. Dis.* **2007**, *43*, S47–S50.

40. Smith, G.J.D.; Fan, X.H.; Wang, J.; Li, K.S.; Qin, K.; Zhang, J.X.; Vijaykrishna, D.; Cheung, C.L.; Huang, K.; Rayner, J.M.; *et al.* Emergence and predominance of an H5N1 influenza variant in China. *Proc. Natl. Acad. Sci. USA* **2006**, *103*, 16936–16941. [CrossRef] [PubMed]

41. Songserm, T.; Jam-on, R.; Sae-Heng, N.; Meemak, N.; Hulse-Post, D.J.; Sturm-Ramirez, K.M.; Webster, R.G. Domestic ducks and H5N1 influenza epidemic, Thailand. *Emerg. Infect. Dis.* **2006**, *12*, 575. [CrossRef] [PubMed]

42. Webster, R.G.; Hulse-Post, D.J.; Sturm-Ramirez, K.M.; Guan, Y.; Peiris, M.; Smith, G.; Chen, H. Changing epidemiology and ecology of highly pathogenic avian H5N1 influenza viruses. *Avian Dis.* **2007**, *51*, 269–272. [CrossRef] [PubMed]

43. OIE. Follow-Up Report No. 45. Available online: http://web.oie.int/wahis/reports/en_fup_0000010005_20101204_123300.pdf (accessed on 15 August 2014).

44. Pfeiffer, J.; Suarez, D.L.; Sarmento, L.; To, T.L.; Nguyen, T.; Pantin-Jackwood, M.J. Efficacy of commercial vaccines in protecting chickens and ducks against H5N1 highly Pathogenic Avian Influenza viruses from Vietnam. *Avian Dis.* **2010**, *54*, 262–271. [CrossRef] [PubMed]

45. Tran, C.C. *Public Policy Instruments for Risk Management of Highly Pathogenic Avian Influenza Subtype H5N1 in Vietnam*; University of Kentucky: Lexington, KY, USA, 2010.

46. Tran, C.C.; Yanagida, J.F. Computational economic analysis of duck production at the farm household level in the context of highly Pathogenic Avian Influenza subtype H5N1 in the Red River Delta, Vietnam. *Asian J. Agric. Ext. Econ. Sociol.* **2015**, *6*, 172–184. [CrossRef]

47. Hinrichs, J.; Sims, L.; McLeod, A. Some direct costs of control for avian influenza. In Proceedings of the 11th International Society for Veterinary Epidemiology and Economics, Cairns, Australia, August 2006.

48. Beato, M.S.; Toffan, A.; de Nardi, R.; Cristalli, A.; Terregino, C.; Cattoli, G.; Capua, I. A conventional, inactivated oil emulsion vaccine suppresses shedding and prevents viral meat colonisation in commercial (Pekin) ducks challenged with HPAI H5N1. *Vaccine* **2007**, *25*, 4064–4072. [CrossRef] [PubMed]

49. Alhaji, N.B.; Odetokun, I.A. Assessment of biosecurity measures against highly Pathogenic Avian Influenza risks in small-scale commercial farms and free-range poultry flocks in the northcentral Nigeria. *Transbound. Emerg. Dis.* **2011**, *58*, 157–161. [CrossRef] [PubMed]

50. FAO. Bio-Security for Highly Pathogenic Avian Influenza: Issues and Options. Available online: ftp://ftp.fao.org/docrep/fao/011/i0359e/i0359e00.pdf (accessed on 26 May 2012).

51. FAO. FAO Recommendations on the Prevention, Control and Eradication of Highly Pathogenic Avian Influenza (HPAI) in Asia. Available online: http://web.oie.int/eng/AVIAN_INFLUENZA/FAO recommendations on HPAI.pdf (accessed on 26 May 2012).

52. FAO. The Importance of Biosecurity in Reducing HPAI Risk on Farms and in Markets. Available online: http://www.fao.org/docs/eims/upload//236621/ah691e.pdf (accessed on 26 May 2012).

53. EAP-AP. Land Cover Assessment and Monitoring. Available online: http://www.rrcap.ait.asia/lc/cd/html/vietnam.html (accessed on 8 January 2015).

54. Gilbert, M.; Xiao, X.; Chaitaweesub, P.; Kalpravidh, W.; Premashthira, S.; Boles, S.; Slingenbergh, J. Avian influenza, domestic ducks and rice agriculture in Thailand. *Agric. Ecosyst. Environ.* **2007**, *119*, 409–415. [CrossRef] [PubMed]

55. Edan, M. *Review of Free-Range Duck Farming Systems in Northern Vietnam and Assessment of Their Implication in The Spreading of The Highly Pathogenic (H5N1) Strain of Avian Influenza (HPAI)*; Agronomes et Veterinaires sans Frontieres: Lyon, France, 2006; p. 101.

PERMISSIONS

All chapters in this book were first published in VS, by MDPI AG; hereby published with permission under the Creative Commons Attribution License or equivalent. Every chapter published in this book has been scrutinized by our experts. Their significance has been extensively debated. The topics covered herein carry significant findings which will fuel the growth of the discipline. They may even be implemented as practical applications or may be referred to as a beginning point for another development.

The contributors of this book come from diverse backgrounds, making this book a truly international effort. This book will bring forth new frontiers with its revolutionizing research information and detailed analysis of the nascent developments around the world.

We would like to thank all the contributing authors for lending their expertise to make the book truly unique. They have played a crucial role in the development of this book. Without their invaluable contributions this book wouldn't have been possible. They have made vital efforts to compile up to date information on the varied aspects of this subject to make this book a valuable addition to the collection of many professionals and students.

This book was conceptualized with the vision of imparting up-to-date information and advanced data in this field. To ensure the same, a matchless editorial board was set up. Every individual on the board went through rigorous rounds of assessment to prove their worth. After which they invested a large part of their time researching and compiling the most relevant data for our readers.

The editorial board has been involved in producing this book since its inception. They have spent rigorous hours researching and exploring the diverse topics which have resulted in the successful publishing of this book. They have passed on their knowledge of decades through this book. To expedite this challenging task, the publisher supported the team at every step. A small team of assistant editors was also appointed to further simplify the editing procedure and attain best results for the readers.

Apart from the editorial board, the designing team has also invested a significant amount of their time in understanding the subject and creating the most relevant covers. They scrutinized every image to scout for the most suitable representation of the subject and create an appropriate cover for the book.

The publishing team has been an ardent support to the editorial, designing and production team. Their endless efforts to recruit the best for this project, has resulted in the accomplishment of this book. They are a veteran in the field of academics and their pool of knowledge is as vast as their experience in printing. Their expertise and guidance has proved useful at every step. Their uncompromising quality standards have made this book an exceptional effort. Their encouragement from time to time has been an inspiration for everyone.

The publisher and the editorial board hope that this book will prove to be a valuable piece of knowledge for researchers, students, practitioners and scholars across the globe.

LIST OF CONTRIBUTORS

Jyotika Varshney and Subbaya Subramanian
Masonic Cancer Center, University of Minnesota, Minneapolis, MN 55455, USA
Department of Surgery, University of Minnesota Medical School, Moos Tower, 11-212420 Delaware Street,S.E.; MMC 195, Minneapolis, MN 55455, USA

Milcah C. Scott
Masonic Cancer Center, University of Minnesota, Minneapolis, MN 55455, USA
Animal Cancer Care and Research Program, University of Minnesota, St. Paul, MN 55455, USA
Department of Veterinary Clinical Sciences, College of Veterinary Medicine, University of Minnesota,St. Paul, MN 55108, USA

David A. Largaespada
Masonic Cancer Center, University of Minnesota, Minneapolis, MN 55455, USA
Department of Pediatrics, University of Minnesota, Minneapolis, MN 55455, USA

Christine Böhmer
UMR 7179 CNRS, Muséum National d'Histoire Naturelle, CP 55, 57 rue Cuvier, 75231 Paris CEDEX 05, France

Estella Böhmer
Chirurgische und Gynäkologische Kleintierklinik ,Tierärztliche Fakultät, Ludwig-Maximilians-Universität München, Veterinärstr 13, 80539 München, Germany

Panditharathnalage Nishantha Kumara Wijesekara
Human Recourse Department, University Grants Commission, 20, Ward Place, Colombo 07 10000, Sri Lanka

Wikum Widuranga Kumbukgolla
Department of Biochemistry, Faculty of Medicine and Allied Sciences, Rajarata University Mihintale, Mihintale 50008, Sri Lanka

Jayaweera Arachchige Asela Sampath Jayaweera
Department of Microbiology, Faculty of Medicine and Allied Sciences, Rajarata University Mihintale, Mihintale 50008, Sri Lanka

Diwan Rawat
Department of Chemistry, University of Delhi, Delhi 110007, India

Rick B. Meeker
Department of Neurology, University of North Carolina, Chapel Hill, NC 27599, USA

Lola Hudson
Department of Molecular Biomedical Sciences, College of Veterinary Medicine, North Carolina State University, Raleigh, NC 27607, USA

Sahatchai Tangtrongsup
Department of Companion Animal and Wildlife Clinic, Faculty of Veterinary Medicine, Chiang Mai University, Chiang Mai 50100, Thailand
Animal Population Health Institute, Department of Clinical Sciences, College of Veterinary Medicine and Biomedical Sciences, Colorado State University, Fort Collins, CO 80523, USA

Mo D. Salman
Animal Population Health Institute, Department of Clinical Sciences, College of Veterinary Medicine and Biomedical Sciences, Colorado State University, Fort Collins, CO 80523, USA

A. Valeria Scorza and Michael R. Lappin
Center for Companion Animal Studies, Department of Clinical Sciences College of Veterinary Medicine and Biomedical Sciences, Colorado State University, Fort Collins, CO 80523, USA

John S. Reif
Department of Environmental and Radiological Health Sciences, College of Veterinary Medicine and Biomedical Sciences, Colorado State University, Fort Collins, CO 80523, USA

Lora R. Ballweber
Department of Microbiology, Immunology and Pathology, College of Veterinary Medicine and Biomedical Sciences, Colorado State University, Fort Collins, CO 80523, USA

Marcello Trevisani, Rocco Mancusi, Matilde Cecchini and Claudia Costanza
Dipartimento di Scienze Mediche Veterinarie, Università degli Studi di Bologna, Alma Mater Studiorum, via Tolara di Sopra 50, Ozzano Emilia 40064, Italy

Marino Prearo
S.S. Laboratorio Specialistico Ittiopatologia, Istituto Zooprofilattico Sperimentale del Piemonte, Liguria e Valle d'Aosta, Torino 10154, Italy

O. Lynne Nelson and Rachael M. Wood
Department of Veterinary Clinical Sciences, Washington State University, Pullman,WA 99164, USA

Jens Häggström
Department of Clinical Sciences and Anatomy, Physiology and Biochemistry, Swedish University of Agricultural Sciences, Uppsala 750 07, Sweden

Clarence Kvart
Faculty of Veterinary Medicine and Animal Science, Swedish University of Agricultural Sciences, Uppsala 750 07, Sweden

Charles T. Robbins
School of the Environment and School of Biological Sciences, Washington State University, Pullman, WA 99164, USA

MariaMagana and Stylianos Chatzipanagiotou
Department of Biopathology and Clinical Microbiology, Aeginition Hospital, Athens Medical School, Athens 15772, Greece

Angeliki R. Burriel
Department of Nursing, Faculty of Human Movement and Quality of Life Sciences, University of Peloponnese, Sparta 23100, Greece

Anastasios Ioannidis
Department of Biopathology and Clinical Microbiology, Aeginition Hospital, Athens Medical School, Athens 15772, Greece
Department of Nursing, Faculty of Human Movement and Quality of Life Sciences, University of Peloponnese, Sparta 23100, Greece

Martin Kramer and Kerstin von Pückler
Department of Veterinary Clinical Science, Clinic for Small Animals (Surgery), Justus-Liebig University (JLU), 35392 Gießen, Germany

Ahmed Abdellatif
Department of Veterinary Clinical Science, Clinic for Small Animals (Surgery), Justus-Liebig University (JLU), 35392 Gießen, Germany

Animal Surgery Department, Assiut University, Assiut 71515, Egypt

Klaus Failing
Unit for Biomathematics and Data Processing, Veterinary Faculty, Justus-Liebig University (JLU), Gießen 35392, Germany

Christopher D. Crowder, Arash Ghalyanchi Langeroudi, Azadeh Shojaee Estabragh, Eric R. G. Lewis, Renee A. Marcsisin and Alan G. Barbour
Departments of Microbiology & Molecular Genetics and Medicine, University of California Irvine, Irvine, CA 92697, USA

Florian R. L. Meyer and Ingrid Walter
Department of Pathobiology, Institute of Anatomy, Histology and Embryology, University of Veterinary Medicine, Veterinaerplatz 1, Vienna 1210, Austria

Lorraine C. Backer
National Center for Environmental Health, Centers for Disease Control and Prevention, 4770 Buford Highway NE, MS F-60, Chamblee, GA 30341, USA

Melissa Miller
Office of Spill Prevention and Response, Department of Fish and Wildlife, Marine Wildlife Veterinary Care and Research Center, 1451 Shaffer Rd, Santa Cruz, CA 95060, USA
School of Veterinary Medicine, University of California at Davis, Davis, CA 95616, USA

John F. Yanagida
Department of Natural Resources and Environmental Management, University of Hawaii at Manoa, 1910 East-West Road, Honolulu, HI 96822, USA

Chinh C. Tran
Department of Natural Resources and Environmental Management, University of Hawaii at Manoa, 1910 East-West Road, Honolulu, HI 96822, USA
East-West Center, 1601 East-West Road, Honolulu, HI 96848, USA

Sumeet Saksena and Jefferson Fox
East-West Center, 1601 East-West Road, Honolulu, HI 96848, USA

Index